The Medical War
against
Chiropractors

The Untold Story
from Persecution to Vindication

ISBN-10: 1453744878
EAN-13: 9781453744871
LCCN: 2010918374

The Medical War
against
Chiropractors

The Untold Story
from Persecution to Vindication

JC Smith

Other books by the author:

A Chiropractic Paradigm
How to Avoid Back Surgery
Poisoned Love: When a Chiropractor and an Orthopedist Fall in Love
The Path to Mastery in Chiropractic

Chiropractic Legends

The McAndrews Brothers

Dr. Jerry McAndrews and his brother, George, the lead attorney in the *Wilk* antitrust trial, were legends in the chiropractic profession years before I had the pleasure of meeting them. By then Jerry was in semi-retirement from his days as president of Palmer College of Chiropractic, as well as the former executive vice president of the International Chiropractors Association and as spokesman for the American Chiropractic Association.

Whenever this profession needed a savvy response to any issue, it turned to Jerry McAndrews. He had an encyclopedic knowledge of the history, research, academia, people, and political events affecting this profession because he was usually directly involved. For many years, Jerry was the face and voice of the chiropractic profession.

As a budding writer reaching out for advice, I ingrained myself on Jerry by sending my articles to him for review and, to my amazement, he responded each and every time. Apparently chiropractors-turned-writers were a rare lot, and that was the beginning of our pen-pal relationship that fortunately blossomed into a mentorship for me over the last many years.

I met Jerry at the National Chiropractic Legislative Conference in Washington, DC. One evening, I saw him in the hotel restaurant alone. He was relaxing after a long day of speaking to the large assembly of chiropractors, students, and the leadership of the American Chiropractic Association. As usual, he was enjoying his dessert; anyone who knew Jerry recalls how he loved a bowl of vanilla ice cream.

I took the opportunity to pick his mind about the many issues facing our profession. Jerry spoke with me freely about many political and historical events, but when I asked

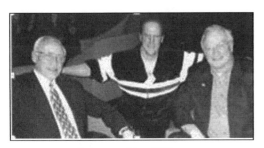

Between Two Pillars
Jerry McAndrews, JCS, George McAndrews

him about his brother, George, the lead attorney in the famous *Wilk v. AMA* antitrust trial, he became quiet and tears began to swell in his eyes. I was afraid that I had upset him.

Jerry sat silently for a few moments staring straight ahead, undoubtedly reflecting on the historical feat his brother had accomplished to save this profession from medical annihilation. Finally, he returned to the present, apologized for being so emotional, and said, "I love my brother, not just because he's my brother, but for what he's done for this profession."

I was touched by his sentiment. In fact, I felt honored to have witnessed his heart-felt gratitude for his brother that only added to his Lincolnesque presence. Indeed, this profession was fortunate to have had brethren of this stature fighting our legal and political battles.

Jerry mentioned, "George once told me that he was born to try the *Wilk* case," and was motivated by his father's personal experience with chiropractic. "We'll make this a present to Dad for what they did to him."

George tells the family story how their father, Patrick McAndrews, initially entered the chiropractic profession first as a patient. He suffered so badly from asthma as a young man that, despite standing well over six feet tall, he weighed only 140 pounds. After the first spinal adjustment where "his heels touched the back of his head," his father finally enjoyed a full night's sleep.

This experience so motivated McAndrews senior that he moved his young family to Davenport, Iowa to begin his chiropractic education at the Palmer School of Chiropractic from which he graduated in 1933. They later settled in Clinton, Iowa, a quaint nineteenth-century riverside town along the Mississippi River, just forty miles upstream from Davenport.

George also spoke of the trauma his father experienced as a chiropractor. Like many early chiropractors, he suffered constant humiliation. George recalled the medical bigotry and public ignorance that affected his father's life; how his father was hospitalized with a nervous breakdown, and how this stress led to his subsequent premature death as another victim of the medical war on chiropractors.

Thus began the McAndrews' ascension into the annals of chiropractic history that, to date, has led to twenty-nine family members becoming chiropractors.

The McAndrews brothers' present to their father has now become a gift to the entire chiropractic profession and to the millions of people who utilize chiropractic care daily because if they had failed, the fate of this profession would have been doomed—the war between the chiropractors and the AMA would have been lost or relegated to the ghetto with once-popular but defeated professions like homeopathy, naturopathy, and many other alternative health care professions destroyed or defamed by the AMA.

I often urged Jerry and George to record their story. Apparently they tried to do so a few times, reminiscing about untold events like George's office being burglarized during the *Wilk* trial and having their phones tapped, forcing them to speak in the corn fields behind Jerry's home—anecdotes that will never be included in the history books.

Jerry told me how the principal characters in the *Wilk* case once met at George's vacation home on Lake Michigan to write their book. Instead of getting down to the serious business of writing about this historic event, they watched George's passion, Notre Dame football, had a good time, and then fell asleep.

Alas, they never did produce a manuscript. Afterwards, Jerry told me that he was now in his 70s and becoming forgetful; on June 9, 2006, he passed away. Afterwards, George told me, "We'll leave that task up to people like you." Indeed, I hope I have met their high professional standards and have done them justice with this book.

It has been a labor of love to recount the trials and tribulations of the chiropractic war with the medical profession. Both Jerry and George have helped me in this process with firsthand information, especially George who sent me some never before seen original *Wilk* trial transcripts. I cannot say how many times I troubled this very successful attorney who interrupted his practice to answer my questions. Only once did he seem perturbed when he told me, "You are quickly becoming my biggest client."

Undeniably, the McAndrews brothers' gift to this profession will endure for generations to come, and for that reason I dedicate this book to Dr. Jerome F. McAndrews and his younger brother, Mr. George P. McAndrews, both legends as victorious leaders in the medical war against the chiropractic profession.

Table of Contents

The Unknown War

*"They have given every single one of their tomorrows
so we can have our today."*

Army Staff Sgt. Salvatore Giunta,
2010 Medal of Honor recipient

T he tomb of the Unknown Soldier at Arlington National Cemetery is a solemn tribute to those faceless heroes who fought for the cause of freedom. Unlike that famous tomb in Washington, DC, there is a little known bell tower in Georgia dedicated to the thousands of unknown chiropractors who fought for freedom in healthcare in a virtually unknown war between medicine and chiropractic that has lasted over a hundred years.

At stake was not only the survival of the chiropractic profession, but the survival of an ageless healing art that has helped millions of people suffering with musculoskeletal pain, which happens to be the single largest cause of disability today.[1]

There is a related story that the American public has never been told—what it was like being a chiropractor during this war. Few people understand

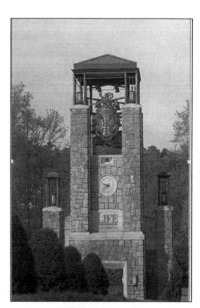

Bell Tower honoring
imprisoned chiropractors,
Life University, Marietta, GA.

---

1 AD Woolf, B Pfleger, "Burden of Major Musculoskeletal Conditions," *Bull World Health Organ* 81/09 (2003):646-656.

how tough it was since chiropractors, due to the imposed taboo stigma, are rarely the subject of examination. Not only did chiropractors have a special knack with their skilled hands to adjust their patients' spines, but the foremost requirements to be a chiropractor were a strong backbone, a thick skin, and a resolute spirit.

For over a century an unwavering attitude has been woven into the chiropractic character that remains an untold story of grit and survival. Certainly this profession has never been for the weak of mind or body—just ask the thousands of chiropractors who have fought in this medical war. When the inevitable salvos began to fly, many who were less dedicated soon sought another line of work. Many chiropractors died of a broken spirit; many more were left gravely wounded financially or buried beneath the burden of bias.

From New York to Louisiana to California, chiropractors were routinely harassed, extorted, arrested, often ran out of town, and beaten up by the local police. During the first half of the twentieth century, over 12,000 American chiropractors were prosecuted over 15,000 times, and some 3,300 were sent to jail for practicing medicine without a license.[2]

This was a bogus charge—by no means did they practice medicine since they never used drugs and surgery. Their only offense was helping sick people get well with their healing hands. Their real misdeed was competing with the medical profession for patients.

Fortunately, there were those dedicated chiropractors who carried the torch despite the overwhelming odds. Imagine yourself in the medical war as a chiropractor before state licensing laws were passed to protect you and your patients. There's a knock at your office door and everyone inside freezes with fear. Like Anne Frank hiding from the Nazis or the runaway slaves on the Underground Railroad to the North during the Civil War, chiropractors and their patients felt the same terror before state laws legalized this type of care.

Your office resembles a speakeasy during Prohibition with a doorman looking through a peephole in the front door when patients knock to be let in. The lookout makes sure they were not the undercover police who often posed as patients to make an arrest. Being busted was a routine event by the authorities to appease the local medical society and to earn a few extra bucks for themselves. Preying upon defenseless chiropractors was easy money.

Every so often the unofficial taxman from City Hall, dubbed the Juice Man, comes unannounced to *squeeze* you for protection money. The local police look the other way as long as you can pay the extortion money. When he finally comes knocking at your office door, he brings a couple of his thugs as enforcers to encourage you to pay.

Sometimes you can pay, but when you can't, the Juice Man is troubled. If he throws you in jail, you won't be able to pay him in the future. So he has his thugs rough you up with a good beating, leaving you with a few sore ribs, a swollen face, perhaps a black eye, maybe a few days in the hospital, and plenty of public humiliation—a clear warning to pay next time or else worse will happen.

---

2 Russell W Gibbons, "Go to Jail for Chiro," *Journal of Chiropractic Humanities* 4 (1994): 61–71.

Chiropractors were not the only victims of this medical war. This warfare has also taken a toll on millions of innocent patients who were collateral damage of the medical fire.

They were told by their local MDs, "Whatever you do, don't go to a chiropractor." Many were ridiculed when they asked about seeing a chiropractor before surgery, "If you're stupid enough to go to a chiropractor, don't come crawling back to me after that quack paralyzes you." Many were even told never to return to their MD's office if they ever used chiropractors as if they would become lepers tainted by the reviled chiropractors.

Many finally caved in to their back pain or succumbed to the verbal maltreatment, and acquiesced to a surgery that would forever change their lives. Not only were patients verbally abused, many were physically abused as victims of millions of ineffective back surgeries, and many were financially exploited who paid thousands of dollars for these unnecessary surgeries.

Yet still they came, literally limping into chiropractic offices with frowns of hopelessness, seeking the proverbial "last resort" because traditional medicine had failed them. Many already had had back surgeries that failed to help despite the promises of their spine surgeons. Most were living in constant pain and disabled, some addicted to drugs. Most of all, they all had lost hope.

Adding to their despair, many felt torn like traitors who reluctantly changed sides in the medical war when their medical treatments failed them. But, after they got relief with chiropractic care, their entire disposition changed from fear and skepticism to relief, support, and then to anger.

They would ask questions that every chiropractor has heard many times: how can this be quackery when it helped me get well? Why didn't my medical doctor refer me to you before he wanted me to have back surgery? Why did he let me suffer so long without telling me chiropractic might help me? These are all good questions that this book will answer.

Indeed, the truth eventually has a way of overcoming propaganda, as it has for millions of patients over the past century who have discovered chiropractic care, including those who waited in fear of the Juice Man.

Just like the chiropractors of yesteryear who lived in fear, maybe that anxious person today is you, someone who lives in pain needing chiropractic care. Like millions of other Americans, you may be living in apprehension of your own Juice Man who takes on many different forms—the skeptical neighbor who condemns chiropractors although she's never been to one, the biased MD who ridicules you just for asking about chiropractic care, the co-worker who had a back surgery but won't admit it failed despite the constant pain, the insurance company that excludes or severely restricts chiropractic care, or anyone who discourages you from seeking a chiropractor's help.

It is past time for the medical war to end and allow the wounded bystanders to seek chiropractic care. It is time to recognize these unknown forces at work that impede the use of chiropractors' good hands to help millions of suffering people. Like the chiropractor hiding behind the locked door, perhaps you are also hiding from possible ridicule from the Juice Man. It is time to end this fear.

DD Palmer, the founder of chiropractic, also felt the wrath of the original Juice Man. Over one hundred years ago, he was prosecuted and jailed, as were thousands of his protégés who gave up many tomorrows to keep alive the benefits of this healing art today. Let their sacrifice be your pathway to a better life.

Learn why generations of the brave men and women inexplicably continue to dedicate their lives to carry the tarnished banner of chiropractic care against overwhelming odds in this medical war. Hear their untold story from legal persecution and professional defamation leading to satisfied patients and scientific vindication.

This exposé is similar to other illuminating portrayals of social injustice, such as Betty Freidan's *The Feminine Mystique* or *Uncle Tom's Cabin* by Harriet Beecher Stowe. It is past time for America to learn of the century of conflict chiropractors have endured to bring people an ageless healing art that has now been shown to be more effective than medical care for most back pain problems.

This exposé fills the void in this dark chapter of medicine that has gone virtually unspoken for decades now. Professors of medical history and their medical and chiropractic students will find this textbook essential to understand the past warfare and present tension between the professions—the proverbial 800-pound gorilla that few have exposed for what is is—an assault on the chiropractic profession. Only a chiropractor/author could write about the unknown plight of chiropractic from persecution to vindication. Only a chiropractor would divulge much of what is publically known is a direct result of medical propaganda.

Plus, every wounded physician and chiropractor who have fought in this medical war will appreciate this perspective in order to understand the historical events, the prominent issues, the leading players, and the overall history that have shaped the prevailing tension between the medical and chiropractic professions that affects nearly every patient as well, certainly the 90 percent who will be struck with an acute low back attack sometime in their lives.

This book will also have cross-over appeal to those lay people and the media who want to know more about the biggest rift among healthcare professionals from the chiropractic perspective. This book will have great appeal to many Americans who can feel the existing cold war between MDs and DCs, but have no idea how this war developed.

Indeed, this book will answer the *how* and *why* this medical war against chiropractors began and has prevailed for over a century. Most assuredly, it will explain why someone polled about chiropractors once answered, "I wouldn't want my daughter to marry one."[3]

---

3 "Attitudes Toward Chiropractic Health Care in Oklahoma," Welling & Company and Oklahoma Chiropractic Research Foundation in cooperation with the Chiropractic Association of Oklahoma (1984)

This compelling story will changed your attitude about chiropractic, astonish your better senses to learn of the crimes committed by the American Medical Association, and will give you a new perspective of the sacrifices of these men and women whose only crime was getting sick people well with only their hands.

JC Smith, MA, DC
January 2011

et al.

"Clear writing requires clear thinking.
One cannot convey clearly to others
what is vague and indistinct in his own mind."

DD Palmer, Founder of Chiropractic[4]

It has been an aggravating experience to write an exposé on the history of the medical war against the chiropractic profession. Actually, I am not sure if "war" is the proper term to use since it suggests a fight between foes of similar size and power. Certainly the medical profession is substantially larger in numbers, funding, and its ability to disseminate propaganda against the outnumbered chiropractors who were more victims than foes. Indeed, a battle between a medical Goliath versus the chiropractic David is more appropriate in this situation.

Nonetheless, this is the story of chiropractic from the early era of intense medical persecution creating an era of pervasive public skepticism to the present era of evidence-based healthcare that has finally vindicated chiropractic care—a huge victory that has escaped the public and the press. It is my goal as a 32-year chiropractic practitioner to explain this unknown struggle for social justice over the past century.

Of course, I could not have written this history alone. I am proud to say there have been a few people who have helped me with this literary effort that has taken years to research and to write. I have always told people that I am not a writer by training, but I do have something to say.

---

4 DD Palmer, *The Chiropractor's* Adjuster, p. 813.

Fortunately, a few people in particular helped me do just that with clarity—Reed Phillips, DC, PhD, past president of the Southern California University of Health Sciences, James Edwards, DC, past chairman of the American Chiropractic Association, and John Gantner, DC, all veteran chiropractors who have fought in this war for up to forty years. Their professional insights into the issues I discuss in this book were invaluable and much appreciated.

The late Joseph C. Keating, Jr., PhD, former president of the Association for the History of Chiropractic, was a treasure trove of historical facts with his many publications that he shared with me before his death. He will also be remembered for his witty expression, "gobbledygook," which he often applied to those personalities within the chiropractic profession who crossed the line from fact to hyperbole. His voice has never been replaced as the most notable chiropractic curmudgeon.

In addition, I received insightful polish from line editors Irene Palmer and Anne Phillips. I must also thank my wife, Christy Smith, a fifth grade teacher who taught me that writing is re-writing is re-writing—a good lesson for any writer to learn.

All of my helpers should be listed as the *et al.* in the byline for their able assistance in the production of this book. They are the "others" who helped me create a manuscript worth the sacrifice of the many chiropractors over the past century whose lives made the storyline of this book.

Lastly, I must thank my courageous predecessors—the thousands of pioneers in chiropractic who were jailed, beaten, humiliated, and ghettoized for the crime of getting sick people well with only their hands and certainly without drugs or surgery. They would be pleased to learn today after a century of conflict that Dr. William Morgan was the first chiropractor to receive hospital privileges at the National Naval Medical Center in Bethesda, Maryland, which includes taking care of members of Congress and the U.S. Supreme Court.[5]

Without their spirit and determination, the art, science, and philosophy of the profession of chiropractic would be lost today. Their plight must be told, and I pray that I have done a commendable job in telling their story.

---

5 Peggy Peck, "Chiropractor Deals With Congress' Pains In Neck," MedPage Today Managing Editor, *MedPageToday.com,* (March 1, 2006)

The Chiropractic Paradox

"...'I wouldn't want my daughter to marry one.'"

1984 Oklahoma poll on chiropractic[6]

S ir Winston Churchill, prime minister of Great Britain during most of World War II, said during a radio broadcast on October 1, 1939: "I cannot forecast to you the action of Russia. It is a riddle wrapped in a mystery inside an enigma."[7]

Undoubtedly, chiropractic must appear just as baffling to most people—its Greek name is confusing; its baffling neurogenic theory of health/disease and mode of treatment via spinal manipulations are unlike medicine's germ theory, drugs, and surgery; and its vitalistic philosophy of health only confounds the mystery behind this enigmatic profession.

The chiropractic profession is, most notably, a paradox concerning its image. Without question, chiropractors have been the most maligned professionals in healthcare by their medical rivals, yet at the same time, the polls show they are praised by the vast majority of their patients. Although many medical partisans swear *at* chiropractors, many patients swear *by* chiropractic care. Certainly, this is a riddle that needs an explanation.

This paradox of the chiropractic profession is a glimpse into a little known era of medical history that began at the turn of the twentieth century, and one that is rarely discussed in classroom textbooks or scrutinized by journalists. The history behind the bias and skepticism is a fascinating exploration that few people understand and few in the

---

6 "Attitudes Toward Chiropractic Health Care in Oklahoma," Welling & Company and Oklahoma Chiropractic Research Foundation in cooperation with the Chiropractic Association of Oklahoma (1984)
7 http://www.chu.cam.ac.uk/archives/gallery/russia/CHAR_09_138_46.shtml

media have chosen to investigate. This revelation is a story the medical profession would prefer kept in the dark.

Without a doubt, the debunking of a cultural icon like the medical profession is not a pleasant task considering its Good Samaritan image held by the public, but it is an essential task to understand the medical war on chiropractors. This challenge will unearth much of the skepticism that is the root cause of the chiropractic paradox. It is a fascinating yet unknown mystery.

The notorious defamation campaign by the American Medical Association (AMA) essentially portrayed chiropractors as the "modern-day equivalent of snake-oil salesmen," according to a 1992 study by the RAND Corporation.[8] No mention was given by these investigators *why* this image existed; however, they did acknowledge this image is changing.

"In the last decade of the twentieth century, chiropractic has begun to shed its status as a marginal or deviant approach to health care and is becoming more mainstream," said Paul Shekelle, MD, director of RAND Corporation's Southern California Evidence-Based Practice Center.[9]

This RAND study revealed that people made around 280 million visits each year to chiropractors and went twice as often as they did fifteen to twenty years before.[10] These statistics shocked many since the study of chiropractic was off the research radar and considered taboo in medical enclaves; indeed, chiropractic had been the radical science profession. These statistics indicated that, despite the effect of a century of abuse from the medical profession, the chiropractic profession was growing.

The "hocus-pocus" image of chiropractic portrayed by the AMA was rattled after a landmark study by Dr. David Eisenberg from Harvard's Osher Institute that revealed more Americans were seeking non-drug, non-surgical solutions and made more visits to complementary and alternative (CAM) providers than MDs.

Baby Boomers made 427 million office visits to non-MDs in 1990 compared to 388 million visits to MDs; the follow-up survey in 1997 revealed that the numbers to non-MDs rose to 629 million while the numbers to MDs went down to 386 million.[11]

These two studies stunned the medical world, and it was shocked that Americans would choose alternative "quacks" over "modern medicine." Apparently the threat to the monolithic medical profession was bigger than anyone had imagined once the researchers took a closer look.

Dr. Eisenberg noted how his own view of chiropractic has changed from his early days to the present. He was taught in medical school that chiropractic was "irrelevant, worthless, a waste of money, and dangerous." In the 1980s it was "unproven, unorthodox,

---

8 PG Shekelle, A Adams, *et* al. "The Appropriateness of Spinal Manipulation for Low-Back Pain: Indications and Ratings by a Multidisciplinary Expert Panel." RAND Corporation, Santa Monica, California (1991)
9 "Changing Views of Chiropractic," RAND Highlights, ttp://www.rand.org/pubs/research_briefs/RB4539/index1.html
10 Shekelle, ibid.
11 DM Eisenberg, RC Kessler, C Foster, FE Norlock, DR Calkins, TL Delbanco, "Unconventional Medicine In The United States--Prevalence, Costs, And Patterns Of Use," *N Engl J Med* 328 (1993):246-252.

and unconventional." After his study showing the huge usage of CAM, he noted that the terminology has changed from "complementary and alternative" in the 1990s, to "integrative" in 2000-05, and "comprehensive" in present-day.[12] Upon seeing the huge number of Americans using CAM practitioners, Dr. Eisenberg concluded, "Maybe 'alternative' isn't so alternative anymore."[13]

Considering that chiropractic is now the third-largest physician-level health profession in the world, only behind medical physicians and dentists, it is more bewildering why so little is known about chiropractors. This snub can only be explained as a result of the medical boycott and propaganda that chiropractors have fought for over a century.

Despite the obvious trend to alternatives, the stigma against chiropractors lingers. To the millions of people who have used chiropractic care, the prejudice against chiropractors made no sense because they knew firsthand the benefits from chiropractic care. These satisfied patients were responsible for the growth of chiropractic care by referring their family and friends over the objections of their MDs.

Throughout the years, chiropractic patients have always been very loyal and supportive, such as those who picketed outside jails when their local chiropractors were imprisoned, the millions who petitioned Congress to include chiropractic care in Medicare, and those to this day who willingly pay out-of-pocket for this brand of health care.

These early chiropractic pioneers and patients would be pleased to learn their struggle against social injustice has resulted in the first Capitol Chiropractor, Dr. William Morgan, to receive hospital privileges at the National Naval Medical Center, which includes taking care of members of Congress and the U.S. Supreme Court.[14] Indeed, chiropractors have come a long way since the days of being jailed.

Yet the stigma continues because it has been engrained into the public consciousness after a century of defamation from medical propaganda. Just as racism and sexism had undesirable roots in American history, so has the medical prejudice against chiropractors been a weed in the social justice of our country.

Perplexing Polls

The paradox of chiropractic's public image has been reflected in various polls. On the positive side, chiropractors are rated very highly for their work with back pain. In fact, according to a 1991 Gallup poll of attitudes and behaviors of both users and non-users of chiropractic services, chiropractors were rated three times more patient-friendly than medical care. [15]

---

12 DM Eisenberg, "Practicing within Mainstream Healthcare," seminar held at the Massachusetts Medical Society headquarters, Boston, Nov. 18, 2006.

13 Ibid.

14 Peggy Peck, "Chiropractor Deals With Congress' Pains In Neck," MedPage Today Managing Editor, *MedPageToday.com,* (March 1, 2006)

15 The Gallup Organization, *Democratic Characteristics of Users of Chiropractic Services* (Princeton, NJ: The Gallup Organization (1991)

The Gallup poll also found of the *users* of chiropractic services:

- 90% felt chiropractic treatment was effective,
- More than 80% were satisfied with their treatment,
- Nearly 75% felt most of their expectations had been met during their visits,
- 68% would see a chiropractor again for treatment of a similar condition, and
- 50% would likely see a chiropractor again for other conditions.

Of the *non-users* of chiropractic services, the Gallup poll concluded:

- 62% responded they would see a doctor of chiropractic for a problem applicable to chiropractic treatment,
- 25% reported that someone in their household had been treated by a chiropractor, and
- Nearly 80% of those had been satisfied with the chiropractic treatment received.

In 2009, another positive poll of 14,000 back pain patients by *Consumer Reports* magazine rated chiropractors at the top. Hands-on therapies were rated above any other type of medical care. 58 percent of those who tried chiropractic manipulation said it helped a lot, and 59 percent were "completely" or "very" satisfied with their chiropractor. Massage and physical therapy were close runners-up, but *medical physician care was at the bottom of the list.*[16]

Also in 2009, in another Gallup poll on Honesty and Ethics Standards of Professions, the image of chiropractors' ranked eighth of twenty two professionals: higher than bankers, state governors, senators, congressmen, stockbrokers, and HMO managers who were all ranked lower than chiropractors. The downside of this survey was chiropractors were ranked among the lowest of health professionals, only above psychiatrists.[17]

Despite the low image among health professionals, in regard to actual treatments rated by chiropractic patients, 34 percent rated chiropractors as VERY HIGH/HIGH and 47 percent rated them AVERAGE, which equates to 81 percent of people who rated chiropractors in a favorable light. Only 19 percent rated chiropractors as LOW/VERY LOW or had no opinion.

Chiropractic care was recently introduced into the military health services selectively at a few TRICARE facilities and scored enormously high patient satisfaction rates in a 2009 poll that ranged from 94.3 percent in the Army; the Air Force tally was also high with twelve of 19 bases scoring 100 percent; the Navy also reported ratings at 90 percent or higher; and the TRICARE outpatient satisfaction surveys (TROSS) rated chiropractors

---

16 "Relief for Aching Backs: Hands-on Therapies were Top Rated by 14,000 Consumers," *Consumer Report* (May 2009)

17 L Saad, "Gallup: Honesty and Ethics Poll Finds Congress' Image Tarnished," (December 9, 2009)

at 88.54 percent, which was 10 percent "higher than the overall satisfaction with all providers" that scored at 78.31 percent.[18]

This Chiropractic Care Study also commented on the Unit Commanders and military treatment facilities (MTF) personnel concerning chiropractic care. "The responses were overwhelmingly a five (the highest rating available); MTFs that offer chiropractic care are pleased to do so."

Another congressionally mandated pilot project conducted from April, 2005, to March, 2007, testing the feasibility of expanding chiropractic services in the Medicare program, patients again gave a high rate of satisfaction with the care they received from doctors of chiropractic.[19] When asked to rate their satisfaction on a 10-point scale, 87 percent of patients in the study gave their chiropractor a level of 8 or higher. What is more interesting is that 56 percent of those patients rated their chiropractor with a perfect 10.

Contributing to that satisfaction was the attention given to patients' needs and the accessibility of chiropractic care. Patients reported that doctors of chiropractic listened to them carefully and spent sufficient time with them. Some 95 percent said they had to wait no longer than one week for appointments.

So, the paradox is evident: on one hand, the majority of actual chiropractic patients are "very satisfied" with their treatments in the *Consumer Reports,* Gallup, TRICARE, and Medicare polls; on the other hand, the public image of the chiropractic professional in the other Gallup poll on image leaves a lot to be desired when only 34 percent of the public rates chiropractors' image as VERY HIGH/HIGH.

Another public survey taken in 1984 in Oklahoma also illustrated the paradox many people have about their mixed attitudes toward chiropractors.

> The fact that *chiropractors are an acceptable part of the health care scene* is the number one attitude which is agreed with in a list of eleven offered to respondents. Number two is the fact that most people do not have a good opinion of chiropractic. *Seventy-one percent feel chiropractors probably suffer under a stigma which may not be deserved.*
>
> The third most agreed with factor is the opinion that *chiropractors are highly underestimated regarding their benefit to the community and their patients.* Sixty percent hold or agree with this opinion to one extent or another...to many respondents, chiropractors are seen as being fine for many people in the community, but *'I wouldn't want my daughter to marry one.'*[20] (emphasis added)

This poll was very insightful: People feel chiropractors are an acceptable part of the health care scene, they realize chiropractors suffer with a stigma which may not

---

18 Chiropractic Care Study, Senate Report 110-335 accompanying the National Defense Authorization Act for FY 2009; letter sent to Congressmen by Ellen P. Embrey, Deputy Assistant Secretary of Defense (September 22, 2009):2.

19 WB Stason, G Ritter, DS Shepard, C Tompkins, TC Martin, S Lee, "Report to Congress on the Evaluation of the Demonstration of Coverage of Chiropractic Services Under Medicare," (June 16, 2009)

20 "Attitudes toward chiropractic health care in Oklahoma," Welling & Company and Oklahoma Chiropractic Research Foundation in cooperation with the Chiropractic Association of Oklahoma (1984)

be deserved, and that chiropractors are highly underestimated regarding their benefit to the community and their patients. These are very astute observations by the public concerning the chiropractic paradox.

However, when someone opines, "I wouldn't want my daughter to marry one," something remains terribly amiss.

I still recall a similar comment made by a good friend of mine while we were graduate students at Rutgers University. We both were satisfied patients of the local chiropractor, but when I announced to my friends I was transferring to chiropractic college, one told me, "It's okay to see a chiropractor, but do you really want to *be* one?"

We both were aware of the stigma against chiropractors, but we also understood its benefits. This is the paradox every chiropractor lives with daily—good results under the cloud of skepticism.

However, the facts today reveal that *being* a chiropractor is much better than most people realize. In 1997, the U.S. Public Health Service conducted an investigation, *"Chiropractic in the United States: Training, Practice and Research,"* that admitted "chiropractic has undergone a remarkable transformation" as well as other very positive conclusions:

> Spinal manipulation and the profession most closely associated with its use, chiropractic, have gained legitimacy within the United States health care system that until very recently seemed unimaginable.
>
> In the past several decades, chiropractic has undergone a remarkable transformation. *Labeled an "unscientific cult" by organized medicine as little as 20 years ago, chiropractic is now recognized as the principal source of one of the few treatments recommended by national evidence-based guidelines for the treatment of low-back pain, spinal manipulation.* In the areas of training, practice, and research, chiropractic has emerged from the periphery of the health care system and is playing an increasingly important role in discussions of health care policy.[21]

In fact, despite the need for a thick skin and a strong back bone, chiropractors today enjoy a professional lifestyle better than many in the healthcare profession.

According to the Occupational Outlook Handbook from the Bureau of Labor Statistics, the top 200 professions were compared in terms of work environment, physical demands, stress, income, and hiring outlook.[22] According an article in *The Wall Street Journal*, "The Best and Worst Jobs," in the latest 2011 jobs outlook the rank of chiropractic has improved from #56 in 2010 to #32 in 2011.[23] The data comes from a survey by CareerCast.[24]

---

21 DC Cherkin, RD Mootz, eds. "Chiropractic in the United States: Training, Practice And Research." Rockville, Maryland: Agency for Health Care Policy and Research, Public Health Service, U.S. Department of Health and Human Services, (1997); AHCPR Publication No. 98-N002.

22 U.S. Department of Labor Bureau of Labor Statistics Occupational Outlook Handbook @ www.bls.gov/oco/ocos071.htm

23 Joe Light, "The Best and Worst Jobs," *The Wall Street Journal*, (January 4, 2011)

24 Andrew Strieber, "Jobs Rated 2011: Ranking 200 Jobs From Best to Worst," (January 5, 2011) CareerCast.com

Chiropractors scored higher than several other professionals as well as other health care professionals, ahead of civil engineer (#33), pharmacist (#36), school principal (#41), physical therapist (#45), nuclear engineer (#49), judge (#53), mechanical engineer (#62), dentist (#75), electrical engineer (#78), attorney (#82), physician (#83), physician assistant (#85), psychiatrist (#92), registered nurse (#94), teacher (#100), surgeon (#101), and in last place, a roustabout (#200).

One can only imagine that chiropractors would be rated higher if the AMA had not waged a war to slander the chiropractic profession. Indeed, if the medical discrimination against chiropractors were a non-issue, being a chiropractor is a rather enjoyable job as most chiropractors realize. As well, if the medical monarchists were not in sole control, in other words, if there were a level playing field in healthcare where free enterprise was the rule, the chiropractic profession would be among the top jobs in America.

According to this report on chiropractic, "Employment is projected to grow much faster than average. Job prospects should be good." Its description of chiropractic in the future is also encouraging for both patients and future chiropractors who will enjoy the fruit sown by the chiropractic predecessors who fought to keep this ancient healing art alive.

> Employment change: Employment of chiropractors is expected to increase 20 percent between 2008 and 2018, much faster than the average for all occupations. Projected job growth stems from increasing consumer demand for alternative healthcare. Because chiropractors emphasize the importance of healthy lifestyles and do not prescribe drugs or perform surgery, chiropractic care is appealing to many health-conscious Americans. Chiropractic treatment of the back, neck, extremities, and joints has become more accepted as a result of research and changing attitudes about alternative, noninvasive healthcare practices. Chiropractors who specialize in pediatric care will be in demand as chiropractic spinal treatment is very gentle and children enjoy subsequent visits. The rapidly expanding older population, with its increased likelihood of mechanical and structural problems, also will increase demand for chiropractors.

Although chiropractic has an image problem among non-users tainted by the medical propaganda as well as a persistent medical foe waging a war that never seems to end, chiropractors have lifted themselves from their humble beginnings to make a comfortable occupation today.

Moreover, recent spine research into the epidemic of back pain has confirmed what chiropractors and their patients have always known—chiropractic care works better than medical care for most back pain cases. This irony is the compelling yet untold story of chiropractic from persecution to vindication—the paradox of chiropractic that begs to be examined.

J. Michael Flynn, DC, the 2011 president of the World Federation of Chiropractic and a past chairman of the American Chiropractic Association, noted the improvement of the chiropractic profession despite these hardships:

> We are maturing as a profession, and I believe that by the end of this decade our advances will find doctors of chiropractic among the most respected of the healing arts for the services they provide. Continued research, legislative success, a growing public relations effort, and the profession coming together harnessing our collective strengths as a profession are excellent signs.
>
> From the office of attending physicians in the U.S. Capitol to the Medical Director of the US Olympic Committee that are manned by chiropractors, and much in-between, there are indications that our profession is on the cusp of greatness for patients in need of chiropractic care. Yes, today we are not fulfilling our capacity and we have been part of the problem by our immaturity and our failure to organize in significant numbers. One of the AMA's covert strategies was to "encourage disunity" and watch them "wither on the vine." We have not withered, but we have yet to fully bloom.[25]

Like the classic tale of the ugly duckling, after a century of torment, chiropractic is slowly transforming into a beautiful swan—albeit long over-due and with a few ruffled feathers.

---

25 M Flynn via private communication with JC Smith (9-13-2010)

Century of Conflict

The medical war began during the first decade of the twentieth century. Within thirty years thousands of chiropractors were arrested and imprisoned. Eighty years later an historic federal court decision stopped the open warfare. Currently a cold war exists.

The Medical War

*"Scientific medicine absorbs from them that which is good,
if there is any good, and then they die."*

Morris Fishbein, MD, former AMA Executive Director[26]

The medical profession has waged a number of highly publicized wars, such as the early wars against small pox and polio, and then the less successful wars against cancer and heart disease. However, these were mere skirmishes compared to the biggest battle of them all.

Unquestionably, the American Medical Association (AMA) has fought its longest, most aggressive, and most illegal war against chiropractors. They were essentially the last survivors after the AMA's wars against other competitors were victorious. Chiropractors reluctantly became the most prominent resistance fighters for freedom of choice in healthcare and, for nearly a century, it was a war chiropractors were to fight alone.

According to historian Russell W. Gibbons, chiropractors felt the brunt as one of the first grass roots movements in America:

> …like abolitioinists, chiropractors were systematically persecuted and driven from town to town. Like the feminists and suffragettes, chiropractors were made objects of ridicule. And like the civil rights workers of more recent times, chiropractors were intimidated and subverted by agents and provacateurs. In the finest tradition of reform movements, they were imprisoned for their beliefs. [27]

---

26 M Fishbein, *Medical Follies,* New York, Boni & Liveright, (1925): 43.

27 R Gibbons, ibid. p. 67.

To place this warfare into historical perspective, America was still in the throes of civil injustice in many arenas when the medical war began. Civil rights and political diversity were not championed during this era. Residual racism from the Civil War was still rampant with the *Ku Klux Klan* and *Jim Crow* mindset prevalent in many communities; women had not yet achieved voting rights; anti-Semitism was brewing internationally; and the power of an emerging medical monarchy in American was taking hold.

Certainly a conflict of ideas between these different approaches was inevitable, but this medical war turned malicious from the beginning because it was never fought in a professional manner with scholarly seminars, comparative clinical research studies, or inter-professional debates. Instead, political medicine used the courts to prosecute chiropractors, lobbied the state legislatures to resist licensing of chiropractors, fought against chiropractic educational improvements, and influenced the media to disparage the reputations of chiropractors. No leaf was left unturned in this campaign to destroy the chiropractic profession.

Early twentieth century medical science refused to investigate the embryonic neurobiological science of chiropractic care or recognize the value of the ageless art of manipulative therapy to help the pandemic of back pain. Historically, the art of spinal manipulation is not a new healing method—over 3,000 years ago the great Egyptian doctor, Imhotep, wrote of this healing art.[28]

In ancient Greece, Hippocrates provided more evidence in his book, *On Joints,* written in the fifth century BC. This described the practice of spinal manipulation by physical means such as traction or local pressure to correct spinal deformities. [29]

During the Renaissance, Leonardo da Vinci (1452-1519) accurately described the anatomy of the spine and was perhaps the first to investigate spinal stability. The first comprehensive treatise on biomechanics, *De Motu Animalium,* was published in 1680 by Giovanni Borelli, who is often called the "Father of Spinal Biomechanics."[30]

The term "bonesetter" first appeared as an English word in 1510 and this skill was an art taught via hands-on training, not in schools, and generally kept secret by family members.[31] One medieval European bonesetter, Sir Herbert Atkinson Barker, was knighted by the King George V of England.[32] Early bonesetters such as the families of Sweets and Tieszens immigrated to the United States long before AT Still began osteopathy in 1874 or DD Palmer began chiropractic in 1895. [33,34,35]

---

28 NM Hadler, *Stabbed In The Back; Confronting Back Pain In An Overtreated Society*, University of North Carolina Press, (2009):6-7

29 Haldeman, Ibid. p. 7.

30 S Abhay, S Setti Rengachary, "The History of Spinal Biomechanics," *Neurosurgery* 39 (1996):657-69.

31 Abhay ibid. p. 657.

32 Unifiedbonesetter.com/page5.htm

33 AT Still, *Autobiography —With a History of the Discovery and Development of the Science of Osteopathy.* (New York: Arno Press, 1972; *New York Times*).

34 MR McPartland, "The Bonesetter Sweets of South County, Rhode Island," YANKEE (January 1968)

35 AT Still, *Autobiography—With a History of the Discovery and Development of the Science of Osteopathy.* (New York: Arno Press, 1972; *New York Times*).

Rather than searching for the truth how this ageless art has helped patients, political medicine instead chose to behave more like a ruthless monarchy persecuting its competitors rather than a professional society seeking scientific truths to help the sick and infirmed.

How the AMA became this medical monarchy required important political maneuvers. First would entail gaining authority and power by petitioning the government. The medical society had to convince politicians as well as the courts that they were the only ones capable to determine their own technical standards. A U.S. Supreme Court decision (*Dent v. State of West Virginia*, 129 U.S. 114, 122-123) in 1888 enabled this concept when Justice Stephen Field wrote that "comparatively few" could comprehend the "subtle and mysterious" nature of medical work.[36] *Trust Regulating Itself and all competition*

The ploy by the medical society to regulate its competition fell under the guise of "public safety." The AMA, as the "guardians of health," created practice regulations based solely on its own allopathic principles and educational standards, excluding all other types of healing arts as "unscientific."

According to Carl Ameringer, author of *The Health Care Revolution*:[37]

> Professionalism was a response to the perceived chaos of the nineteenth century, in which quacks, pretenders, and poorly trained practitioners proliferated for lack of educational standards and government regulation. Medical licensing, which took hold in the late 1800s, was a prime example. On the one hand, politicians gained from having professionals solve societal problems without having to expand the size of government; on the other, *professionals furthered their own interests by wielding governmental authority to control competition.* (emphasis added)

By 1901, all states had delegated authority to the medical profession to set standards and to police itself with a medical code of ethics. The code also demanded physicians "to bear testimony against quackery in all its forms," which included homeopathy, naturopathy, eclectics, and Christian Scientists. Later osteopaths and chiropractors became targets of physicians and their medical societies.[38] Not only were snake oil salesmen a target of this anti-quackery effort, so too were non-allopathic, drugless practitioners who disdained drugs of any sort. The medical society also deplored those allopaths who advertised for patients, their action being perceived as a "divisive" behavior.[39]

The strategy in the medical war against quackery embraced a new tactic after the demise of patent medicines. Ironically, those now branded as "quacks" were no longer just the "snake oil" salesmen associated with patent medicines. Many victims in this emerging medical war were principally the complementary and alternative medicine (CAM) practitioners.

---

36 C Ameringer, ibid. p. 23, (*Dent v. State of West Virginia*, 129 U.S. 114, 122-123 [1888])

37 C Ameringer, *The Health Care Revolution*, UC Press Foundation, (2008):22.

38 Ibid.

39 Ibid.

DD Palmer, the founder of chiropractic, was in good company when the AMA began the witch hunt on the new quacks. In 1906, Palmer found himself in this anti-quackery hysteria led by the AMA that was sweeping the country, so it would come as no surprise that was he was the first chiropractor convicted and sent to jail for practicing medicine without a license.[40]

In view of the fact that no layman was hurt or complained about Palmer's treatment, this trial was really a sham that became the first act of war against chiropractic. Like the shot heard around the world at Lexington, it was the first blow from the AMA's heavy handiness to stop chiropractic's healing hands, and it would not be the final one.

According to historian Russell Gibbons, Palmer "waxed eloquent in his defense" during the trial and after his conviction gave his own closing remarks:

> The jury was not to blame for rendering the verdict they did. Behind the jury was the judge, who gave his instructions. Behind the judge was the medical law. This law was not made by the people, but by the medical profession. It was made for the purpose of protecting that profession. Not for protecting you and I.
>
> I, as DD Palmer, the discoverer and developer, the originator of Chiropractic...feel that I have a constitutional liberty to the discovery that I have made and the people have the right to it.[41]

Palmer spoke of the basic rights in healthcare—the freedom of choice by patients seeking health care was not protected by the Constitution nor is it today. Neither is the right of any type of practitioner to practice healthcare. Simply the laying of hands to help suffering is considered legally the practice of medicine and it was this legal loophole that enabled the medical monarchy to wield the authority of government.

The rights of patients to use chiropractors and the right of chiropractors to help patients without legal persecution would only be guaranteed when the last state law was passed in Louisiana nearly three-quarters of a century after DD Palmer's conviction. Thousands of other chiropractic martyrs would continue to be incarcerated until those scope laws were individually passed in each state to establish and protect the chiropractors' scope of practice.

Palmer after his conviction pointed out one bit of irony at his trial:

> When Con Murphy (the assisting prosecuting attorney) came in here yesterday, he did not offer his services as prosecuting attorney. He was brought into my office, suffering excruciating pain from sciatica rheumatism, and was cured with one adjustment. It was a crime to tell it.[42]

---

40 Gielow, *Davenport Democrat* publishes story of DD's conviction and refusal to pay fine (Mar 28, 1906), (1981):106,

41 R Gibbons, ibid. p. 62.

42 Gibbons, ibid. p. 62. (found in *The Chiropractor*, 3/4 (April 1906).

The scene of a prosecuting district attorney or arresting officer in a defendant's office would be replayed many times by local police officers who were also patients of the chiropractors they were arresting. Often many imprisoned chiropractors were allowed to adjust patients and jailers while incarcerated.

When the medical monarchy's prosecution of chiropractors spread throughout the country, out of legal necessity the chiropractic profession had to develop a defense, and the unique philosophy of chiropractic became its cornerstone.[43]

DD Palmer in his writings made it clear that the science and philosophy of chiropractic was distinctly different than osteopathy or allopathic medicine—nerves vs. blood—and this became the foundation for its legal defense. The landmark legal case that rescued chiropractors from continued persecution would feature a most unlikely man—a Japanese immigrant by the name of Shegetaro Morikubo—who attended Palmer School of Chiropractic (PSC) in 1906.

He was a learned man having previously earned a PhD from the Tokyo Academy of Science, was fluent in German and English, and while a student at PSC was involved with DD Palmer in the development of his book, *The Chiropractor's Adjustor*. In fact, many of the photo illustrations in the book were of him as DD's patient.[44]

In 1907, Morikubo settled in the Midwestern town of LaCrosse, Wisconsin, where he encountered not only a hostile medical society, but anti-Oriental racism and conservative opposition to liberal immigration sentiments. When he was arrested for practicing medicine without a license, *The LaCrosse Tribune* newspaper headline proclaimed, "Jap Chiropractor Arrested."

According to historian William S. Rehm, "The *Tribune's* race-baiting was obvious as it characterized Morikubo's reaction to being arrested. 'I am an American citizen duly naturalized and insist upon my American rights and liberties,' said the little Jap with flashing eyes to this reporter."[45]

To Morikubo's rescue came BJ Palmer and famed liberal attorney Tom Morris, formerly the LaCrosse County district attorney from 1900 to 1904, who had a reputation for opposing what he considered to be selfish interests—the railroads, the rich, the "stalwarts" of the Republican Party, including the medical society.[17]

Morris found a winning defense when he introduced two essential differences between chiropractic and his opponents—osteopathy and allopathic medicine—a different "philosophy" and different healing techniques. He found his supportive research not from anything either DD Palmer or BJ Palmer had written, but from a textbook by Solon M. Langworthy, a staunch rival of the Palmers with his school in Cedar Rapids, Iowa,

---

43 D Seaman, "A Cure for the Curse of Chiropractic, Part One," *Dynamic Chiropractic* 25/3 (January 29, 2007).

44 Gibbons, ibid. p. 64.

45 Gibbons, ibid. p. 65.

with his journal, *The Backbone,* and with his new textbook, *Modernized Chiropractic,* also published in 1906.[46]

Morris showed the court that, according to Langworthy's propositions, chiropractic was concerned with nerves while osteopathy and medicine were primarily focused on blood. He also showed that chiropractic techniques were more specific and specialized compared to the more general osteopathic manipulation.

DD Palmer wrote about this important trial that "it took the jury but twenty minutes to decide" in favor of Morikubo. [47] This huge victory established chiropractic as a separate and distinct health profession. Morris was retained by BJ Palmer and the Universal Chiropractors Association (UCA) and they established a Chiropractic Health Bureau as a legal defense group to defend chiropractors elsewhere by creating a network of regional attorneys throughout the country.[48]

From 1907 until his death in 1928, attorney Tom Morris was the chief legal counsel for the UCA and principal "defender of chiropractic." Headquartered in La Crosse, Morris' law firm defended thousands of DCs charged with unlicensed practice, and won a reputed 75-80 percent of their cases, especially when the verdict was rendered by a jury rather than a judge.[49]

BJ Palmer and John Fitz Alan Howard (who founded in 1906 the National School of Chiropractic (NSC) and now known as the National University of Health Sciences in Chicago), agreed that chiropractic needed to create distinctive terminology and a unique philosophy for the purpose of legal protection.

In his 1934 *Memoirs,* Howard stated:

> In the early days it was necessary to protect the 'child' (as DD was wont to refer to his Chiropractic) by evasive terminology in order to avoid the chill and ice of the law and 'analysis' was used for diagnosis, 'adjustment' was employed for treatment, 'pressure on the nerve' was used for reflex stimulation or inhibition, etc. These terms were garments to protect the child until legal clothing could be secured.[50]

Unfortunately, as author R.P. Beideman noted, too many chiropractors took this "legal clothing to be gospel, rather than a temporary semantic means to one end–legal protection."[51] From this would later evolve the evangelistic branch of the chiropractic tree.

In 1908 Howard moved his NSC to Illinois so as to obtain the "legal clothing" instantaneously of drugless physicians through the Medical Practice Act which was

---

46 Rehm, ibid. p 53.

47 Palmer, ibid. p. 389.

48 Rehm, ibid. p 53.

49 JC Keating, "The Gestation & Difficult Birth of the American Chiropractic Association," National Institute of Chiropractic Research, A Presentation to the Association for the History of Chiropractic (June 2006)

50 RP Beideman, *In the Making of a Profession: The National College of Chiropractic, (1906-1981),* National College of Chiropractic, Lombard, IL (1995):28.

51 Beideman, ibid. p. 38

already in place since 1899. Illinois chiropractors were licensed as doctors to diagnose and treat human ailments without the use of drugs, medicine and operative surgery.[52] This legal coverage prevented the mass arrests in Illinois experienced by chiropractors in other states.

While the National School of Chiropractic favored the drugless, non-surgical aspect of Palmer's brand of "straight" chiropractic, the National brand had a much broader, "liberal platform" of chiropractic. More shocking to the Palmers was Howard's difference that chiropractic could cure all disease:[53]

> Before taking up the application of Chiropractic, or "Chiropractic in Practice," we desire that the student shall have a thorough understanding of the comprehensive and liberal platform for which our school stands. We do not claim that it is a panacea for all ills, *nor that it is potent in all cases to the entire exclusion or depreciation of other agencies.* [54] (emphasis added).

Dr. Howard refrained from DD Palmer's belief that 95 percent of all disease stemmed from the spine and, instead, constructed a holistic drugless *therapeutic* system including the essential features characterizing the practice of chiropractic as it would become more widely accepted and practiced today.[55]

In 1906, these two branches that sprouted from the chiropractic tree would lock horns in a bitter civil war and remain rivals to this day—the fundamentalist Palmer "straight" branch and the Howard "mixer" branch.

In battles in state legislatures, progress was slowly being made to protect chiropractors and their patients. Dr. Anna M. Foy, seven other Kansas chiropractors, and BJ Palmer founded the Kansas Chiropractic Association on January 28, 1911. That led to Kansas passing the first chiropractic licensing law in the world. In recognition of her efforts, Dr. Anna M. Foy received Kansas license Number 1.[56]

In 1913, legislation similar to that of the Illinois Medical Practice Act passed in the states of Pennsylvania and Michigan. It consisted of Drugless Practitioners amendments to their Medical Practice Acts, which included chiropractors. This was followed by rather generous inclusions of broad scope chiropractic practice in the Medical Practice Acts of the States of Virginia, West Virginia, Ohio and Alabama.

This legal precedent did not stop the prosecutors in other states. Until 1922, when a referendum was passed in California to protect chiropractors, roundups were used to jail chiropractors en masse as this account testifies:

---

52 RP Beideman, "Chiropractors Are Physicians (And Almost Always Were)," *Journal of Chiropractic Humanities* The National College of Chiropractic (1999): 7.

53 JFA Howard, "Home Study Course," 15 (1910): 391

54 Ibid. p. 10.

55 Ibid. p. 3

56 WS Rehm, "Kansas Coconuts: Legalizing Chiropractic in the First State, 1910-1915." *The Archives and Journal of the Association for the History of Chiropractic*, Centennial Issue, (December, 1995)

In just one year [1921] 450 of approximately 600 chiropractors were hauled into court and convicted of practicing without a license. They were given jail sentences or the alternative of a fine. They chose to go to jail.[57]

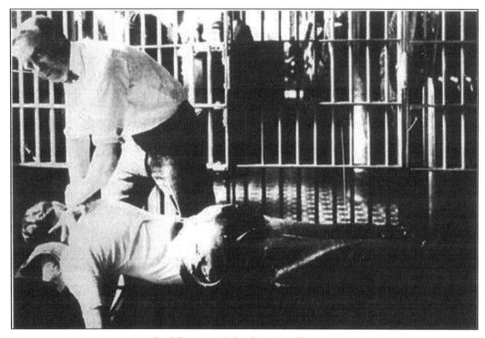

Fred Courtney, DC, adjusting cell mates
in LA County jail, Feb. 1921
Used by permission of Palmer College of Chiropractic

Convictions became more difficult as patients refused to testify against them. In 1922, after four chiropractors were jailed in Taft, California, the judge asked the sheriff why there were so few witnesses in view of the many subpoenas issued. The Sheriff said:

> Your Honor, the sheriff's office has been unable to catch the witnesses. They hide under beds and run out the back doors. They won't testify against these chiropractors. The Sheriff's office has a lot of important business, so if you want these witnesses, you'll have to catch them yourself.[58]

The nastiness of the medical profession was evident not only by these legal persecutions, but by many uncivil acts. For example, in 1926, a medical society spokesman debating Lyndon Lee, DC, a 1915 Palmer graduate and former Amherst student, snarled at Lee during a legislative fray in New York State:

> "Yes, we are against you. We are against chiropractic and all other fakers. If this legislature will give us this bill, we will drive you and your ilk out of this state! What do think about that?"

---

57 B Inglis. *The Case For Unorthodox Medicine,* New York: GP Putnam (1963)
58 Ibid. p. 67.

"First, sir," Lee responded, "I'd like to see your driver's license."[59]

The warning to "drive you and your ilk out of this state" was not merely a blowhard speaking, but it was a real threat that happened to many chiropractors. Like the KKK terrorizing African-Americans, the medical society was powerful in the courtrooms, in the churches, and in the streets.

Evon Barvinchack, a second-generation chiropractor, spoke of a childhood event in the 1940s when he first experienced the "Juice Man" from the local police department in Binghamton, New York. The Juice Man came to *squeeze* his father for extortion payoff:

> In 1945 my dad graduated from Palmer Chiropractic College and opened his first practice at 38 Baxter Street, Binghamton, New York. This is where the "Juice Man" roamed. He was usually accompanied by two other enforcers. Chiropractic was not licensed in New York State at this time. Therefore, my dad was guilty of practicing medicine without a license. Thus the Juice Man. It is my understanding that in order to not go to jail, chiropractors paid the Juice Man to "look the other way" (equivalent to a modern day protection racket). As with all "protection" scams, the price kept going up and it became harder and harder for the chiropractors to come up with the money.
>
> So now the Juice Man had a quandary: if he jailed the chiropractors he lost his cash stream. Thus, the beatings began; I remember my mother crying and screaming and my Dad being knocked around his office. Once he was dragged out into the front yard and publically beaten. I still have a picture in my mind of his severely swollen face and a black eye—a very grotesque picture to a young boy. This was the first black eye I had ever seen. My mother said I had nightmares about it for several months. Another local DC was hospitalized after one of his beatings.
>
> Evidently, the Juice Man was someone of authority or had connections to someone of authority, because he scared my parents and other chiropractors. How much did he collect I don't know and I don't think my parents ever said. But I remember my mother telling me that "the Juice Man" stole our Christmas. My dad soon closed his office in Binghamton and moved to Marathon, New York. No Juice Man there.[60]

Dr. Barvinchack's experience was not the only example of this medical persecution in New York. In 1949, the saga of two chiropractic "jailhouse martyrs" occurred in New York. Katherine "Kitty" Scallon and her husband, Mack Scallon, also a chiropractor in Manhattan (their patients included Ambassador Joseph Kennedy), were jailed simultaneously when they refused to desist in the practice of medicine without a license.

Kitty Scallon said from the Women's House of Detention in 1949:

> Being here [in jail] is sometimes like a bad dream…but I'd throw my shoulders back and be ready and willing to make any sacrifice to help free our beloved science.[61]

---

59 Gibbons, ibid, p. 67.

60 E Barvinchack via private communication with JC Smith, 9-9-10.

61 Gibbons, ibid. p. 27.

The same battles were fought in every unregulated state until 1974 when the last state, Louisiana, passed the state law to create a separate scope of practice for chiropractors. The law now protected chiropractors from charges of practicing medicine without a license, but these legislative victories did not come without a price.

It is difficult for Americans to imagine such skullduggery would occur simply because chiropractors chose to help people get well with only their hands, without drugs or surgery. Today people do not understand the dedication by many activists in the long fight to preserve the chiropractic profession.

Dr. James Edwards, former chairman of the American Chiropractic Association, spoke about one such warrior, Dr. Lyndon Lee, who led the chiropractors in New York in the half-century struggle for licensure. He was 95 years old when he died and had practiced in Mt. Vernon, New York, for 65 years. He retired in 1979 at the age of 91 only due to a fractured hip.

> Dr. Lee's passing brought the finish to one of the more remarkable personal histories of the chiropractic profession. He graduated from Palmer School of Chiropractic in 1915 and was a charter member of the reorganized New York State Chiropractic Society and became one of the profession's best known figures. He helped draft every licensing bill presented to the New York legislature between 1915 and 1963 when a favorable vote was finally obtained. During his career he had many roles including serving as vice-president-at-large of the American Chiropractic Association in the late 1920s and was all everything for the state of New York for decades.

> But I want to tell you what I consider Dr. Lee's greatest achievement. In 1933, Dr. Lee was arrested and cited for "practicing medicine without a license." Although he would finally be acquitted, his case was in and out of the courts 30 times within the next three years. Dr. Lee and others like him were singled out and tested by those who were trying to destroy chiropractic during those early years. We have this great profession today because the Lee pioneers were willing to pay the price for what they believed in.[62]

---

62 J Edwards, DC, Logan College of Chiropractic Commencement Address, (August 23, 2008)

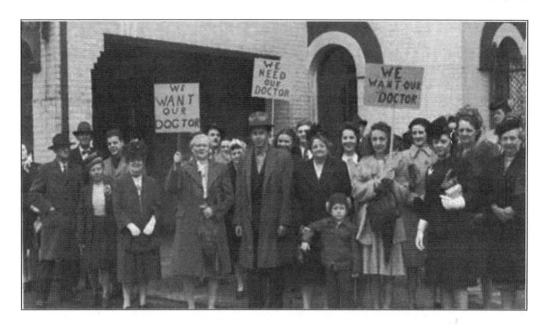

Patients protest outside the Ohio jail where their doctor, Herbert
R. Reaver, D.C., was imprisoned. Circa 1920s.

JC Keating, CS Cleveland III, M Menke, "Chiropractic History: a Primer,"
(c) 2004, Association for the History of Chiropractic, Davenport, Iowa

History books will never mention that 12,000 chiropractors were jailed, collectively, over 15,000 times in the first thirty years of the twentieth century for allegedly practicing medicine without a license, resulting in 3,300 convictions, even though chiropractors never used drugs or surgery.[63] Ironically, their real crime was getting people well *without* drugs or surgery. No matter what healing method used, the AMA was against any and all competition and used its political might to maintain their monarchy, including mass arrests.

Although a cascade of victories in state legislatures won the chiropractic profession legal recognition and protection from medical harassment, the acrimonious, dominating medical monarchy—aided by a medical-friendly media—would continue to battle chiropractors in the war for public opinion and in federal/state legislative conflicts. Although chiropractic had dodged one bullet with licensure, it was certainly not out of the line of fire in the medical war.

The AMA was poised to continue the fight on other battle fronts, and they needed a strong leader to maintain control of the healthcare market by fostering public skepticism of chiropractic practitioners with a multi-year campaign of dirty tricks, public propaganda, legislative obstruction, and other coercive legal tactics. Such deliberate tactics were to become the hallmark of the AMA's leadership under its most notorious leader.

---

63 Gibbons, ibid. pp.61–71.

The Medical Mussolini

History is replete with political or industrial leaders plotting to "contain and eliminate" their competitors. At the turn of the twentieth century, many believed that big businesses, referred to as "trusts," were harmful to the nation's economy and to consumers. By eliminating competition, trusts could charge whatever price they chose. Corporate greed, rather than market demands, determined the price for products.[64] This opportunity became the model for the medical monarchy.

Progressives advocated legislation that would break up these trusts, known as "trust-busting." Although trust-busting was popular during the Theodore Roosevelt administration after the Sherman Anti-Trust Act was passed in 1890, the AMA eluded such regulation due to its privileged position after the U.S. Supreme Court decision (*Dent v. State of West Virginia*, 129 U.S. 114, 122-123) in 1888. This enabled the AMA to become a ruthless and unregulated trust falling outside of the antitrust laws until the law was changed after a U.S. Supreme Court ruling in 1975.[65]

The building of the medical trust and the defamation of chiropractors can be traced back to one man—the original medical demagogue by the name of Morris Fishbein. If it had not been for his conniving character and devious strategy, the image of chiropractic would be dramatically different today.

Chiropractic historian, Russell Gibbons, recognized the singular impact of Fishbein and concluded he was "the most important non-chiropractor to influence the chiropractic profession."[66]

Fishbein's tyranny essentially began in 1910 after the Flexner Report[67] resulted in the closing of many medical, homeopathic, and osteopathic schools. Two years later the fledging medical monarchy went on the offensive through the establishment of its Propaganda Department that was specifically dedicated to attacking any and all unconventional medical treatments and anyone (including MDs) who practiced them, namely the chiropractors, naturopaths, homeopaths, and original osteopaths.

The Flexner Report used the nonprofit, federally subsidized university hospital setting as the new teaching facility of the medical profession, with Johns Hopkins as the model school, eventually gaining control of federal healthcare research and student aid.[68] This was the insidious second step by the AMA to become an invisible branch of government with the Flexner Report in one hand and the purse strings for healthcare in the other hand.

64 "Trust Busting", *Ohio History Central*, (July 1, 2005) http://www.ohiohistorycentral.org/entry.php?rec=1520

65 US Supreme Court: *Goldfarb v. Virginia State Bar*, 421 U.S. 773 (1975)

66 RW Gibbons, "From Quacks To Colleagues?" Viewing the evolution of orthodox tolerance of deviant medical practice, *Journal of Chiropractic Humanities* 4/1 (1994):61-71.

67 The Flexner Report was published in 1910 under the aegis of the Carnegie Foundation and called on American medical schools to enact higher admission and graduation standards, and to adhere strictly to the protocols of mainstream medical science in their teaching and research.

68 C Lerner, 'Report on the history of chiropractic' L.E. Lee papers, Palmer College Library Archives

Medical sociologist Paul Starr wrote in his Pulitzer Prize-winning book, *The Social Transformation of American Medicine*,[69] that as a result of the Flexner Report, the AMA presumed to have cultural authority to invoke its force upon both the medical profession and competing health professions like homeopathy, osteopathy, and chiropractic.

> The AMA Council became a national accrediting agency for medical schools, as an increasing number of states adopted its judgments of unacceptable institutions...*Even though no legislative body ever set up...the AMA Council on Medical Education, their decisions came to have the force of law.*[70] (emphasis added)

The Flexner Report referred to chiropractors only once in a very derogatory light, stating that they were:

> ...not medical sectarians, though exceedingly desirous of masquerading as such; they are unconscionable quacks, whose printed advertisements are issues of exaggeration, pretense, and misrepresentation of the most unqualifiedly mercenary character. The public prosecution and the grand jury are the proper agencies for dealing with them.[71]

In this same year, Morris Fishbein, MD, was hired as a publicity man for the AMA. By 1913, he was promoted as the assistant to the editor of the *Journal of the American Medical Association*, and in 1924, Fishbein became editor of the *Journal* and of *Hygeia*.[72]

In 1925, Fishbein wrote in *Medical Follies* his disparaging view of chiropractic care:

> *Scientific medicine absorbs from them that which is good, if there is any good, and then they die.* Perhaps osteopathy has taught us something by its stress on massage...Others, such as chiropractic...teach only the ease with which delusions may be foisted on the public.[73] (emphasis added)

Fishbein lived during the era when fascism was growing in Europe and in North America. This undoubtedly fueled the fire of Fishbein to use similar techniques on medicine's rivals. Just as Hitler condemned any and all non-Aryan people, Fishbein took the same attitude toward anyone who practiced differently than his medical brethren.

As the spokesman for the AMA, his "personality" was so embedded in mainstream media that he was honored in 1937 on the cover of *TIME* magazine as the AMA's guardian of health. Lest we forget, *TIME* also honored Adolf Hitler as Man of the Year in 1938 and Joseph Stalin in 1939. Fishbein was in appropriate company of demagogues.

---

69 P Starr, *The Social Transformation of American Medicine*, New York: Basic Books, (1982).

70 Ibid.

71 RP Beideman, *In the Making of a Profession: The National College of Chiropractic 1906-1981*, The National College of Chiropractic, Lombard, Ill. (1995):3

72 D Ullman, *How the American Medical Association Got Rich*, City: Publisher, year, www.Natural News. com.

73 M Fishbein, *Medical Follies*, New York, Boni & Liveright, (1925): 43.

TIME magazine recognized the power of Morris Fishbein in a 1937 article:

> At various times, various types of doctors have personified the American Medical Association. At one time it was William Osler, a learned, sympathetic bedside physician. At another time it was an austere, didactic experimenter like Simon Flexner. Now it is worldly, alert Dr. Morris Fishbein who writes 15,000 words a week, makes 130 speeches a year, edits the A.M.A. *Journal* and *Hygeia*, manages nine A.M.A. special journals, is publishing a book on Syphilis next month, and is finishing *Diet & Health and Curiosities of Medicine* for publication this autumn. He syndicates a health column to 700 newspapers.[74]

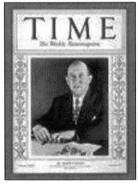

Dr. Morris Fishbein
1937
"Medical Mussolini"

Fishbein became the foremost medical politician of his time; he understood the importance of print and broadcast media, and utilized it to the fullest. His frequent, loud attacks on health fraud were broadcast far and wide, in part through his own syndicated column as well as a weekly radio program heard by millions of Americans.

According to a 1938 issue of *Fortune*, over the next fourteen years he "promoted the AMA from a mild academic body into a powerful trade association."[75] In effect, he was the first king of the medical monarchy.

He was a frequent contributor to popular magazines such as the *American Mercury, Collier's, Cosmopolitan, Good Housekeeping, McCall's, Reader's Digest,* and the *Saturday Evening Post,* and he was able to spread his demagoguery through articles they published. Fishbein authored twenty-two books between 1924 and 1947, three of which—*The Medical Follies, The New Medical Follies* (specifically, osteopathy, homeopathy, and chiropractic) and *Fads and Quackery in Healing*— sold three million copies.[76] As a result, his anti-chiropractic message reached millions.

"The AMA had no public or press relations when I came," Fishbein admitted. Fishbein gave the AMA a public voice, and it was an angry one, especially for those who crossed swords with him.[77]

Fishbein ultimately took control of the AMA in 1924 when his predecessor at the AMA headquarters, George "Doc" Simmons, was dismissed due to a sex scandal. In his new position, Fishbein was able to assume dictatorial control of the state licensing boards and made it as difficult as he could for any doctor who did not join his AMA. He, and the three doctors who formed the corporation, were little more than extortionists who made millions by using the power of the State to suppress competition. The AMA, which started out as a legitimate organization, rapidly became corrupt with Fishbein at its head.[78]

---

74 No author, "Nationalized Doctors?" *TIME* (June 21, 1937): 26-30. http://www.time.com/time/magazine/article/0,9171,757971,00.html

75 "The A.M.A. Voice," *Fortune*, November 1938: 152+

76 Ibid.

77 M Mayer, "The Rise and Fall of Dr. Fishbein," *Harper's Magazine*, 199/1194 (Nov. 1949): 81.

78 B Wallace, "Morris Fishbein - AMA Enemy Of American Health," Rense.com, Copyright © 2002 LewRockwell.com.

In 1949, writer Milton Mayer in *Harper's* magazine recognized Fishbein's growing influence as a power broker:[79]

> "Some people believe I run the AMA," he often said. Some people certainly did. In the course of thirty-seven single-minded and single-handed years, *he had converted a panty-waist professional society into the most terrifying trade association on earth.*"[80]

> Fishbein held all the strings, knew everything, was everywhere and everything... Morris Fishbein not only had an American Dream; he was one. In his square-fingered hands he held the priestly power of 140,000 Men in White. (There are 165,000 practicing physicians, but most Negroes are excluded from the AMA by their exclusion from local medical societies.) [81] (emphasis added)

Morris Fishbein was dubbed the "Medical Mussolini" by his opponents for his campaign to destroy any and all non-allopathic healers.[82] He even attacked ethical physicians who did not toe the line of his medical fascism when they referred patients to chiropractors or practiced non-traditional treatment methods themselves. He used the Flexner Report to destroy perceived enemies who stood in his way. In effect, he was the sole judge and jury in the decision to absorb or to kill.

It is essential to understand how this one man in his role as executive director of the AMA and editor for the *JAMA* could attack, contain, and demean the development of a competing healthcare profession with total immunity. To reframe this, it would be equivalent to Henry Ford sabotaging Chevrolet by telling the public that Chevy's cars were dangerous, deadly, and built by incompetents, then declaring only Fords can drive on America's roads.

Of course, that would have been immediately deemed slanderous and monopolistic, but the AMA used the same tactics to defame the chiropractic profession for nearly eighty years before a federal court intervened. Fishbein used his media power to slander all other competitors as quackery. Propaganda, not the truth, was his specialty. Demagoguery, not scientific debate or research, was his style. His moniker was well-earned.

In his 1925 book on quackery, *The Medical Follies*, Fishbein described chiropractic as a "malignant tumor." He belittled chiropractic theory as "so simple that even farm-hands can grasp it."[83] Because chiropractic colleges did not follow the medical school guidelines of the Flexner Report, he ridiculed chiropractic education despite having no personal awareness of the curriculum:

> [T]he blacksmiths, barbers, motormen, and beauty specialists who sought an easy road to healing turned by the thousand to the chiropractic schools, which demanded no

79 Wallace, ibid.
80 M Mayer, ibid. p. 76.
81 Ibid. p. 77.
82 JH Donahue, "Morris Fishbein, MD: The 'Medical Mussolini' and Chiropractic," *Chiropractic History*, 16/1 (1996): 39-48.
83 M Fishbein, *The Medical Follies*, New York: Boni & Liverright, (1925): 61.

preliminary education for matriculation and guaranteed a diploma to any aspirant who could pay their fees.[84]

Just a few years later, Fishbein's 1928 assessment of chiropractors became more degrading when he suggested they were thieves:

> It has been said that osteopathy is essentially a method of entering the practice of medicine by the back door. Chiropractic, by contrast, is an attempt to arrive through the cellar. The man who applies at the back door at least makes himself presentable. The one who comes through the cellar is besmirched with dust and grime; he carries a crowbar and he may wear a mask.[85]

This public safety ploy would be used by Fishbein and his followers for decades afterwards despite its glaring irony that those allopathic practitioners who used drugs and surgical methods were far more dangerous than those of natural healers.

Undeterred, by the late 1930s, Fishbein estimated the AMA had been tracking over "300,000 charlatans, patent medicines, and nostrums."[86] In fact, any non-allopathic practitioner became his target. This power far exceeded his role as the head of a trade association since it is the state governments' responsibility to govern the practices of health providers, but that legal point did not stop his pursuit to harass and demean the AMA's competitors.

By 1939, Fishbein was considered worse than Mussolini by Joseph Ambrose Jerger, MD:

> Mark Twain told me that this was a land of free speech and liberty. Well, so it is, but Dr. Fishbein [Morris Fishbein, A. M. A. spokesman and *Journal* editor] is a dictator, a Hitler...But the trouble here is too much concentrated power, power that will not stand for criticism of thought or action in American medicine.[87]

In 1939, MA Bealle, author of *Medical Mussolini*, described the vast power of Morris Fishbein:

> Of doubtful medical credentials, but undoubted business acumen and vulpine cunning, the new prince and potentate establishes valuable tie-ups, makes brilliant connections, solidifies weak lines, compels monied interests to pony up, hammers falterers into submission, excommunicates 'non-conformists' with ridicule and vilification, *employs guerrilla tactics as blandly as he'd light a cigarette* and keeps everlastingly at tying up the loose threads until a potent medical trust assumes shape.[88] (emphasis added)

---

84 Ibid, p. 63

85 M Fishbein, ibid, p. 98

86 M Fishbein, "Modern Medical Charlatans." *Hygeia* 186/21-4 (Jan/Feb 1938):113-5+

87 No author, "Medicine: Here's Your Hat!" *TIME* (Apr. 03, 1939):46-7.

88 MA Bealle *Medical Mussolini*, Columbia Publishing Co. third ed. Washington, DC. (1939)

AMA, Inc.

Despite appearing as a fourth branch of government, neither the AMA nor Fishbein were elected to public office or appointed by government to act as a type of a medical watchdog; they assumed this role in order to create a medical monopoly by eliminating all competition.

Michael Shadid revealed the transformation of the AMA from a useful medical association to protect the public into a political machine:

> Like so many political parties, [the AMA] originated as a forward-looking association that fought for much-needed improvements, only to degenerate into a bureaucracy upholding the status quo. Many years ago the A.M.A. forced out of existence the "diploma mills" and raised standards of medical schools throughout the country; it brought about an increase in the amount of training required of physicians; it combated the spread of quacks, false cures, and patent medicines making misleading claims. *It established a code of ethics that was originally drawn up for the protection of the public against unscrupulous doctors but which now is twisted so as to serve for the protection of unscrupulous physicians against the public.*[89] (emphasis added)

As a result, today America has one trade association—the AMA—that virtually controls the entire healthcare system. Even government agencies designed to regulate the healthcare industry are manned primarily by medical doctors who are members in proper standing with the politics of the AMA.

Of course, the reality of having just one school of thought is dangerous–particularly in healthcare. Imagine the problems that would arise from having a single religion or political party. It would be impossible, yet that is exactly what we have in healthcare today.

According to author Kenny Ausubel:

> The AMA came to dominate medical practice through brute financial force, political manipulation, and professional authority enhanced by rising public favor with "scientific" medicine. The AMA emerged as the supreme arbiter of medical practice, making binding pronouncements regulating even the most picayune details. American medicine surged forward as a profit-driven enterprise of matchless scope. By the time Dr. Morris Fishbein assumed the mantle of Dr. Simmons, who had himself started out as a homeopath, the AMA was at the helm of a strapping new industry flying the allopathic flag. The code word for competition was quackery.[90]

Looking at the history of the AMA, its main goal has been to serve its own economic interests rather than patients. As authors Howard Wolinsky and Tom Brune mentioned in their book, *The Serpent on the Staff: The Unhealthy Politics of the American Medical Association,* Americans had best realize the AMA is not an altruistic medical organization dedicated

---

89 Ameringer, ibid. pp. 28-9.
90 K Ausubel, *When Healing Becomes A Crime*, Rochester, VT: Healing Arts Press, (2000):291

to the betterment of patients; in fact, it is a virtual monopoly that should be branded as "AMA, Inc."[91] Indeed, to "AMA, Inc." its main concern is money, not free enterprise or patient welfare.

The AMA had a number of selfish motivations for attacking their competitors according to the authors of *The Serpent on the Staff.* These included protecting the financial interests of orthodox practitioners and supplying the divided factions within mainstream medicine with a common enemy against whom they could rally. Chiropractors became the target for both purposes. [92]

Fishbein's crusade to eliminate competing providers and his control of the *JAMA* advertising revenues played a big part in the AMA's financial success and in Fishbein's power. in effect, he had become "the tail that wagged the dog" in the medical profession:

> While member dues accounted for half the AMA's revenues, the balance flowed from the *Journal,* now the most profitable publication in the world. Flush with revenues, it soon became known as "the tail that wagged the dog." In addition, the *Journal* owned or controlled another half-dozen medical journals along with the thirty-five state society journals, with advertising revenues of over $2 million, a huge sum in those days.[93]

Fueling the Medical War

Under Morris Fishbein, the AMA flourished and he became much more than his title of managing editor would suggest. As its chief executive and business manager, he brought in the money and he decided how it was spent. His investments on behalf of the Association were extremely profitable, so the grateful membership dared not complain. One of the reasons for this investment success was that over ten million dollars of the organization's retirement fund had been put into tobacco and leading drug companies.[94]

Every war needs to be funded, and so too did the medical war against chiropractors. Since the AMA had only dues and journal subscriptions for revenue, it needed outside sources of income. While Fishbein's AMA was demonizing any and all efforts by competing healthcare providers to corner the healthcare market, it was up to its neck in spurious moneymaking efforts, most notably, accepting tobacco ads in its journals to fuel his warfare.

According to author Mike Adams, Fishbein was a "racketeer" who masterminded a scam where he alone determined what products were fit to be advertised in his *Journal* and other medical publications or to carry the AMA's "seal of acceptance." Of course, this seal was better than the *Good Housekeeping* stamp of approval since it came with the weight of the prestigious medical society; however, the "seal of acceptance" did not come without a steep price to the manufacturers of those products.[95]

---

91 H Wolinsky and T Brune, *The Serpent on the Staff: The Unhealthy Politics of the American Medical Association*, Putnam Book, New York, (1994): viii.

92 Wolinsky and Brune, ibid. p.xiv.

93 K Ausubel, ibid. p 89

94 GE Griffin, *World Without Cancer*, (2006):274

95 M Adams, "FDA Fraud, Abuse, FDA Scandals that Cause Death," NewsTarget.com, (June 23 2005)

Ironically, the AMA had no facilities in which to conduct tests of foods, appliances, or drugs to evaluate these products. Gaining the seal was merely a matter of paying Fishbein for advertisements in AMA publications. As editor of *JAMA*, Fishbein had full control over what information reached the public and what did not, including advertisements. Consequently, the AMA became "financially dependent on Fishbein."[96]

These lucrative ads also made the *JAMA* the most profitable magazine in the world, and from this profit stemmed the increasing power of the AMA. Fishbein commented on this easy money, and suggested it was only a fraction of what he could earn:

> The *JAMA* netted a non-taxable $1,400,000 in 1948…the 1948 accounting showed revenue of $4,858,000 from "periodical subscriptions and advertising" out of $5,166,000 from all sources. "I turn down as much advertising as I accept—over a million a year," the editor [Fishbein] said. [97]

One of the most notable—and ultimately embarrassing—advertising deals arranged by the AMA was with leading tobacco companies. Though it was a cash cow for the medical corporation, it ultimately revealed the AMA's true intentions—to make money by exploiting the image of the medical profession as "guardians of health" at the expense of patients and the truth.

Apparently the ploy of "public safety" was only a smokescreen to attack other health professionals since the AMA obviously had no real concern for public safety by endorsing the tobacco industry.

Indeed, as *Harper's Magazine* described in 1949, it was tobacco money that initially transformed the AMA from a "panty waist" organization that promoted education and research into "the most terrifying trade association on earth."[98] Under Fishbein's reign, the tobacco companies became the largest advertiser in *JAMA* and in various local medical society publications. The AMA allowed the image of physicians in these ads, as well as that of actor Ronald Reagan.[99]

The irony of a healthcare association relying upon the tobacco industry to fund its war may seem odd by today's standards, but Fishbein and the AMA would go to bed with anyone who would pay the price. The cigarette industry was eager to link its product with health benefits, and Fishbein saw a vast new opportunity for revenues from nonmedical products, despite the fact that by this time in the 1930s medical journals were already publishing studies associating smoking with lung cancer.[100]

Fishbein was instrumental in helping tobacco companies conduct supposedly "scientific" testing to substantiate their claims. Some of the ad claims that Fishbein approved for inclusion in *JAMA* were:

---

96 Ameringer, ibid. p. 29.

97 MS Mayer, "The Rise and Fall of Dr. Fishbein," *Harper's Magazine*, (Nov. 1949): 76-85.

98 Mayer, ibid. p. 78.

99 D Ullman, *How the American Medical Association Got Rich*, Berkeley: North Atlantic Books (2008)

100 K Ausubel, ibid. p.90

- "Not a cough in a carload" (Old Gold cigarettes).
- "Not one single case of throat irritation due to smoking Camels".
- "More doctors smoke Camels than any other cigarette."
- "Just what the doctor ordered" (L&M cigarettes).
- "For digestion's sake, smoke Camels" (Allegedly the magical Camel cigarettes would "stimulate the flow of digestive fluids").

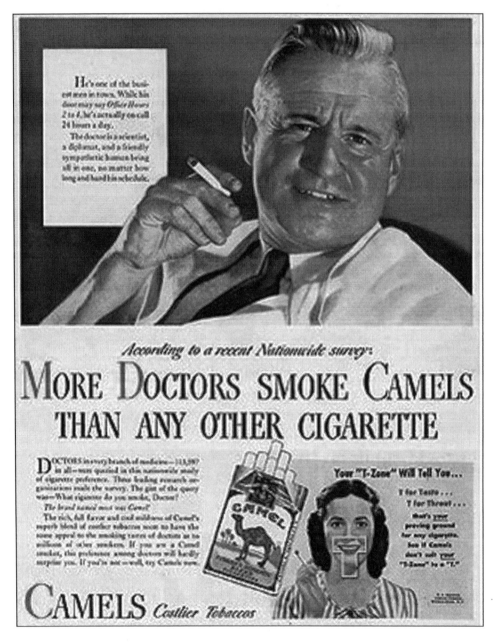

The *JAMA* published its first cigarette advertisement in 1933, stating that it had done so only "after careful consideration of the extent to which cigarettes were used by physicians in practice."[101] The same year, Chesterfield began running ads in the *New York State Journal of Medicine*, with the claim that its cigarettes were "Just as pure as the water you drink... and practically untouched by human hands."[102]

This ruse exemplifies the deceitfulness of the AMA to do whatever it could to make money to fuel its political war chest. For the AMA to lie to the public about the safety of cigarettes and actually suggest tobacco was healthy while at the same time defame chiropractic as dangerous seriously questioned the integrity and intelligence of Fishbein and the AMA executives. Yet no one in the media questioned this obvious skewed logic, illustrating the infallibility of the medical monarchy to lie.

By the time Fishbein was ousted in 1949, the AMA's advertising revenue exceeded $9 million annually, thanks mostly to the tobacco industry. Through its Members' Retirement Fund, the AMA continued to own tobacco stock in the seven figures until the mid-1980s.

In the 1950s when overwhelming evidence of the causation of lung cancer by smoking reached the public did the *Journal* stop accepting tobacco ads, though Fishbein was by then serving as a highly paid consultant to the Lorillard tobacco company after his ouster from the AMA.[103]

Three decades after medical research demonstrated the dangers of cigarettes, the AMA finally issued a statement on smoking, calling it "a serious health hazard" and sold its $1.4-million investment in tobacco stocks in 1986, and urged medical schools to do the same in 1987. The reason why medical schools were the last to distance themselves from the tobacco industry was due to the huge research monies they were given to prove tobacco was safe.[104]

Certainly Morris Fishbein must be rolling over in his grave knowing that his AMA, Inc. is willing to reject millions of dollars simply due to ethical or health reasons. Perhaps Fishbein's infamous statement about competing health professions might be appropriate in regards to tobacco advertisers: "Scientific medicine absorbs from them [advertisers] that which is good [money] ...and then they [the public] die."[105]

Think of the millions of suffering and deceased Americans who were misled by the AMA's endorsement of tobacco and its cover-up as a link to cancer and heart disease. In a similar fashion, Americans have been misled on chiropractic and the proper care of back pain, which is currently the leading cause of work disability in the world. Under the leadership of the AMA, the facts are clear that millions of Americans have been misled, exploited, and even killed by the policies of the medical monarchy.

101 NaturalNews.com: "American Medical Association Promoted Tobacco, Cigarettes in its Medical Journal," http://www.facebook.com/note.php?note_id=44588419945
102 Ibid.
103 K Ausubel, ibid. p. 90
104 Staff Editorial, "Smoke-out tobacco from portfolio," Student Life, Washington University, St. Louis, November 19, 2004
105 M Fishbein, *Medical Follies*, New York, Boni & Liveright, (1925):43.

Unfazed by the taint of tobacco, in a brief twenty years, Fishbein established himself as the editor of the most widely read and profitable medical journal in the world. He also learned how to extend his editorial opinions nationwide with his many books and syndicated newspaper columns. He became, as the saying went in those years, a "personality."[106]

The following excerpt from a 1947 *TIME* magazine article fairly summarizes the career of Morris Fishbein:

> 'And this, ladies and gentlemen,' trumpets the guide as he conducts his sightseeing party past an impressive, eight-story structure on Chicago's North Dearborn Street, 'is the American Medical Association, founded by Dr. Morris Fishbein.' Officials of the century-old AMA are no longer amused by this glorification of noisy Dr. Fishbein, 58. *He is the nation's most ubiquitous, most widely maligned, and perhaps most influential medico.* U.S. medicine has many anti-Fishbeinites, and the AMA has lately been trying to soft-pedal its best-known doctor...The AMA's huge Chicago headquarters is largely the house that Fishbein built...
>
> Fishbein has one absorbing interest—medical research—and *two absorbing hatreds—quacks and socialized medicine.* His special fame has come from his slam-bang crusading in all three fields.[107] (emphasis added)

Fishbein's career came to an end in 1949 when the AMA board finally tired of his autocratic manner and voted him out of office. However, the amount of success he had created for the AMA and the damage he inflicted on the public's perception of chiropractic were both immeasurable.

When Fishbein died in 1976 at the age of 87, his obituary noted that he thrived on opposition and libel actions from those he described as "charlatans, qualified and unqualified."

> "The quacks of various professions, like birds of a feather, flock together—lawyers, journalists, and doctors. The birds they resemble most are vultures."[108]

Without question, it was Morris Fishbein, the Medical Mussolini, who caused the demise of many healthcare providers, and it was he, like the vulture, who feasted on their remains.

Historian JH Donahue spoke of the long-lasting impact of Morris Fishbein has had upon the chiropractic profession:

> He is long dead but Fishbein's legacy lives on in the culture. Yet today, the working chiropractor often has a patient express surprise that chiropractic schooling is not just eighteen months. In discussing a health problem, chiropractors often have patients tell him they had to go to their "real" doctor. That's the "Medical Mussolini" talking.[109]

---

106 JE Pizzorno and Michael T Murray *Textbook of Natural Medicine* Volumes 1-2, (2006):35
107 No author, "Angry Voice," *TIME* magazine, (June 16, 1947): 61-2. http://www.time.com/time/magazine/article/0,9171,855763,00.html
108 Obituary notices, *British Medical Journal*, October 23, 1976.
109 JH Donahue, ibid. p.39-49.

The Medical Bastille

Ironically, the call for healthcare equality initially began with Dr. Benjamin Rush, a Founding Father and signer of the Declaration of Independence, who warned of the rise of a medical monarchy. Dr. Rush, the father of American medicine, believed in the separation of powers as it applied to the exercise of the professions. He wrote:

> The Constitution of this Republic should make specific provision for medical freedom as well as for religious freedom. To restrict the practice of the art of healing to one class of physicians and deny to others equal privileges constitutes the Bastilles of our science. All such laws are un-American and despotic. They are vestiges of monarchy and have no place in a republic. [110]

Not only did Rush call for medical equality, he was apologetic for the ineffectiveness of medical care:

> I am insensibly led to make an apology for the instability of the theories and practice of Physic. Those physicians generally become the most eminent in their profession who soonest emancipate themselves from the tyranny of the schools of physic. What mischief have we done under the belief of false facts and false theories! We have assisted in multiplying diseases; we have done more, we have increased their mortality.[111]

Dr. Rush also decried the exclusion of other health care practitioners:

> Conferring exclusive privileges upon bodies of physicians, and forbidding men of equal talents and knowledge from practicing medicine within certain districts of cities and countries are inquisitions—however sanctioned by ancient charters and names— serving as the Bastilles of our profession.[112]

As a Founding Father and Signer of the Declaration, Dr. Rush foresaw what has happened today in American healthcare—the formation of a medical "undercover dictatorship" that aptly came to describe his own profession and AMA, Inc.:

> Unless we put medical freedoms into the Constitution, the time will come when medicine will organize into an undercover dictatorship.[113]

Ironically, the Medical Mussolini himself was a graduate of Rush Medical School in Chicago that was named after Dr. Benjamin Rush. To be a graduate of the namesake of a Founding Father who expressed the need for medical freedom, Fishbein certainly lost that message as the driving force behind the AMA for a quarter of a century.

The war against chiropractors was not the only war fought by the AMA against competition; homeopathy and naturopathy had already been defeated by the first turn of the twentieth century. Fifty years later another battle in the medical war was waged

---

110 ER Booth, *History of Osteopathy and Twentieth Century Medical Practice*, Cincinnati: Caxton Press, 1905 (1924):312.
111 Ibid.
112 Ibid.
113 Ibid.

between optometrists (OD) and the AMA. Just as the AMA would do with chiropractors, it stigmatized optometric care as inferior to medical care for the eye, which was motivated more by financial considerations than by concern for the patients' welfare.

In 1955, the American Medical Association passed several resolutions against the profession of optometry that were similar to those passed against chiropractors in the early 1960s, such as prohibiting members of the AMA from associating professionally with optometrists. Resolution 77, adopted by the AMA in June, 1955, stated:

> Resolved, that it is unethical for any doctor of medicine to teach in any school or college of optometry, or to lecture in any optometric organization, or to contribute scientific material to the optometric literature, or in any way to impart technical medical knowledge to nonmedical practitioners.[114]

In addition to this boycott of optometry, the AMA made the public believe that only medical doctors could examine eyes properly and ophthalmologists were not allowed to hire optometrists to work for them.

This resolution and boycott resulted in a $90 million lawsuit, *Dr. Cyrus Bass et al. v. the American Medical Association et al.*, seeking triple damages by the principal plaintiff, Dr. Cyrus Bass, and a group of optometrists filed in the U.S. District Court of Northern Illinois. This suit was brought against the AMA and eight Chicago ophthalmologists on July 24, 1964, charging them with violation of the Sherman Antitrust Act.[115]

The complaint alleged, in short, that the defendants conspired to monopolize the examination of the eyes and the production, marketing, and sale of ophthalmic eye-wear, and to restrain trade and commerce in the dispensing of eye-glasses.

Two important court decisions were decided in favor of the optometrists, forcing the AMA to dissolve its resolutions against optometrists. In 1967, when the boycott against optometry was removed, the lawsuit against the AMA was dismissed.

Although relations between optometrists and ophthalmologists have improved somewhat since then, according to Donald S. Rehm, OD, author of *The Myopia Myth*, "the AMA would undoubtedly prefer to eliminate optometry as a profession or at least to make optometrists subservient to ophthalmologists."[116]

As time would tell, the AMA had the same motivation for the role of chiropractors— either be eliminated or become subservient to MDs—when war was formally declared within a decade. And it would take another antitrust lawsuit to defend chiropractors from a much more formidable medical attack.

The AMA remains the dominant power in healthcare today by suppressing all competitors. Without question, the AMA has been the proverbial wolf in sheep's clothing masquerading as the guardian of health when, in reality, it has been the guardian of

---

114 Donald S. Rehm, "The Myopia Myth: The Truth about Nearsightedness and How to Prevent It," copyright 1981, 2001
115 Ibid.
116 Ibid.

its own wealth. It is time for the public to see the AMA for what it really is: "the most terrifying [and wealthiest] trade association on earth."[117]

Finally in 1976, the wolf's clothing would be stripped away when a few courageous chiropractors took the AMA to task in a federal antitrust trial in Chicago. After decades of warfare tormenting the chiropractic profession and its patients, it was time to hold the AMA's feet to the fire in courtroom cross-examination. This trial would blow the AMA's cover of Big Lies to disprove their allegations against chiropractic, making for one of the most interesting trials in medical history, and a trial the AMA would prefer remain untold.

---

117 Mayer, ibid.

The Medical Watergate

"Rabid dogs and chiropractors fit into about the same category...
they killed people."

Joseph A. Sabatier, MD, chairman of the Committee on Quackery [118]

The medical war has been fought on many fronts, but the most intense battles were at the doors of the medical fortresses–this nation's public hospitals. The strategy by the medical profession was to ban chiropractors from entering its sanctuary, even though it was a *public* facility paid from public taxes. This epitomized the complete domination by the medical community that preferred strict segregation rather than integration for its own benefit over the needs of the patients in public hospitals.

Even though chiropractors were licensed in every state of the Union, and in spite of the fact that public hospitals were owned by the *public taxpayers*, not by the medical professionals, the AMA devised a plan to prevent chiropractors from using hospitals in order to monopolize these facilities for their sole profit. This segregation was obviously unfair and a violation of civil rights, but it would take a federal court case to prove it.

An equivalent historical event that changed civil rights in America began in Montgomery, Alabama, on December 1, 1955, when pioneer activist Rosa Parks refused to obey the city bus driver's order to give up her seat to make room for a white passenger and move to the back of the bus. Her refusal changed our society.

Just as Rosa Parks was unfairly told to sit in the back of the bus, chiropractors were figuratively thrown under the medical bus. Finally, five brave chiropractic activists in

---

118 Minutes from the "Chiropractic Workshop," Michigan State Medical Society, held in Lansing on 10 May 1973, exhibit 1283, *Wilk*.

1976 stiffened their backs to challenge *the most terrifying trade association on earth* when they were refused access to *public* hospitals due to the medical discrimination against chiropractors. These chiropractic activists would fight in a federal courtroom in Chicago for their civil rights and your right as a patient to have a freedom of choice in your healthcare treatments.

As Dr. Benjamin Rush predicted, the era of the medical dictatorship had finally arrived, and this medical Bastille was about to be attacked by the chiropractic peasantry.

Think of the enormity of the Constitutional violation of one trade association to walk into a public facility and take complete control to keep out all competitors. In any enterprise, this is purely antitrust activity, anti-competitive, and anti-American, but this disreputable activity has occurred for decades under the auspices of the American Medical Association, and continues to this day.

This injustice was about to change when many serendipitous events occurred among the most unlikely characters, including chiropractors in bed with Scientologists. Along with the highly motivated McAndrews brethren to champion the chiropractic cause, a timely U.S. Supreme Court ruling in the *Goldfarb* case, a flood of new research findings, and truthful medical expert witnesses—a perfect storm came together to vindicate the chiropractic profession.

The chiropractors were able to unmask the illegal conspiracy of the AMA and the major medical organizations in the United States whose admitted goal was to *"contain and eliminate"* the chiropractic profession. As loud as the cannons firing on Fort Sumter to declare the War Between the States, this is the untold story every American needs to hear how the medical generals were unmasked by a few brave chiropractors.

"This is the first time anywhere in any trial where the *Marcus Welby, MD,* [a popular television show from 1969 to 1976] mask has been stripped away from them and they have been revealed for what they are," said the chiropractic-plaintiff's attorney, George P. McAndrews.[119]

As the evidence in this trial would soon prove, *Marcus Welby* was revealed to be more like Joseph Goebbels than the altruistic family doctor portrayed on television.

Medical Segregation: The Iowa Plan

By the early 1960s, the AMA had in place a secretive multi-faceted plan to contain chiropractic, including a massive anti-chiropractic defamation PR campaign, tactics to deter chiropractic colleges from gaining federal accreditation, underhanded political shenanigans to exclude chiropractic from Medicare and insurance programs, and, most of all, an illegal plan to keep chiropractors out of public hospitals by denying staff privileges. No stone was left unturned by the AMA to thwart the growth of chiropractic.

The first step in the segregation of chiropractors began in 1962 when the AMA conspired to use its influence to persuade the Joint Commission on Accreditation of

---

119 United Sates District Court, Chicago, Illinois, *Wilk et al. v. AMA et al.,* (June 26, 1987):3397.

Hospitals (JCAH) to make its "The Principles of Medical Ethics" a part of its Standards for accreditation of hospitals. JCAH was a phantom organization that regulated American hospitals and was comprised of four other organizations, the American Medical Association (AMA), the American Hospital Association (AHA), the American College of Physicians (ACP), and the American College of Surgeons (ACS).

JCAH responded to this AMA request with Standard Ten that stated, "A hospital, for accreditation, in effect, will require all medical physicians to comply with 'The Principles of Medical Ethics.'"[120] At the heart of these ethics was Principle 3 that simply stated:

> "A physician should practice a method of healing founded on scientific basis; and he should not voluntarily associate professionally with anyone who violates this principle."[121]

This meant members were prohibited from all forms of exchange with chiropractors, including referring to or accepting referrals from medical doctors–a common professional courtesy among practitioners seeking the best care for their patients. Additionally, medical physicians were prohibited from teaching at a chiropractic college or speaking at a chiropractic seminar. A total boycott was in place to drive chiropractors out of business.

Despite being a phantom, the JCAH was a powerful organization. Any hospital could be closed if it lost JCAH accreditation, and an individual physician could lose hospital privileges and be deemed unethical if found working with a chiropractor. The medical boycott not only prohibited referrals between physicians and chiropractors; any hospital itself could run the risk of losing JCAH accreditation if medical staff gave assistance, x-ray or laboratory services, or consultations to a chiropractor.

If hospitals lost their Joint Commission accreditation, they lost their nursing affiliation; they lost residency programs, internship programs, Medicare affiliation, Blue Shield status, and it might lose its state license–"a whole bundle of adverse consequences flow from the loss of accreditation," according to Mr. McAndrews.[122]

The American Hospital Association (AHA), another member of JCAH, published its book, *Hospital Accreditation References*, which was mailed to 21,000 hospitals and stated in no uncertain terms: "The Commission looks on chiropractors as *cultists*. A hospital that encourages *cultists* to use its facilities in any way would very probably be severely criticized and lose its accreditation."[123]

The AMA's reasoning for the exclusion of chiropractors from public hospitals was, in reality, financially motivated to have more spine surgeries by not offering chiropractic services as an option to patients. This financial ploy was well hidden behind the smoke screen of its allegations of "scientific basis," "patient care," and "unscientific cult."

Nonetheless, the medical professionals, the media, and much of the public had bought this propaganda hook, line, and sinker without any consideration of the obvious

---

120 G McAndrews closing argument, *Wilk v. AMA,* p. 69.

121 PX-56, 156A

122 Ibid. p. 6782.

123 G McAndrews closing argument, p. 6787

discrimination. The medical demagoguery was well planned and enforced with an iron hand by the AMA, and with the prevailing stigma against chiropractors, like racism in the South, people just accepted that chiropractors were not allowed in these public facilities just as blacks were not allowed in white restaurants.

The battle for the medical domination began formally in 1962, when the Iowa Medical Society, through its General Counsel Robert B. Throckmorton, devised a plan to contain chiropractic in the state of Iowa, the home of Palmer School of Chiropractic and considered the Fountainhead of chiropractic.[124] If the growth of chiropractic could be contained in Iowa, his plan would work elsewhere.

Based on his efforts in Iowa, Throckmorton urged that the crusade against chiropractic be expanded; hence his Iowa Plan became the war plan nationally. On November 11, 1962, at the North Central Medical Conference, Throckmorton issued a call to arms–medicine's equivalent to the Final Solution–to organize medicine against the "menace of chiropractic." He stated that medical societies had to address "the chiropractic problem" through comprehensive programs at the county, state, and national level. His tone and message were eerily reminiscent to European demagogues of a few decades earlier.

To his torment, Throckmorton found most medical doctors had not considered chiropractic as a serious threat to patients nor to themselves as the AMA's propagandists would have wanted, so he made a concerted effort to enforce his planned boycott:

> To physicians, chiropractic is utterly ridiculous. Consequently, physicians have either ignored or ridiculed chiropractic and let it go at that…the public is entitled to have facts, figures, and scientific information about this cult and its practices and limitations. *The public does and should look to the medical profession for unbiased and authoritative information on this subject.* Medicine has not fully met this responsibility.[125] (emphasis added)

In 1963, Throckmorton was invited to become General Counsel of the AMA and to implement a national medical physician "unity" program to contain and eliminate chiropractic.[126] Since the removal of Fishbein, the AMA had not had a strong personality to lead its charge in the war against chiropractors, and Throckmorton eagerly filled that role when he suggested his Final Solution to the chiropractic problem.

Throckmorton recommended that each state medical society and each county medical society consider the formation of a special committee on chiropractic with a focused goal. According to court records, Throckmorton clearly spelled out his Iowa Plan, "What Medicine Should Do about the Chiropractic Menace:"[127]

---

124 RB Throckmorton, legal counsel, Iowa Medical Society, "The Menace of Chiropractic," an outline of remarks given to the North central Medical Conference, Minneapolis, plaintiff's exhibit 172, *Wilk*, 6: (November 11, 1962):126.

125 Ibid. Throckmorton Dep. 131-32.

126 G McAndrews, "Plaintiffs' Summary of Proofs as an Aid to the Court," Civil Action No. 76 C 3777, *Wilk*, (June 25, 1987) Throckmorton, Howard, Taylor, and Monaghon Deps.

127 Ibid. PX-172 (November 11, 1962)

1. Encourage chiropractic disunity.
2. Undertake a position program of 'containment'...If this program is successfully pursued, it is entirely likely that chiropractic as a profession will 'wither on the vine' and the chiropractic menace will die a natural but somewhat undramatic death. This policy of 'containment' might well be pursued along the following lines:
   a. Encourage ethical complaints against doctors of chiropractic.
   b. Oppose chiropractic inroads in health insurance.
   c. Oppose chiropractic inroads in workmen's compensation.
   d. Oppose chiropractic inroads into labor unions.
   e. Oppose chiropractic inroads into hospitals.
   f. Contain chiropractic schools.

...Any successful policy of 'containment' of chiropractic must necessarily be directed at the schools. To the extent that these financial problems continue to multiply, and to the extent that the schools are unsuccessful in their recruiting programs, the chiropractic menace of the future will be reduced and possibly eliminated.

Action taken by the medical profession should be persistent and behind the scenes whenever possible.

   g. Never give professional recognition to doctors of chiropractic.
   h. A successful program of containment will result in the decline of chiropractic.

Throckmorton sought to cut chiropractic off at every point where it might improve its professionalism. He urged the AMA as well as local medical groups to form anti-chiropractic committees. He emphasized a point that would be the cornerstone of future AMA public relations efforts: "Action taken by the medical profession should be firm, persistent and in good taste *behind the scenes whenever possible*." [128] Like the KKK, this clandestine tactic would characterize the deceptive nature of the AMA throughout the medical war and to the present.

After fomenting anti-chiropractic attitudes among its members to garner support for its professional segregation, on September 24, 1963, Robert Youngerman, AMA's Department of Investigation lawyer, reported to Throckmorton on the AMA's official announcement of its goal:

> It would seem from certain declarations of the House of Delegates and the Judicial Council, that the ultimate objective of the AMA theoretically, is *the complete elimination of the chiropractic profession.* [129]

Perhaps the AMA attorney failed to recognize the similarity of language, or he just did not care that his choice of words calling for "the complete elimination of the

---

128 Ibid. p. 127.
129 Memo from Robert Youngerman to Robert Throckmorton, 24 September 1963, plaintiff's exhibit 173, *Wilk.*

chiropractic profession" sounded reminiscent to Nazi propaganda, yet Youngerman continued to demonize chiropractors:

> ...present a clear and present danger to the health and welfare of the public, and it would seem that as guardians of our nation's health, doctors of medicine should be dedicated to the total elimination of any such unscientific cult. [130]

Despite the lack of scientific or legal proof that chiropractors were a danger, in 1963, Youngerman suggested the formation of a "Committee on Chiropractic" that was changed by the AMA Board of Trustees to "Committee on Quackery (COQ)."[131] Apparently the AMA Board was a bit more discreet than the Youngerman, although it certainly had the same intention to eliminate chiropractors.

By 1964, the AMA formally implemented its plan by establishing the COQ. The court record is replete with documentary and testimonial proof that this Committee had two goals: "contain chiropractic" and then "eliminate" it.[132] Dr. David Stevens, a COQ member from 1967 to 1974, testified in no uncertain terms that the goal of the AMA was to "eliminate" and to "destroy" the entire chiropractic profession.[133]

Little did the public, the media, or the chiropractic profession realize the secretive fascist attitude that prevailed in the medical association. Although most Americans realized there was a great deal of animosity between the two health professions, no one knew the goals of the AMA were to "eliminate" and to "destroy" the entire chiropractic profession.

Despite its stated goals, in 1964-66, the AMA was shocked to find its Final Solution had stalled because there was a degree of collegiality between some MDs and chiropractors. "One of the more surprising items brought to the attention of the Committee is reported to be professional cooperation and association between doctors of medicine and these cult practitioners."[134] This should not have been surprising. The defendants' own internal documents would later reveal they knew there was significant value in chiropractic care.[135]

To assist the new Committee on Quackery, in January, 1965, Throckmorton hired as department director H. Doyl Taylor, an attorney by training and former city editor of the *Des Moines Register* newspaper. His brother, Don Taylor, was then executive director of the Iowa Medical Society. In his new post, Taylor enthusiastically pursued all manner of quackery, from psychic surgeons in the Philippines to arthritis and cancer quackery in Mexico. But his main target was chiropractic since it posed the largest financial threat.

---

130 Ibid.
131 Memo from Robert Youngerman to Robert Throckmorton, 24 September 1963, plaintiff's exhibit 173, *Wilk*.
132 G McAndrews, ibid, PX-464.
133 Ibid. Tr. 2104, 2117, 2122, 2162, 2170, 2185.
134 G McAndrews, *et al.,* (PX-550A).
135 Ibid. PX-241, PX-139, PX-194.

The namesake chiropractor-plaintiff in the antitrust trial, Chester Wilk, DC, later portrayed Taylor as "the AMA's Adolf Eichmann,"[136] the architect of the Holocaust who followed orders to destroy undesirables in Nazi Germany.[137] Considering the AMA's penchant to "contain and eliminate" chiropractors, it is obvious why Dr. Wilk harbored such animosity:

> The AMA Committee on Quackery gave the illusion that its primary function was policing its own members from inappropriate and unprofessional conduct which would be a noble responsibility. However, its real function was about as nebulous as the "Showers of Auschwitz." It stated its "prime mission was the containment and ultimate elimination of chiropractic." The AMA worked covertly behind the scenes using negative propaganda to aggressively discredit and ultimately plan to eliminate the chiropractic profession. [138]

Despite his Iowa roots, Taylor professed to know nothing about chiropractors until he joined the AMA staff. "I didn't know a chiropractor from an antelope," he would later testify. But when his superiors told him chiropractic was a menace, he reconsidered his admitted ignorance and immediately recognized chiropractic as the "greatest hazard to the public health." Like a good Storm Trooper, he carried out his duty unmercifully. "I opposed whatever the Committee instructed me to oppose."[139]

In 1967, the AMA needed to put teeth into its policy to boycott chiropractors, so its Judicial Council issued an opinion under Principle 3 specifically holding that it was unethical for a physician to associate professionally with chiropractors. "Associating professionally" would include accepting or making referrals of patients to chiropractors.[140] This would become the focal point of the antitrust trial.

In 1971, H. Doyl Taylor, now the Director of the AMA Department of Investigation and Secretary of its Committee on Quackery, submitted a memo on his equivalent "Showers of Auschwitz" policy to the AMA Board of Trustees stating:

> Since the AMA Board of Trustees' decision, at its meeting on November 2-3, 1963 to establish a Committee on Quackery, *your Committee has considered its prime mission to be, first, the containment of chiropractic and, ultimately, the elimination of chiropractic.* (emphasis added)
>
> Your Committee believes it is well along with its first mission and is, at the same time, moving toward the ultimate goal. This, then, might be considered a progress report on developments in the past seven years. [141]

---

136 C Wilk, "A Format to use on Radio, TV and Press," http://www.nmchiroassoc.com/articles/wilk percent20article.pdf.

137 H Wolinsky and T Brune, *The Serpent on the Staff,* Putnam Book, New York, 1994. p. 128.

138 C Wilk, *Living a Prophesy: A Chiropractor's Incredible Story*, published by Chester A. Wilk, (2008):25.

139 Material relating to H. Doyl Taylor is based on a deposition in the case of *Wilk et al. v. AMA et al.*, in Phoenix,(April 28, 1987):15.

140 Ibid, p.39

141 G McAndrews, "Plaintiffs' Summary of Proofs as an Aid to the Court," Civil Action No. 76 C 3777, *Wilk*, (June 25, 1987):21.

For more than twelve years, and with the full knowledge and support of their executive officers, the AMA, under the leadership of H. Doyl Taylor, paid the salaries and expenses for a team of more than a dozen medical doctors, lawyers, and support staff for the expressed purpose of conspiring with others in medicine to "destroy the profession of chiropractic" in the United States and elsewhere.

Doyl Taylor also spoke of the problem of cooperation between MDs and "these cult practitioners," and his intent was to end this cooperation by any means, including threatening their own members. Rather than accept what the medical practitioner thought was in the best interest of his patient, the AMA leadership was unfazed when the COQ suggested threatening its own members when it proclaimed:

> It is the position of the medical profession that chiropractic is an *unscientific cult* whose practitioners lack the necessary training and background to diagnose and treat human disease.[142]

Taylor and the COQ knew by injecting "unscientific cult," they could invoke Principle 3 of the Medical Code of Ethics to stop the ongoing cooperation between chiropractors and MDs and to prevent the admission of chiropractors to any hospitals. Both individual MDs and hospitals were afraid of losing accreditation if found to violate this Principle 3.

Taylor and his AMA allies could not wage a successful war if their own members were collaborating with the enemy. The AMA had to play hardball and threaten these MDs who worked in the patients' behalf with chiropractors. To put pressure on its members, the AMA passed another frantic policy, Principle 4, that required each member to spy on his colleagues. Principle 4 stated:

> "The member should expose without hesitation unethical conduct of fellow members of the profession."[143]

This principle was not aimed at preventing unethical conduct more commonplace such as unnecessary surgeries or dispensing controlled substances and narcotics to drug abusers, nor was it aimed at sexual abuse or insurance fraud, the most widespread unethical conduct done by physicians.

This Principle 4 was solely aimed at those MDs who referred patients to or accepted patients from chiropractors. In effect, this principle was in total defiance of ethical patient care to refer patients to the appropriate type of doctor's office. Indeed, it became obvious that political policy would now supersede proper patient care.

In 1966, the AMA sent letters to medical societies, medical schools, medical boards, and state and county medical associations telling them it was "unethical" for medical physicians to professionally associate with chiropractors. The warning was also published in the *AMA News* of May 2, 1966, and sent to all members of the AMA. The headline read: "AMA Letter Denies Association Between Physician, Chiropractor."[144]

---

142 Ibid. p. 6750-51.
143 Ibid. p. 7090.
144 G McAndrews Aid to the Court, PX-1467

The AMA Code of Ethics even forbade an MD from being a member of the Rotary Club, a church, or a golf club if a chiropractor was also a member, illustrating the boycott extended into every phase of life. Of course, it was the chiropractor who came up on the short end of the stick in these confrontations. During the medical war against chiropractors, the medical societies around the country not only boycotted chiropractors professionally, they also took every opportunity to personally humiliate them publically.

J. Michael Flynn, DC, recalls such a story about his father:

> Upon graduating from Palmer School of Chiropractic in 1954 and on the insistence of BJ who told the graduates that four states had yet to license the profession, my dad took his wife and four children to Louisiana which would prove to be the last state to grant licensure. He was the president of the state association when the "day" finally arrived.
>
> My older brother, an army helicopter gunman, was killed in Vietnam—the first from Louisiana and the 100th of the "conflict" in 1964. I recall vividly months after the military burial when my dad was able to get my mom out of the house for the first time since my brother was KIA and she accompanied him to his weekly bowling league game.
>
> Within 30 minutes they were back and mom was crying as she entered our home. "Is it Raymond?" I asked Dad. "No," he replied, "there was an MD on the other team who made a big stink that he would not bowl if a chiropractor was on the opposing team and it embarrassed your mom so we just left."
>
> Mom was in no frame of mind to take this abuse after losing her son in service to our country. In the weeks before she passed on this last year (2010) at age of 85, she recounted this story again to me about how callous those MDs could be.[145]
>
> On another occasion in 1968 while a high school senior, I was cutting the grass in front of my dad's clinic when two television vans pulled up and out jumped news reporters with camera crews. I would later find out that charges had been made by a patient claiming my dad could cure his cancer. It made the local news in New Orleans and Baton Rouge which happened to be during the legislative session when a bill was once again introduced to license the profession.
>
> I learned later that it was common for such "dirty tricks" to be played out against high profile chiropractors to influence the legislature and society on how "unscrupulous those chiropractors were." Minos Simon represented my dad and once the legislative session was over the charges were dropped.

Despite the few "flowers in the desert" that did refer to chiropractors, the vast majority of MDs followed the AMA's Principle 3 to discriminate against chiropractors. This blind allegiance had nothing to do with any proof that chiropractic was unscientific, dangerous, or ineffective, but it had everything to do with outright bigotry and to deny free enterprise in healthcare—issues Americans still face today.

---

145 J. Michael Flynn, DC, via private communication with JC Smith (1-21-11)

Masters of Deception

Though well aware of the emerging record of successful chiropractic treatment for back and neck problems, the AMA leadership never provided this information to its members. Attorney McAndrews mentioned that the AMA also failed to inform its members of the New Zealand Report[146], or the California[147] and Oregon[148] workmen's compensation studies, or the report by its own former trustee, Dr. Irwin Hendryson,[149] or any of the credible research showing chiropractic's effectiveness.

In effect, the AMA steadfastly lied to its own members about chiropractic care in order to maintain its charade that chiropractic was an "unscientific cult." This Big Lie also extended to the public in an effort to "educate" them and other people within the medical profession. The Committee on Quackery produced "Quack Packs" and organized "quackery conferences" around the country to focus on the "menace of chiropractic." The AMA distributed anti-chiropractic literature by the gross, purchasing 10,000 copies of journalist Ralph Lee Smith's book, *At Your Own Risk: The Case Against Chiropractic*, which was clearly a biased attack on the profession of chiropractic; in fact, records revealed the author was paid by the AMA.

Smith's book exposed the few random tragic accidents at the hands of chiropractors, revealed the greed of some chiropractors, and ridiculed chiropractic training and treatments.[150] The AMA gave the book, which was partially based on the AMA's Department of Investigation files and Smith's earlier writings in an AMA magazine for consumers, to one thousand of the nation's largest libraries.[151]

Another medical PR deception also occurred during the Medicare/Medicaid legislative debate in the early 1960s. It is a little known fact by the public that the AMA has opposed Medicare since its inception. Actually, the AMA and Republican Party, along with their celebrity spokesman, Ronald Reagan, were able to kill President John F. Kennedy's original legislation in a covert campaign that came to be known as *Operation Coffee Cup*. Reagan used Red-baiting fear tactics to scare Americans into thinking these national health programs for seniors and the poor were a "slippery slope to Communism." Apparently this scare tactic worked since the initial legislation was defeated.

Reagan's efforts against Medicare were revealed in a scoop by Drew Pearson in his *Washington Merry-Go-Round* column of June 17, 1961. Pearson titled his item on Reagan, "Star vs. JFK," and he told his readers:

> Ronald Reagan of Hollywood has pitted his mellifluous voice against President Kennedy in the battle for medical aid for the elderly. As a result it looks as if the old folks would lose out. He has caused such a deluge of mail to swamp Congress that

146 Ibid. PX-1829.
147 Ibid. PX-194
148 Ibid. PX-193
149 Ibid. p.42.
150 RL Smith, *At Your Own Risk: The Case Against Chiropractic*, New York: Trident Press, (1969)
151 H Wolinsky and T Brune, ibid. p.129.

Congressmen want to postpone action on the medical bill until 1962. What they don't know, of course, is that Ron Reagan is behind the mail; also that the American Medical Association is paying for it.

Reagan is the handsome TV star for General Electric...*Just how this background qualifies him as an expert on medical care for the elderly remains a mystery.* Nevertheless, thanks to a deal with the AMA, and the acquiescence of General Electric, Ronald may be able to out-influence the President of the United States with Congress.[152]

Little did the public realize the AMA was adamantly opposed to Medicare; in fact, it spent $950,570 alone on "legislative interests"[153] during the first three months of 1965 as it fought the Johnson administration's program to provide health care for the elderly and, specifically, chiropractic care, which was not included until 1972.

In 1967, the AMA Committee on Quackery released its anti-chiropractic Final Solution campaign goals that included blocking the inclusion of chiropractic under Title 18 of the original Medicare legislation. The COQ was afraid that inclusion of chiropractors into Medicare would facilitate their inclusion into public hospitals.

Aside from *Operation Coffee Cup*, AMA resorted to other dirty tricks that many had never been revealed to the public to accomplish its goal to prevent the inclusion of chiropractic into Medicare. In 1968, HEW Secretary Wilburn Cohen was authorized by Congress to make recommendations of alternative healthcare into Medicare, and the AMA began to thwart the will of Congress.

Keep in mind this mid-1960s political battle in Congress came at the height of the AMA's Iowa Plan to obstruct chiropractic's involvement in any insurance program. However, many of the AMA's clandestine efforts to sabotage chiropractic's inclusion in Medicare began to surface during this period while direct evidence from the *Wilk* trial confirming this political sabotage would not come to light for another ten years.

Testimony later revealed this was a sham study engineered by biased panel members who were recommended by the AMA and appointed by loyal medical personnel within the Public Health Service. *Wilk* trial evidence showed the AMA secretly coached these panel members and suggested how they should vote. In fact, testimony revealed *the outcome was decided five months before the study commenced.*

In a February, 1968, letter, Doyl Taylor told Dr. Samuel Sherman, a member of HEW's Health Insurance Benefits Advisory Council, of the need to keep the AMA's involvement clandestine and to lie to the committee:

I'm sure you agree that the AMA hand must not 'show' in this matter at this stage of the proposed chiropractic study...We must guard against the possibility that HEW may decide to do only what is politically expedient and include chiropractic 'as

152 D Pearson, "Attorney General Gets Scolding, The Washington Merry-Go-Round," *The Washington Post*, (June 17, 1961): C15.
153 DE Biser, "AMA Spends $950,570 on Fight against Medicare," *Texas Chiropractor* 22/10 (Aug 1965):14 reprint from the *Dallas Times Herald*

licensed at the state level'; or *if a study is undertaken, admit chiropractic's totally unscientific testimonials*.[154] (emphasis added)

Months before the study actually began, Sherman assured Taylor in a letter on March 1, 1968, that the final decision would be based upon chiropractic's "lack of scientific merit."[155] On October 2, 1968, six weeks before the chiropractors were due to testify before the Panel, Dr. John Southard of HEW told Dr. Samuel Stevens of the AMA Committee on Quackery that "Testimony by the AMA or the medical profession is unnecessary as the final answer has already been determined."[156] (emphasis added)

This predetermined decision did not sit well with a few members of the HEW committee. Sociology professor Walter Wardwell, PhD, was a participant in the investigation. He was an objective and knowledgeable source as indicated in his dissertation, *Social Strain and Social Adjustment in the Marginal Role of the Chiropractor*. Later in 1992, his pivotal work on chiropractic was published: *Chiropractic: History and Evolution of a New Profession*. In his book, Dr. Wardwell mentioned that the 22-member committee of scholars, professionals, and businessmen assembled by HEW would have no actual voice in the final report, which had already been prepared by staff members of the US Public Health Service.[157]

Dr. John McMillan Mennell, another HEW panelist, was a distinguished orthopedist, professor, and expert on manipulative therapy who had taught at eight medical schools. In a letter dated October 28, 1968, to the HEW panel on Medicare coverage for chiropractic in which he participated, he mentioned the value of chiropractic care:

> Manipulative therapy relieves symptoms of pain arising from mechanical joint dysfunction and restores lost joint function. No other modality or physical treatment can do this as effectively. This is clear from personal experience, from assessing the value of manipulative therapy in my practice, from experiences related by intelligent, well-educated people in all walks of life including other doctors...from the best figures available to me I would suspect that *nearly 20 million Americans today could be spared suffering and be returned to normal pain-free life were manipulation therapy as readily available to them as empirical nonspecific drug treatment is.*[158] (emphasis added)

Dr. Mennell also complained of receiving phone calls "indirectly, but clearly inspired by the AMA, implicitly suggesting what the tenor of my paper should be."[159] Dr. Mennell complained of the AMA's coaching:

> I was disturbed in the past four weeks to receive two telephone calls indirectly from, but quite clearly inspired by, the AMA implicitly suggesting what the tenor of

154 SR Sherman, letter from H. Doyl Taylor, director, AMA Dept. of Investigation, 20 February 1968, Plaintiff's exhibit 220, *Wilk*.
155 Letter from Sherman to Taylor (March 1, 1968)
156 Ibid. PX-332
157 WI Wardwell, "Chiropractic: *History and Evolution of a New Profession*," St. Louis, Mosby, (1992):165.
158 Null, ibid.
159 Deposition of Mennell, in *Wilk*, p. 75

my paper should be. I can only assure the Consultant Group that my conclusions are arrived at through my independent research, thinking and experience unaffected by extraneous pressure.[160]

Certainly *Doctors of Chiropractic should not be penalized simply because of the bitter bias of the AMA when there is substantial evidence that manipulative therapy brings relief to sufferers from mechanical pain which only manipulative therapy can relieve.*[161] (emphasis added)

The final vote of the panel was four to four. This was changed, after an informal procedure, to five to three against inclusion of chiropractic in Medicare. Though it asked for a response to the charges of AMA involvement, Congress was never told that:

- The results of the study had been concluded five months before the study even commenced;
- The AMA had secretly "coached" the members of the panel;
- The AMA had suggested how the panel members should vote;
- The AMA had provided the panel members with AMA materials; that the AMA had procured and copied confidential documents from the panel during the study,
- Biased members had been selected for the panel;
- A 4 to 4 vote (changed 5 to 3) under these circumstances had supported the negative report;
- The Principles of Medical Ethics of the AMA had been considered as a barrier to inclusions of chiropractic under Medicare; and
- A HEW medical physician had been in private contact with the AMA during the study.

Not only did the AMA, through its Committee on Quackery, thwart the wish of Congress to include chiropractic in Medicare, it also broadened its deceptive war against chiropractic by distributing such propaganda to the nation's teachers and guidance counselors as a part of the Quack Pack. The COQ also called for the elimination of the inclusion of chiropractic from the U.S Department of Labor's Health Careers Guidebook, and establishing specific educational guidelines for medical schools regarding the "hazards to individuals from the unscientific cult of chiropractic." Indeed, the AMA was willing to lie to everyone about chiropractic care, even Congress, and they were eager to use celebrities to do their bidding, including the most prominent newspaper journalist in America.

The Mistress of Medical Misinformation

"Just possibly, Ann Landers was the most influential American woman of the second half of the twentieth century. Her claim rested not on political achievement or pioneering

160 G McAndrews, p. 52
161 Ibid. PX-1529

social reform—but on her unchallenged status as the most widely read agony aunt of her age," read her obituary when she died on June 22, 2002, at the age of 84.[162]

Over her 47-year career, she was awarded more than 30 honorary degrees. The Ann Landers column appeared in over 1,000 US newspapers—in some of them for seven days a week—and she was considered the most prominent newspaper columnist in America.

Unbeknown to most people, she was also used by the AMA to ridicule chiropractors in her *Ask Ann Landers* syndicated advice column in exchange for compensation from the AMA, including a paid vacation to China. The AMA used her to show that "third parties" were attacking chiropractors, not just the AMA spin doctors like Doyl Taylor who supplied her and the media with the Quack Packs informational kits.

In deposition for the *Wilk* trial, Landers admitted she had been paid by the AMA to write articles condemning chiropractic as an "unscientific cult." When confronted by intelligent rebuttals to her columns from readers and chiropractors who refuted her misinformation, she admitted she turned to the AMA for help in writing responses with talking points written by Taylor.

Under oath during the *Wilk* trial, Dr. Ernest K. Howard, the AMA president, admitted, "It is possible I would prepare something, not for her to print, but to look at... We sent her material to prepare the article...Ms. Landers is very prominent in medical circles and programs relating to health."[163] Considering she had no academic training in any health profession, her only prominent role was as a propagandist for the AMA agenda in the syndicated newspapers.

Dr. Howard admitted he and Landers often met together "once every two or three weeks for lunch to discuss innumerable subjects." He admitted, "Ann Landers is probably the most prominent writer in the country in terms of columns with a daily audience of about 50 million."[164]

Landers knew her cover was blown and was belligerent at being deposed. On the elevator going to McAndrews' office for deposition, Ms. Landers was heard by a paralegal from his office saying "their (chiropractors') attorney must be an ambulance chaser" because no one else would represent them. Actually, today the law firm of McAndrews, Held, and Malloy, LTD, has 104 lawyers and a total of 230 employees and an additional 14 scientists and engineers.[165]

Landers acknowledged in deposition she had been a member of the AMA Advisory Committee and admitted she had regular luncheons with Howard; both resided in Chicago where the AMA's headquarters and Lander's *Chicago Sun-Times* newspaper were located.

While Ann Landers hoodwinked millions of Americans with her anti-chiropractic columns, occasionally some upset readers would respond and accuse her of "being in

---

162 R Cornwell, *The Independent* (June 22, 2002)
163 Deposition of Ernest K. Howard by G McAndrews, (Dec. 15, 1980):1053.
164 Ibid. p. 1054
165 G McAndrews via private communication with JC Smith, (December 14, 2010)

cahoots with the American Medical Association." Although this allegation proved to be true, Landers publicly denied it in her column:

> Many who wrote to express shock and anger accused me of being in cahoots with the American Medical Association. This is an interesting accusation in the light of the fact that I have repeatedly said in print and from the lecture platform that I am appalled by the degree of incompetence in some sectors of medicine, that some physicians are a disgrace to their profession, that every day someone dies from an unnecessary or botched operation, that one reason for pill-popping and drug abuse is that some physicians find it easier to prescribe medicine than to make a house call.[166]

Rather than admitting her cozy relationship with the AMA, Landers continued to mislead her readership by using the Dr. Howard's tactic suggesting that any benefits from chiropractic care was simply psychosomatic, likening it to faith healing and witchcraft[167]:

> To all who wrote in praise of chiropractors, I say, "help is where you find it." Many people keep well through religious faith alone, and I have no quarrel with them either. But in the name of common sense *I urge my readers to recognize that the power of suggestion can play an enormous part in the success of any cure*. Through the centuries faith healers have restored sight to the blind and hearing to the deaf and exhorted the crippled to throw away their crutches. Miracles? The cured will say "yes," but *medical authorities know these disorders were psycho-generated, and not organic*...so in conclusion, I repeat, to each his own—be it religion, chiropractic, witch doctor or whatever. Just don't wait so long that a medical doctor can't help you.[168] (emphasis added)

One would expect a nationally known newspaper columnist would get her facts straight; however, not only were Ann Landers' columns without scientific merit, she often resorted to ridicule to make her point, such as in her infamous "goofus feathers" comment in 1971:

> Chiropractors are wonderful—if you have a tired back, and nothing else. But if you are sick I hope you will go to a physician who has been licensed by his state's Board of Medical Examiners.
>
> Many illnesses are self-limiting. This means they disappear without treatment. A person who has been massaged by a chiropractor and gets well often credits the chiropractor with having cured him. *The truth is, he'd probably have been cured if he had fanned himself with goofus feathers.*
>
> Massaging the spine will not cure a brain tumor, cancer, diabetes or gallstones. Nor will it cure a skin disease or a throat infection. The following testimony was given to a congressional committee considering the question, "Should chiropractors be included in Medicare?"

---

166 Letter to Mr. Robert U. Brown from Ann Landers, (Oct. 8, 1974): PX-1687.
167 Deposition of Ernest K. Howard by G McAndrews, (Dec. 15, 1980):1052.
168 *Ask Ann Landers*, "Clearing the Air On Chiropractic," *Chicago Sun-Times* (Mar. 9, 1971)

"It is the universal opinion of health experts that chiropractors lack the proper training and background to diagnose and treat human disease. The education of chiropractors is sub-standard and unscientific and the theory on which treatment is based is medically unsound."[169] (emphasis added)

Her column parroted the talking points of the AMA. She wrote that chiropractors had substandard training and were unscientific, but like her AMA mentors, she offered no proof, just her opinion. She cited the Department of Health, Education, and Welfare's (HEW) Report concerning the exclusion of chiropractic into Medicare, but failed to mention the claim by the chiropractic associations that the Medicare committee's conclusion was "fixed" months before the committee convened due to the AMA's intervention behind the scenes.

As a reporter, Ann Landers failed to do her homework on the Medicare fiasco. The chiropractic associations had submitted a White Paper detailing this medical sabotage, but instead Landers acted as a propagandist mouthpiece for the AMA's Committee on Quackery to undermine chiropractic. She repeated the AMA's allegation of patient safety, but offered no proof that patients were unduly harmed by chiropractors. Her reference to chiropractors treating brain tumor, cancer, diabetes, or gallstones was also misleading in that chiropractors did not seek such patients for care; some patients may seek chiropractors for relief of concurrent back pain, but this argument was clearly an incongruent statement in that it was created primarily from the AMA's Committee on Quackery to discredit chiropractors.

She resorted to the standard fear-mongering used by many MDs that patients waste money on "this poppycock" until they "get smart" and seek medical care:

Every year millions of dollars are spent on chiropractors before the patient gets smart and switches to a physician or an osteopath. Unfortunately, too many people keep going to chiropractors until their illness becomes so advanced that an MD or a DO can't help them.

The basic concept of chiropractic is that most illness is caused by spinal misalignments (subluxation) and can be cured by spinal adjustments. *This theory has been greatly discredited, yet millions of people continue to believe in it and they shell out a great deal of money on this poppycock.*[170] (emphasis added)

Never did Landers suggest that patients who were unresponsive to medical care for spinal problems are misdiagnosed, mistreated by drugs and surgery, and should seek treatment by chiropractors. She did admit needing help from the AMA to answer her malicious remarks about chiropractic after receiving thousands of angry letters to her snide remarks:

I know I'll be inundated after my column of August 5th. Can you supply me with a good response, which I will, of course, re-write?[171]

---

169 *Ask Ann Landers,* "Chiropractors Eyed," *The Times-Picayune,* New Orleans, LA. (January 28, 1971)
170 *Ask Ann Landers,* "Dog in Chiropractor's Office?" *The News and Observer,* Raleigh, NC. (August 5, 1974)
171 Letter to Ernest Howard, MD (Executive Vice President of the AMA), (August 12, 1974): *Wilk v AMA* Trial Exhibit 1407

Ann Landers' cozy relationship with the AMA was clearly misleading considering she supposedly represented only her own views rather than those of a paid sponsor. Her conflict of interest did not go unnoticed; a professional trade journal, *Editor & Publisher*, published an editorial critical of Lander's subsidized trip to China. Publishers Hall Syndicate, which was owned by Field Newspapers, employed her.[172] At issue was, first, the subsidization of syndicated writers by outside interest groups and, second, the responsibility of the parent syndicate to inform its subscribers of the subsidization and possible conflict of interest.

Publishers Hall executive vice president Richard Sherry responded that it was "ridiculous" to consider that "an outfit as upright as the AMA" would try "to buy Ann Landers."[173] He also said the syndicate did not find it necessary to notify Landers subscribers of her subsidization, which was an obligation outlined by the National News Council.

She traveled to China with an AMA delegation as "volunteer advisor" although the AMA paid for the trip. When criticized, she responded sarcastically, "I need a free trip like a giraffe needs a sore throat."[174] She did admit she was "the first American journalist to get into The People's Republic in nearly a year and considered herself very lucky, indeed."

She bemoaned the accusation of her conflict of interest in her letter to Mr. Robert U. Brown, publisher of *Editor & Publisher Year Book*.[175] While Landers and her publisher were decrying the conflict of interest allegation, they both knew it was absolutely true.

Lander's cover-up was unhinged when Dr. Howard admitted under oath that:

> "Yes, she was concerned from the beginning that serving on an AMA committee, being identified as serving on the committee might be construed by some as suggesting that she was responsive to AMA thinking. Yes, as a columnist, she was concerned about that."[176]

The reasons why Dr. Howard and the AMA nurtured a relationship with Ann Landers were twofold: first, swaying the most prominent journalist in American to their political viewpoint was helpful to tarnish their chiropractic rivals and, second, as a supposed third-party, using Ann Landers to disseminate misinformation would avoid the equal time and Fair Doctrine issue among newspapers.

One would think Ann Landers had learned her lesson about being a paid mouthpiece for the AMA propagandists, but apparently she did not since she continued her campaign to misinform the public. In 1993, Landers wrote a foreword for the book, *The Health Robbers: A Close Look at Quackery in America*, an anti-chiropractic book written by two known medical misinformers, Stephen Barrett and William Jarvis.[177]

---

172 J Levere, "Editorial Raps Ann Lander for Taking Free Trip," *Editor & Publisher*, (October 5, 1974):25.

173 Ibid.

174 Letter to Mr. Robert U. Brown from Ann Landers (Oct. 8, 1974): PX-1687.

175 Ann Landers letter to Robert U. Brown, president and publisher of *Editor & Publisher Year Book* (Oct. 8, 1974).

176 Deposition of Ernest K. Howard by G McAndrews (Dec. 15, 1980):1517.

177 S Barrett and WT Jarvis, *The Health Robbers: A Close Look at Quackery in America*, Foreword by Ann Landers Amherst, N.Y.: Prometheus Books, 321-335, (1993): vii.

In her foreword, Ms. Landers wrote:

> PT Barnum was right. There's a sucker born every minute…The saddest letters of all come from the relatives of the desperately ill, those who are dying of cancer or kidney disease. "Our family doctor said there was nothing more he could do, so we took mom to this wonderful chiropractor. She seems a little stronger today. Do you think, Ann that *we should have brought her to the chiropractor from the beginning and not wasted all that time and money on a specialist with a fancy diploma from Harvard hanging on his office wall?*"
>
> Every letter gets a personal reply in the mail if there's a name and address. I urge my readers to beware of quacks and phonies. I warn them against the charlatans and fakers. More often than I care to admit, I have received in return a seething reply: *"How dare you take away our hope! I'll bet you are on the payroll of the American Medical Association. The medical doctor didn't do anything but send us big bills…"*
>
> How can the public be protected against phonies, quacks, and unscrupulous money-grubbers who prey on the insecure, the frightened, and the sick? The answer is education. And that is what this book is all about. (emphasis added)

Of course, Landers was aware of the *Wilk* trial and did not directly condemn chiropractors as quacks in her foreword as she might have beforehand, but she did insinuate as much when she failed to answer the writer's question whether it was correct to take her mother to the "wonderful chiropractor." Instead, Landers ignored the woman's comment about her ineffective medical doctor who "didn't do anything but send us big bills," and continued with her inference by attacking "phonies, quacks, and unscrupulous money-grubbers," clearly suggesting chiropractors fall into that category and alluding to the fact that these satisfied chiropractic patients were "suckers."

Although Landers promoted this book, it is imperative to add that the authors of *The Health Robbers* have been denounced by authorities as so-called experts on quackery. Indeed, the team of Stephen Barrett, William Jarvis, and Murray Katz, members of the Lehigh Valley Committee Against Health Fraud, were disciples of Fishbein and Taylor. The chapter on chiropractic in *The Health Robbers* (entitled "The Spine Salesmen") was written by Stephen Barrett, MD, a renowned medical propagandist who periodically raises his voice to disparage chiropractic.

Years after the *Wilk* trial, George McAndrews recalled an interesting encounter with Ann Landers. As an alumnus and contributor to Notre Dame University, he had been invited to attend a black tie banquet engagement where he and Ms. Landers met unexpectedly in the elevator. He said her eyes almost popped out of her head. Later that evening, a very nervous Ms. Landers expressed relief that she had not been further targeted in the successful lawsuit by the chiropractors against the AMA.

Mr. McAndrews had made the decision not to further pursue the damage she had done to the chiropractic profession and its patients because he did not believe she knew what the AMA was conspiring to do. He also lauded her for her columns on other topics that were otherwise useful for the reading public. After this encounter, Ms. Landers ceased her anti-chiropractic diatribes and appeared to be more selective with information obtained from the AMA.[178]

Rabid Dogs & Killers

No leaf was left unturned in the effort to demean chiropractors and to sway public opinion. The AMA did everything it could to blackball chiropractors, from destroying their public image with blatant propaganda, to boycotting their presence in hospitals, and limiting their role in the mainstream healthcare delivery system like workers' compensation programs, Medicare, the Veterans' Administration, and military health programs.

Throughout this period, members of the Committee on Quackery made speeches across the country with disparaging comments to build opposition to chiropractic. Dr. Joseph A. Sabatier, chairman of the COQ, hailed from Louisiana, the only state by the early 1970s that had not yet licensed chiropractors. Chiropractors either had to pass the medical examination to practice or else practice illegally as most did. The chiropractic licensing act was not passed until 1974 that protected chiropractors.

Sabatier told a gathering of the Michigan State Medical Society officials that "rabid dogs and chiropractors fit into about the same category...they killed people."[179] He also said that "it is very important to point out to members of the medical profession that it is considered something less than totally unethical to refer a patient to a chiropractor for any purpose whatever."[180]

The supposed danger of chiropractic care was another issue the AMA promoted but again they could not prove it in court. In fact, the AMA warned witnesses against using this claim in court. An official of Blue Shield wrote "Doyl Taylor...urged that we stay clear of attempts to show [chiropractors'] civil malpractice suits. With the relative weight in numbers against physicians he felt we'd by playing with dynamite."[181]

The statistics prove that chiropractic care was safer than medical care, but this fact did not stop the Committee on Quackery from telling people that chiropractors were *rabid dogs* and *killers*. The masters of deception would not let the facts stand in their way of misinforming the public or their own members with yet another Big Lie.

This war plan included training the impressionable "young physician in his formative years" to boycott doctors of chiropractic. Sabatier stated, "It would be well to get across the point that the doctor of chiropractic is stealing his [the young physician's] money."[182] In essence, this war was always about money, and the COQ used it to frighten their rank and file members.

---

178 George McAndrews via private communication with JC Smith, December 14, 2010.
179 Minutes from the "Chiropractic Workshop," Michigan State Medical Society, held in Lansing on 10 May 1973, exhibit 1283, *Wilk*.
180 Ibid. PX-1288, p. 2
181 Ibid. PX-439.
182 PX-322, p. 16

In an article titled, "Competition: The Surprising Swing to Non-Physicians," from the trade journal, *Medical Economics*, were complaints of competition with chiropractors. It warned physicians of the loss of income to chiropractors:

> It's not enough that the ranks of doctors are ballooning. The numbers and varieties of your non-physicians competitors are also swelling: Doctors of chiropractic… are moving in on what was once your exclusive domain.[183]

Without a doubt, money was the primary motive in this medical war, not patient safety or clinical care as the AMA claimed. Additionally, the AMA's was confident that it would be immune to antitrust action because it was a "learned profession." However, that bubble would soon burst and expose the medical monarchy to legal action.

The decisive moment in culpability occurred in 1975, when the U.S. Supreme Court ruled in the case of *Goldfarb v. The Virginia State Bar* that learned professions are not exempt from antitrust suits. The *Goldfarb* case alleged price fixing among real estate attorneys in violation of Section 1 of the Sherman Antitrust Act. The Supreme Court found that the bar association's activities constituted a classic case of price fixing. It rejected the contention that Congress never intended to include "learned professions" within the meaning of "trade or commerce" in Section 1 of the Sherman Act. Moreover, the Court held that such anticompetitive activities were not exempt from the Sherman Act as "state action."[184]

This landmark decision would open the door to the courtroom for chiropractors to challenge the AMA's boycott, expose their illegal tactics, and reveal their injustices. But it would take a few more essential and coincidental events to make a realistic legal challenge–finding the evidence and the witnesses who would stand up in court to make the case against the medical profession. After all, taking on *the most terrifying trade association earth* was a daunting task.

Operation Sore Throat

At the height of the medical war in 1972, the chiropractic profession experienced a serendipitous windfall from a most unlikely group that would change the course of the medical war by giving chiropractors the ammunition for its first major counterattack. This event was, by today's standard, a "WikiLeaks" incident that implicated the AMA with their own words pilfered from their own files.

Jerry McAndrews, DC, the International Chiropractors Association Executive Director (and brother of George McAndrews), received from an anonymous agent a book, *In the Public Interest,* written by William Trever, believed to be a pen name. Dr. McAndrews also noted that "the book was not truly copyrighted but was printed in someone's basement."[185]

183 "Competition: The Surprising Swing to Non-Physicians," *Medical Economics*, (May 30, 1983)
184 US Supreme Court: Goldfarb v. Virginia State Bar, 421 U.S. 773 (1975), argued 25 Mar. 1975, decided 16 June 1975 by vote of 8 to 0, http://www.answers.com/topic/goldfarb-v-virginia-state-bar-1
185 JF McAndrews email to JC Keating dated July 5, 2005, notes on *Wilk et al. vs. AMA et al. and The Century-Long War Between Chiropractic And Allopathic Medicine.*

Dr. McAndrews personally met with a secret representative of Trever who sold him the rights to the manuscript for $2,500. Adding to the clandestine affair, the carrier would not give McAndrews "a name to make a check out to, so I went to the bank and had a cashier's check made out to cash. I then had 15,000 copies printed and made them available to the International Chiropractic Association membership. The only change I made to the newly printed copies was to remove the swastika from where it overlay the medical caduceus on the cover of the original version."[186]

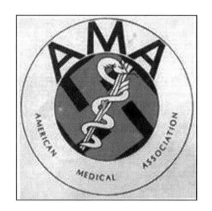

1972: cover photograph
William Trever, author,
In the Public Interest

This book contained actual photocopies directly from the AMA's files revealing its war against chiropractors–the smoking gun needed to pursue legal action. What made this book and its clandestine nature more fascinating was its alleged ties to the Church of Scientology. The animosity between L. Ron Hubbard's Church of Scientology and the AMA began in the 1950s when the AMA attacked his *Dianetics* as psychological pseudoscience. In 1968, the AMA had published an article, "Scientology–Menace to Mental Health,"[187] written by Ralph Lee Smith, the same freelance writer paid by the AMA in 1969 to write *At Your Own Risk, The Case Against Chiropractic.*[188]

Basically, the AMA accused Scientology of practicing psychiatry without a license, so Hubbard simply turned *Dianetics* into a religion to escape medical persecution. He then retaliated with his own investigative department, the Guardian's Office, which carried out numerous covert operations against a range of opponents of Scientology, in particular, the AMA.

Allegedly, members of the Church of Scientology pilfered the secret documents from inside AMA headquarters. The release of this sensitive internal information became known as "Operation Sore Throat," and Scientology's espionage to reveal medicine's conspiracy instigated a medical Watergate.

In The Public Interest proved to be a treasure trove of evidence—a true smoking gun that proved the AMA's campaign to destroy chiropractic with actual internal documents. With this insider information, the chiropractors were finally given the conclusive proof needed to wage a counter attack against the AMA, but the chiropractic profession still needed actual plaintiffs who had been harmed to come forward and withstand the scrutiny expected from the army of medical attorneys.

Chester Wilk, DC, who was to be the lead plaintiff in the antitrust case, wrote of this serendipitous event:

---

186 Ibid.
187 RL Smith, "Scientology—Menace to Mental Health," Today's Health, (Dec. 1968):34-39.
188 RL Smith, *At Your Own Risk: The Case Against Chiropractic*, Simon & Schuster, (1969).

The negative propaganda against chiropractic became more dishonest than ever yet we still did not know its source. And then we got our answer when an underground book surfaced exposing the AMA entitled, *"In the Public Interest"* by William Trever. The book provided photocopies of many of the AMA's secret internal memos exposing its covert and sinister plot to destroy the public image of chiropractic through dishonest negative propaganda for the prime intent of "containing and ultimately eliminating chiropractic." These were frightening words and I was the intended target.[189]

The motivation of the author, William Trever, was very clear in his disgust of the AMA:

Behind the closed, guarded doors of the AMA headquarters there is an elite and secretive group of men who have worked with the diligence, tenacity, shrewdness and deceit of the KGB, Gestapo, and the CIA combined. This book is a chronological, historical, factual outline of this medical government's scheme and activities concerned with misleading the public and legislators in their attempts to do away with chiropractors. [190]

According to Trever, as a result of the Committee on Quackery:

... headed by Doyl Taylor and his assistant William Monaghan, the AMA has lost its true purpose. These two men, along with their department, have subverted the professional organization of medicine and have succeeded in turning it into a medico-intelligence complex. *Instead of being the progressive, humanitarian organization it was founded to be, these men through their secret activities have made the AMA into a Gestapo-type information collection agency.*[191] (emphasis added)

Trever outlined the ill-begotten propaganda strategy used by the AMA's Committee on Quackery to destroy the reputation of the chiropractic profession.

Time and time again the AMA's Merchants of Misinformation have subverted the truth for their own fascist ends. Using these tactics to "build up a case" against chiropractic they have taken objective reports, studies, and individual opinions in favor of chiropractic and reversed them into what appears to be anti-chiropractic views coming from many "non-medical" sources. Done enough, this tactic would give the appearance that *"everybody* knows that chiropractic is an unscientific cult."[192] (emphasis added)

He also found testimonies among the AMA's Committee minutes showing the contradictions among its own members. Despite the Committee on Quackery's misinformation suggesting chiropractic was dangerous, a few brave MDs argued against this tactic. Despite this honesty, the COQ ignored their pleas:

Dr. Richard A. Elmer had been assigned to gather evidence against the chiropractic profession. He went about this project by covertly attending a symposium held by the

---

189 Wilk ibid. p. 25.
190 W Trever, *"in the Public Interest,"* Scriptures Unlimited, Los Angeles, Calif., (1972):1
191 Trever, ibid, p. 146.
192 Ibid. p. 11

American Chiropractic Association…the minutes revealed that the following took place: *"Dr. Elmer answered a variety of questions, and commented that a big problem was documenting our position to the public with substantial proof"*…Dr. Elmer felt that the Committee was in a very difficult position because *"we do not have this documented proof that what they are doing is wrong"*…He said, "they (chiropractors) do read many things in their x-rays accurately." He also stated that "when they talk about the spine, in most cases, *their observations are correct"*…and "that in his opinion, the quality of the pictures (x-rays) exhibited at the (chiropractic) symposium *were excellent*."[193] (emphasis added)

Even the original chairman of the Committee on Quackery warned against the blanket condemnation of chiropractic, but his plea was ignored:

Dr. John G. Thomsen of Des Moines, Iowa, was the first chairman of the Committee on Quackery. Dr. Thomsen stated that he thought *"the Committee on Quackery should not be placed in the position of condemning everything the chiropractors do."* From the minutes, the Committee knew "that many actual maneuvers used by chiropractors are quite similar to those used by physicians."

Another physician, Dr. James Mennell of St. Thomas's Hospital in London, said about manipulative techniques, "So long as the medical profession withholds this method of treatment, so long will patients where operated on or not, seek the advice of manipulators outside the profession; and so long will the *reputations of these manipulators be enhanced by their success in curing where other methods have failed."*

A.S. Blundell, an English orthopaedic surgeon, said, *"Generally, the results of manipulative treatment are most satisfactory. Most of the cases respond readily, and over 90 percent are cured,* or sufficiently improved to be able to resume full work in short order. The medical man and other colleagues cannot afford to ignore the art of spinal manipulation. He will meet it at every turn, and unless he knows something about it he is helpless, both in criticism and in action… for *as a result of manipulation, the cure is sudden and dramatic.* It is exceptional to meet a case which obstinately resists treatment by manipulation."[194] (emphasis added)

The record made clear that the contradictions and problems pointed out by these doctors fell on deaf ears. While the Committee on Quackery claimed chiropractic was an unscientific cult, many of their own members used the same techniques. They admitted they had no scientific proof of what chiropractors were doing was wrong, yet they told the public that chiropractic had been "proven wrong by overwhelming scientific proof."[195] Again, the masters of deception would not let the facts stand in their way of their Big Lie.

Trever noted the disingenuous research obtained by the Committee:

The "scientific evidence" the Committee claims to have, which they say disproves chiropractic claims, is composed of literature and pamphlets which their spies have

---

193 Ibid, p. 9-12.

194 Ibid. p. 10-13.

195 Ibid, p. 11.

gathered. They take these pamphlets and pick them apart, distort their contents...in what the Committee calls "an organized program of gathering scientific data."[196]

In an editorial in *JAMA,* Joseph A. Sabatier, Jr., MD, chairman of the AMA's Committee on Quackery, cited this propaganda that he authorized to propagate the mistaken belief that *"everyone* knows chiropractic is unscientific":

> The rapidly growing accumulation of compelling evidence that chiropractic is a public health hazard has been documented again in a newly published book, entitled *At Your Own Risk: The Case Against Chiropractic.* The book is the result of author-science writer Smith's years of personal, penetrating investigation of chiropractic. And, like others who have taken the time to investigate chiropractic, he concludes that the theory of chiropractic is false, and that treatments given in accordance with the theory bear no relationship to the management or cure of human disease.[197]

Trever regarded Ralph Lee Smith as a "'prostitute writer' turned AMA "mouthpiece" who paraphrases the merchants of misinformation throughout his book. It's no wonder they are seeing to it that the book is distributed all over the country."[198]

This was part of Sabatier's and Taylor's plans to deceive readers into believing outside sources were independently critical of chiropractors:

> We believe this independently written, privately published book will be another major tool that can be used in medicine's continuing attempts to inform the public in general and the legislators in particular, about the evils of chiropractic.[199]

Chester Wilk wrote of his debate with Sabatier about this tactic:

> I had the opportunity to debate Dr. Joseph Sabatier on the radio who was chairman of the infamous AMA Committee on Quackery at that time. I borrowed his copy of this book [Ralph Lee Smith's, *The Case Against Chiropractic*] which he brought into the radio studio and used it to thoroughly discredit him and the AMA. The book became a serious embarrassment to him and the AMA because I brought in solid documents exposing its lies and then suggested that the AMA should send a formal apology to the chiropractic profession. The apology never came. The AMA thereafter abandoned the book.[200]

The Committee on Quackery had no evidence that chiropractic was dangerous or any less scientific than medical care. Without such evidence, it resorted to outright lies and deception despite the testimony of some of their own members. That did not stop Taylor from disseminating Big Lies to the public and press.

---

196 Ibid, p. 26.
197 JA Sabatier, "At Your Own Risk: The Case Against Chiropractic," *JAMA* 209/11 (1969):1712.
198 Trever, ibid, p. 44
199 Ibid, p. 42
200 CA Wilk, *Living a Prophesy: A Chiropractor's Incredible Story*, published by Chester A Wilk, (2008):31

Trever mentioned this ploy when he suggested Taylor used tactics of giving the appearance that *"everyone* knows that chiropractic is an unscientific cult." Taking these "independent" stands against chiropractic coming, supposedly from "outside medicine," and giving them wide exposure would add to the Committee's arsenal of weapons.[201]

Little did the public, press, or legislators realize this so-called evidence was the total fabrication of medical misinformers' intent on the elimination of chiropractic. Trever summarized Taylor's impact on the image of chiropractic in the court of public opinion:

> In an all out effort the Committee on Quackery, with misinformation supplied by Taylor's Department of Investigation, put together literature and saturated state medical societies, state boards of medical examiners, individual physicians, all news media, educators, state legislators, other interested persons and organizations and the general public, thus setting about to accomplish their stated mission…the elimination of chiropractic.[202]

Trever also summarized the overall impact on society as a whole:

> Through the flagrant misuse of their position and influence they have all but eliminated chiropractic from federal and state health-care service programs. They have engaged in spreading mistruths, misrepresented data, misinformation, character assassination, attempting to rig a government study, deception in Congress, misuse of appointed political positions, unwarranted meddling in labor-business negotiations, and every form of political, propagandistic chicanery of which an organization could ever be accused, yet they continue today without censure or restriction.[203]

With these documents pilfered from the AMA, the Scientologists fired the first salvo broadside into the medical Bastille. What the chiropractors could not do through reason or peaceful measures to turn the tide in the medical war, the Scientologist did through espionage and cunning.

The AMA found itself repeatedly embarrassed by leaks of confidential documents to the press by an unknown source who became dubbed "Sore Throat," akin to "Deep Throat" of the Watergate affair who, in 1974, brought down the Nixon administration.

One AMA spokesman characterized the release of these confidential documents as "death by a thousand cuts." The AMA responded by hiring a former Secret Service agent to uncover who was behind these leaks. In their attempt to deflect criticism and demean chiropractic, the AMA representatives continued their misinformation campaign by telling the press that Sore Throat was "a fruity chiropractor in Georgetown whose hobby is hairdressing."[204] In addition, the AMA investigation found that the publisher,

---

201 Trever, ibid, p. 95

202 Ibid. p. 4

203 Trever, ibid, p. 146.

204 R Shaffer, "Scientologists Kept Files on 'Enemies.'" *Washington Post*, (May 16, 1978): A1.

Scriptures Unlimited, was purchased by the Church of Scientology just to publish *In the Public Interest.*[205]

Trever claimed Sore Throat to be "a doctor who worked in the AMA's Chicago office for about ten years," who had become discontent with the AMA's policies; he had moved to Washington, DC, where the clandestine event occurred. [206]

The AMA accused the Church of Scientology of being behind Sore Throat, but Scientology spokesman denied responsibility, accusing the AMA of "grasping in the dark to cover their own crimes."[207] Even after the role of the Guardian's Office was exposed, Scientology spokesmen Jeffery Dubron defended Sore Throat's actions telling the *Los Angeles Times,* "Whoever 'Sore Throat' was should get a medal. I don't know who that person was...If this person went in and lied to get a job in the AMA and exposed crimes and created change, should that person be prosecuted for his or her actions?"[208]

Assistant U.S. Attorney Raymond Banoun, in charge of the Scientology case, testified in Los Angeles federal court that documents seized by the FBI prove that "Sore Throat" was allegedly a Scientologist agent named Michael Meisner,[209] who later became a key witness for the US government against the Guardian's Office leadership.[210] Two secretaries in the AMA's Washington office were also discovered to be Scientologists.

In 1972, the AMA and Doyl Taylor learned that their documents, including those of the Committee on Quackery, had been compromised when many were published without permission in *In the Public Interest.*[211] After learning of the public disclosure of its documents and the public outrage it generated, the AMA covered its tracks by altering its "contain and eliminate" statements.

For example, the "Unit Plan" drafted by Mr. Taylor in 1974, added the underscored phrase "as a health hazard" as a postscript to the goal "eliminate." The evidence would show that this postscript was added in an attempt to "dress up" the actual plan. [212] It was clear the AMA authorities suspected that litigation would probably follow the disclosure of these incriminating documents.

While the phraseology may have changed, the real goals of the AMA and the other defendants did not. Mr. Taylor's deposition and subsequent activities, documents, and testimony made this abundantly clear.[213]

205 R Rawitch, R Gillette, "Church Wages Propaganda on a World Scale," *Los Angeles Times,* (August 27, 1978)

206 "Sore Throat" Attacks". *Time.* August 18, 1975. http://www.time.com/time/magazine/article/0,9171,917737-2,00.

207 R Shaffer, "Scientologists Kept Files on 'Enemies'," *The Washington Post.* (May 16, 1978).

208 R Rawitch, ibid.

209 R Rawitch, ibid.

210 LA Kiernan, "Harsh Penalties Urged In Scientology Case," *The Washington Post,* (December 4, 1979).

211 G McAndrews, ibid. Taylor Dep. p. 72

212 G McAndrews, ibid. PX-1909, pp. 3, 4

213 Taylor Dep. 19 and Stevens Tr. 2104, 2117, 2122, 2162, 2170, 21285.

By 1975, Sore Throat had also sent copies of the AMA papers to consumer advocate Dr. Sidney Wolfe, cofounder with Ralph Nader of Public Citizen Health Research Group. These confidential AMA documents were also sent to congressmen and reporters at major newspapers, including the *New York Times,* the *New York Daily News*, the *Washington Star,* the *Washington Post*, and the *Chicago Sun-Times*.[214]

These internal documents revealed a pattern of nefarious activities, indicating possible postal and tax abuses involving the *Journal* of the AMA, apparent AMA manipulation of certain congressional leaders in the HEW committee on Medicare legislation, and battle plans for the war to "contain and eliminate" chiropractic.

Incidentally, Dr. McAndrews said the same AMA files were hand-delivered to the Subcommittee on Oversight and Investigations of the U.S. House of Representative's Interstate and Foreign Commerce Committee. He noted that:

> I also learned that the House Committee, after a four month study, concluded the documents appeared to represent a violation of the antitrust laws in the avowed attempt to conduct an illegal boycott of the chiropractic profession. The Committee sent its conclusion to the Federal Trade Commission, *which did nothing.*[215] (emphasis added)

The McAndrews Dynasty

With this treasure trove of incriminating information given to him by Sore Throat, Jerry McAndrews, executive vice president of the International Chiropractors' Association, searched for an antitrust attorney in Chicago who would take on the AMA. As he soon discovered, no attorney would take the case for fear of retribution by the AMA, which is headquartered in Chicago.

Dr. McAndrews finally approached his brother, George P. McAndrews, a Chicago patent attorney, who was well versed in the medical war against chiropractors since it included his father as a casualty. Jerry McAndrews recounts at first how many chiropractors criticized the selection of George as the lead counsel in the *Wilk* case citing nepotism. Unbeknownst to most, George did not want to take the case initially.

He had recommended eight Chicago law firms specializing in antitrust. These attorneys politely but firmly turned away the chiropractors, uncomfortable because they feared that if they accepted the chiropractors' case, they might lose business from AMA and the many national medical associations based in Chicago.

When the chiropractors informed him the suit would not be filed unless he represented them, George McAndrews decided to pursue the case himself, obtaining assistance from Northwestern University antitrust expert Paul Slater.[216]

Little did the chiropractic profession as a whole realize the magnitude of the case or of George's skill as a lawyer. According to his brother, George not only graduated number

---

214 Wolinsky, p. 134.
215 Ibid.
216 Wolinsky, p. 136.

one in his law class at Notre Dame, but he also had a dual major—law and engineering—and had the highest academic record in the history of his college. His large and successful law practice in Chicago verifies the fact that the chiropractic profession got a lot more for their money than they realized when George accepted their case.

George afterwards admitted to Jerry that he was "born to try the *Wilk* case." He told his older brother, "We'll make this a present to Dad for what they did to him" because their father had felt the full wrath of Morris Fishbein's medical warfare.

Chester Wilk wrote about George McAndrews' motivation—his father:

> Mr. McAndrews realized that he could not turn his back on chiropractic and refuse to take the case. He could visualize his dad kicking the vault from his grave and telling George, "I put you through law school and you must come to the support of my profession." His dad suffered the agony of knowing that chiropractic could bring health and comfort and save human lives yet chiropractic was isolated from the other health care professionals. He was refused membership to the golf club because he was a chiropractor. He'd make house calls at one AM in the morning in the cover of darkness so that the neighbors could not see they were using a chiropractor.[217] Frustration brought his dad to a nervous breakdown, hospitalization and premature death. This lawsuit had a great personal significance to George.[218]

Just as it required steadfast people like Rosa Parks and Martin Luther King, Jr, to confront the white racists, so it would take committed people like George McAndrews and Chester Wilk to muster the courage and perseverance to tackle *the most terrifying trade association on earth* in what would become a 14-year long legal combat. If there ever was a David versus Goliath battle, this was it.

217 CA Wilk, ibid. p. 26-7
218 Ibid. p.27

The Turning Point

"We weren't out to be fair. We were advocates.
Our job was to destroy chiropractic."

Dr. David Stevens, member of the Committee on Quackery[219]

In 1975, Chester Wilk concluded that to have any hope of success, a lawsuit would need the backing of the entire chiropractic profession. He had been traveling and discussing with various chiropractic associations the AMA's attacks on chiropractic, but he had not had much success in convincing other chiropractors to support his cause.

When Dr. Wilk initially approached the American Chiropractic Association (ACA) and International Chiropractors Association (ICA) for endorsements, the ACA declined. For years the ACA had been prohibited from donating to this worthwhile cause because the Association's books and records could have been subpoenaed under discovery during the suit. The attorneys originally agreed not to involve the American Chiropractic Association as an association, but asked that the Association recommend to its members that they donate what they could to help defray the cost.[220]

The National Chiropractic Antitrust Committee was formed to raise funds for a federal lawsuit and consisted of Allen Unruh of Elkton, South Dakota; Michael Pedigo of San Lorenzo, California; Chester Wilk of Chicago, Illinois as secretary; Clair O'Dell of Southgate, Michigan as chairman; and Collin Haynie from Greensboro, North Carolina, as treasurer.

---

219 G McAndrews closing argument, *Wilk v. AMA,* p. 3055
220 "ACA responds to emergency appeal" *Digest of Chiropractic Economics* 31/6 (May/June 1989):9-10

According to Dr. Unruh, "Any idea has its humble beginnings," and that was certainly true for this monumental undertaking. When asked how the plaintiffs were selected, Dr. Wilk said:

> Actually we did not select the plaintiffs; they came to us because the word got out that we were planning a suit. If they had a legitimate complaint we accepted them. It was that simple. The plaintiffs volunteered on their own. They were courageous chiropractors who had enough and were outraged by the criminal dishonesty and fraud coming from the AMA. As for myself, I believe God led me to pursue it relentlessly until it came to a suit.[221]

The chiropractors each had asked their local hospitals to allow them to send patients for x-rays when necessary. None had asked to be on the medical staff or to admit patients for care. They merely sought to use the services of the public hospital facility, which, of course, was supported by public taxes. In each case they were turned away due to the Medical Ethics policy of the Joint Commission on Accreditation of Hospitals, the AMA, and the American College of Radiology, which prohibited association with chiropractors.

In the case of plaintiff Dr. Patricia Arthur, this boycott required her patients to travel over fifty miles through the Rocky Mountains to the nearest available chiropractor to provide her x-ray services. Eventually she was forced to leave town because she had no x-ray machine of her own. She worked for other chiropractors for a while before she left the profession.

Dr. Michael Pedigo had a successful practice in San Leandro, California. He had asked for the right to have his x-rays reviewed by a radiologist when he suspected pathology. He was turned down by the local hospital, and he never received referrals from MDs due to the boycott. Dr. Chester Wilk was also turned down by three hospitals in the Chicago area.

Dr. James W. Bryden of Sedalia, Missouri, worked on a patient who thought he had back pain that turned out to be a case of myocardial infarction detected from an EKG by a cardiologist. The cardiologist, a Dr. Block, was called before the Bothwell Memorial Hospital ethics committee to explain why he cooperated with Dr. Bryden. He said, "I don't know whether or not there is a scientific basis to chiropractic, but it works." He also told the court he was "afraid because of the opprobrium brought to him by the defendants and his colleagues if he associates with Dr. Bryden."[222]

Mr. McAndrews commented on this relationship:

> Dr. Bryden had asked to be able to work with Dr. Block so that he would not be taking care of cases that he shouldn't take care of. Most chiropractors know the limitations to their practice. It is the medical physician that does not.[223]

But Dr. Block's ethical principles demanded he do what was best for the patient. He was among many "flowers in the desert" who Mr. McAndrews praised for doing what was

---

221 Allen Unruh via personal communication with JC Smith, 6/3/2010
222 G McAndrews closing argument, p. 6814
223 Ibid.

best for patients despite the threats from the medical society. In fact, Dr. Block said he would "work with the devil himself if he thought it would help a patient."[224]

This cooperation presented a problem to the COQ according to McAndrews:

> If there was no fear that medical physicians wanted to associate with chiropractors then the AMA had wasted a great deal of time, effort, and money over a 12 year period to do a useless act. Physicians wanted to associate with chiropractors because physicians were able to fill a void in their educational background, that being the biomechanical problems of patients.

Not only did Principle 3 of the Medical Code of Ethics intimidate those "flowers in the desert," but Principle 4 was just as bad when it promoted outing those ethical MDs who worked with chiropractors and put patient care ahead of the AMA's political agenda.

According to attorney McAndrews:

> The fact of the matter is they [the AMA] threatened the medical physicians across the country with professional disgrace, public humiliation, loss of membership, loss of cross-referrals, loss of consultation, and loss of hospital privileges if they wanted to relate to a chiropractor. And you don't find many medical physicians that are going to commit professional suicide to consult with or refer patients to or from chiropractors.[225]

Mr. McAndrews was bewildered at the obvious lack of ethics and empathy on the part of the medical society:

> How you can say that a licensed professional can be banned from cooperation in the care of a patient defies me. How can you isolate a group of people that the law allows to see patients and say, "We will not talk with them, we will not help them, and we will not counsel with them even though we know they get good results in certain areas that we are incompetent in?"[226]

Like many rational observers, no one had the answer to his questions until the trial began, and what was told would amaze everyone.

In October, 1976, led by George McAndrews, plaintiffs Chester A. Wilk, James W. Bryden, Patricia A. Arthur, Steven G. Lumsden (who soon dropped out of the suit for personal reasons), and Michael D. Pedigo, all licensed chiropractors, came together and filed an antitrust lawsuit against the AMA in the Northern District Court of Illinois; it came to be known as *Wilk et al. v. AMA et al.* [227]

The antitrust lawsuit was brought against a litany of medical organizations that included:

---

224 Ibid. p. 6815.

225 Ibid, p. 7091

226 Ibid

227 [76 C 3777] [671 F. Supp. 1465, 1473 (N.D. Ill. 1987), *aff'd*, 895 F.2d 352 (7th Cir. 1990), *cert. denied*, 498 U.S. 982, 111 S. Ct. 513 (1990).]

American Medical Association (AMA)

American Hospital Association (AHA)

American College of Surgeons (ACS)

American College of Physicians (ACP)

Joint Commission of Accreditation of Hospitals (JCAH)

American College of Radiology (ACR)

American Academy or Orthopaedic Surgeons (AAOS)

American Osteopathic Association (AOA)

American Academy of Physical Medicine and Rehabilitation (AAPMR)

Illinois State Medical Society (ISMS)

H. Doyl Taylor, Director and Secretary of the AMA Committee on Quackery

Joseph A. Sabatier, AMA Committee on Quackery

H. Thomas Ballantine MD, Chairman of Committee on Quackery

James H. Sammons, Executive Vice President of AMA

This legal battle was enormous. It would go on for 14 years—from 1976 to 1990—in two separate federal trials the United States District Court in Chicago, the 7th Circuit Court of Appeals, and, eventually, to the U.S. Supreme Court. This legal marathon revealed characters, facts, tactics, lies, and dirty tricks never known to the public or the media. The unknown medical war against chiropractors was about to be revealed for the first time.

In preparing for the first *Wilk* trial from 1976 through 1980, attorney McAndrews visited 34 states and collected over one million documents and 164 depositions. In all, the first *Wilk* trial included 58 trial days, 78 trial witnesses, 159 individual deponents, and 207 days of deposition testimony.[228] In the second *Wilk* trial, the file record included 3,624 pages of transcript, 1,265 exhibits, excerpts from 73 witnesses and 164 depositions in another two-month session. In the end, the file measured twenty-seven feet in length.[229]

George McAndrews and his legal team consisted of four attorneys, including Paul E. Slater, Robert C. Ryan, and Timothy J. Malloy, while the opposition totaled twenty-two attorneys who entered formal appearances on behalf of the various defendants.[230]

As in every war, there was the requisite propaganda to demean the enemy in order to justify the war. Due to the lack of any real smoking guns to make its case, the AMA manufactured fictitious motives to fuel their war against chiropractors–protecting "patient safety" and halting "unscientific treatments."

At trial, the emerging evidence would refute these Big Lies by the COQ against chiropractors. Issue after issue was proven misleading or totally false by the chiropractors' attorney McAndrews, who submitted evidence that contradicted the propaganda that chiropractors were dangerous, poorly trained, rabid dogs, killers, or utterly ridiculous as the COQ portrayed them.

---

228 Wolinsky and Brune, ibid. p. 137.

229 George McAndrews via personal communication with JC Smith, 12-22-2010

230 Andrew Sunaitis via personal communication with JC Smith, 1-18-2011

Spot On, Down Under

Another serendipitous event occurred just two years after the *Wilk* trial was filed in 1976 and two years before it went to trial in 1980. Half-way around the world, the New Zealand government convened a Commission of Inquiry into Chiropractic in 1978-79 headed by Mr. BD Ingles, QC, BA, JD, and LL.D. This inquiry would be the most in-depth, balanced, and thorough investigation into all aspects of the chiropractic profession ever conducted to this day. Although the *Wilk* trial was the most detailed investigation of the legal aspects of the medical war against chiropractors, the New Zealand Inquiry would surpass the trial material on many battle fronts.

Numerous experts, academicians, legal counselors, patients, and leaders from the main New Zealand stakeholders participated: the Medical Association, the Society of Physiotherapists, the Chiropractors' Association, the Department of Health, and the Consumer Council were involved in this investigation as to whether or not chiropractic services should be included in its national healthcare services.

In 1975, a petition signed by 94,210 citizens was presented to Parliament asking that "Chiropractic services be subsidized under Social Security and Accident Compensation, so that patients of Registered Chiropractors may receive their services on the same basis as they receive other Health services with the community." In July, 1976, the then Minister of Health announced the government's decision to establish a Commission of Inquiry into Chiropractic.[231] But this decision did not happen without open warfare, such as had never been seen before in the hearing room.

It was the first time any commission scoured the research journals, interviewed all parties, heard from scientists, interviewed practitioners, and listened to patients to understand the many issues and complexities of the medical war against chiropractic.

According to a report by Kevin Drew of the Department of Public Health, Wellington School of Medicine, University of Otago:

> There were 136 formal submissions made to the Commission, coming to more than 2,300 pages. Oral evidence amounted to 3,658 pages of transcript presented over a period of 78 days (CIC 179:15). In addition, the Commission received nearly 13,000 completed questionnaire forms from chiropractic patients...The Commission visited the medical schools at Otago and Auckland and the schools of physiotherapy in Auckland and Dunedin. In addition, chiropractic colleges were inspected in Australia, England, Canada and the United States.[232]

Obviously no leaf was left unturned in this two-year investigation. As the Commission admitted:

---

231 BD Inglis, B Fraser, BR Penfold, *Chiropractic in New Zealand, Report of the Commission of Inquiry into Chiropractic*, PD Hasselberg, Government Printer, Wellington, New Zealand. (1979): 55.
232 K Dew, "Apostasy to Orthodoxy: Debates Before A Commission Of Inquiry Into Chiropractic." *Sociology of Health & Illness*, 22/3, (2000):314-15.

The matters with which we had to deal were therefore difficult, both because of their substance and because of their emotional overtones. A careful approach was required. We would need solid facts and concrete evidence.[233]

Unlike the *Wilk* trial that dealt primarily with the illegal antitrust activity of the AMA toward chiropractic in the U.S., this Commission dealt with the social, political, and scientific aspects of chiropractic care in New Zealand. In effect, this inquiry revealed the same medical prejudice sown by Morris Fishbein decades before as illustrated by testimony from the Medical Association's witnesses. As the Commission found, the tentacles of the Medical Mussolini reached worldwide and, just as the *Wilk* trial later found, most of the negative accusations were without merit.

The New Zealand Commission discussed these controversial issues directly, and in the end, its findings were surprising to the medical antagonists and to the committee itself. At the beginning of this investigation the Commission admitted its own naiveté and inherent prejudice:

> We entered upon our inquiry in early 1978. We had no clear idea of what might emerge. We knew little about chiropractors. None of us had undergone any personal experience of chiropractic treatment. *If we had any general impression of chiropractic it was probably that shared by many in the community: that chiropractic as an unscientific cult, not to be compared with orthodox medicine or paramedical services.* We might well have thought that chiropractors were people with perhaps a strong urge for healing, who had for some reasons not been able to get into a field recognized by orthodox medicine and who had found an outlet outside the fringes of orthodoxy.
>
> But as we prepared ourselves for this inquiry it became apparent that much lay beneath the surface of these apparently simple terms of reference. In the first place, it transpired that for many years chiropractic had been making strenuous efforts to gain recognition and acceptance as members of the established health care team. Secondly, it was clear that organized medicine in New Zealand was adamantly opposed to this on a variety of grounds which appeared logical and responsible. Thirdly, however, it became only too plain that the argument had been going on ever since chiropractic was developed as an individual discipline in the late 1800s and that in the years between then and now *the debate had generated considerably more heat than light.*[234] (emphasis added)

And the light of truth is definitely what this Commission shined on this debate unlike any group other than the legal team for the chiropractic-plaintiffs at the *Wilk* trial. This extensive inquiry into chiropractic produced many pros and cons, and perhaps the New Zealand Commission of Inquiry into Chiropractic answered the underlying confusion about how chiropractic works when it said: "Indeed, it is probably true to say that chiropractic is a form of treatment still in search of an explanation for its effectiveness."[235]

---

233 Inglis, ibid. p. 1.
234 Ibid. p.1
235 Ibid. pp. 43-44

Indeed, testimony from all sides showed the complexity of this chiropractic paradox. The opening address for the New Zealand Medical Association, the leading counsel, Mr. JT Eichelbaum, QC, initially parroted Morris Fishbein and the AMA's Committee on Quackery. He said chiropractic was "absurd," "unproven," and will be "completely discredited":

> It is the firm belief of medicine that the theory of disease on which chiropractic is founded will never be proven; that it is incapable of proof; and that in the end it will be completely discredited, if indeed that is not already the position.[236]

The Commission concluded that the medical view of chiropractic is "understandable but unjustified," all the while "ignoring its now well-demonstrated useful contributions to health care. The fact that it remains outside orthodox medicine is probably sufficient reason for most doctors to banish it."[237]

The more the Commission investigated this negative attitude by the Medical Association, the more it found irony in its stance of accusing chiropractic of being unproven and absurd. In fact, the more evidence the Commission brought to light through this inquiry, the more it led to revelations that were judicious and insightful—something the Medical Association never had done in its lengthy war on chiropractors. This would be identical to the testimony at the *Wilk* trial that revealed the lack of investigation by the AMA into chiropractic curriculum or practice.

Indeed, the Commission commented on the "remorseless and unrelenting opposition" of chiropractic by the medical society:

> Chiropractors have for years been claiming that chiropractic treatment may be and in some cases is beneficial for the type of [visceral/organic] disorder we have mentioned. *Yet it is astonishing to find that little if any constructive effort has been made by the medical profession to investigate these claims. In the face of that neglect it would appear unreasonable that organized medicine should be so bitterly and adamantly opposed to chiropractic.* The approach of organized medicine to chiropractic is not one of detached scientific interest and curiosity about a form of treatment that appears to have helped a large number of patients. This is an approach which might have been expected; but *instead it has been one of remorseless and unrelenting opposition.*[238] (emphasis added)

The findings by the Commission were just the opposite of their first Fishbein-laden bias that chiropractic was an "unscientific cult." The Commission confessed that "Anyone who attempts to judge modern chiropractors by what was written or taught about chiropractic in the early 1900s will obtain a wholly misleading picture of what chiropractic is today."[239]

---

236 Ibid. p. 119
237 Ibid. p. 201
238 Ibid, p. 28.
239 Ibid. p. 42.

The Commission summarized its findings:

Summary of Principle Findings[240]
General

- Modern chiropractic is far from being an "unscientific cult."
- Chiropractic is a branch of the healing arts specializing in the correction by spinal manual therapy of what chiropractors identify as biomechanical disorders of the spinal column. They carry out spinal diagnosis and therapy at a sophisticated and refined level.
- Chiropractors are the only health practitioner who are necessarily equipped by their education and training to carry out spinal manual therapy.
- General medical practitioners and physiotherapists have no adequate training in spinal manual therapy, though a few have acquired skill in it subsequent to graduation.
- Spinal manual therapy in the hands of a registered chiropractor is safe.
- The education and training of a registered chiropractor are sufficient to enable him to determine whether there are contra-indications to spinal manual therapy in a particular case, and whether the patient should have medical care instead of or as well as chiropractic care.
- Spinal manual therapy can be effective in relieving musculo-skeletal symptoms such as back pain, and other symptoms known to respond to such therapy, such as migraine.
- In a limited number of cases where there are organic and/or visceral symptoms, chiropractic treatments may provide relief, but this is unpredictable, and in such cases the patient should be under concurrent medical care if that is practicable.

The Commission understood that the actions of the AMA were "unjustifiable" and the "ethics of medical practice in the United States were themselves far from beyond criticism." Recall this conclusion was before the *Wilk* trial had exposed the nefarious misdeeds of the AMA. The Commission also laid blame on the warfare between organized medicine and the chiropractic profession on three main reasons that annoyed the medical establishment:

> The attitude of the medical profession in the United States can be understood although it is clear that at that time the *general standards and ethics of medical practice in the United States were themselves far from beyond criticism.* But chiropractors did not improve their own image among orthodox medical practitioners. First, *they drew in patients.* Secondly, *they claimed cures which orthodox doctors considered impossible.* Thirdly, *they tended to advertise their treatment and its results to a degree which must have acted as a severe irritant.*[241] (emphasis added)

---

240 Ibid. p. 3
241 Ibid. p. 40

This inquiry began in 1978 and took eighteen months to complete. The Commission's findings stood in direct opposition to the position of the medical society regarding chiropractic and condemned MDs as "largely ignorant of those matters simply because he has had no training in them":

> 1. *One of the greatest barriers to integration of doctors of chiropractic into the general health care team has been ignorance.* During this inquiry we have heard a great deal about chiropractic from non-doctors of chiropractic who might well have come within Isabella's category of those "most ignorant of what he's most assur'd' (*Measure for Measure,* a comedy by William Shakespeare)."[242]

> 33. The idea that in some matters a medical practitioner will have to defer to the chiropractor may seem at first outrageous. It is not outrageous at all. It is simply a question of the scope of professional training. You go to a dentist, not a doctor, for repairs to your teeth. There is nothing surprising in that. *Doctors are not experts in dentistry; nor are they experts in spinal manual therapy. So it is right and proper that they should feel the need to defer to those who are experts.*

> 34. The Commission has found it established beyond any reasonable degree of doubt that doctors of chiropractic have a more thorough training in spinal mechanics and spinal manual therapy than any other health professional. *It would therefore be astonishing to contemplate that a chiropractor, in those areas of expertise, should be subject to the directions of a medical practitioner who is largely ignorant of those matters simply because he has had no training in them.* [243] (emphasis added)

More Smoking Guns

Not only did the AMA completely ignore the favorable New Zealand report, the Committee on Quackery (COQ) also overlooked another coincidental and very favorable report by a member of the AMA Board of Trustees, Irwin Hendryson, MD. This report was shocking in its content as was the AMA's decision to ignore it.

Dr. Hendryson was an orthopedic surgeon who conducted research on his own during World War II on the effects of manipulative techniques, which he observed from a chiropractor at work.[244] Dr. Hendryson recalled two interesting experiences of an officer and former All-American football player whose "back went out" and another of a pregnant woman, both of whom were helped by a chiropractor:

> I must say quite honestly that there are still aspects of the manipulative therapy itself which impress me and which I feel practicing clinicians should be using in the management of low back pain.
> In the first place, I have the feeling that since *manipulative therapy is generally well recognized by the public* as being a method of treatment that we, as practitioners should not neglect, it as one of our arms of therapy.

---

242 Ibid. PX-1829, p. 299.
243 Ibid. PX-19-829, p. 5.
244 Ibid. Minutes of Committee on Quackery, May 13, 1969, Drake Hotel, Chicago Illinois. PX-240.

As a final note in this regard, I must cite two cases which I think are of clinical significance. The first is that of an All-American football player who was "down in his back." This man was definitely not in the psychosomatic class nor was he neurotic. He was a Commanding Officer in an Engineer Battalion on Guadalcanal and about as tough a man as I have ever seen in my life. However, in reaching over to pick something out of his footlocker, his back "went out."

Being the type of individual he was, he preferred to perform duty with the help of his medication given by his Battalion Medical Officer but finally reached the place where he was completely incapacitated. Finally, he was sent to us and fell into the class of the next case for manipulation and after the routine million dollar roll…the chiropractic punch…this man was able to get off the table and say, "This is the best I've felt in days."

I was impressed with this case and I still am…this was impressive.

The second case … it is commonly known that in the third trimester of pregnancy unrelenting back pain is one of the prices that is paid for perpetuation of the race. I have learned from personal experience that general manipulations of backs in this particular condition has given these women a great deal of physical relief and has permitted them to go on to term and deliver without having to be bedfast during the latter term of pregnancy.

However, I must say that I am impressed by the many cases who are able to go to term, to manage their households, to lead a comparatively comfortable third trimester without having to be hospitalized or traction, heat, support and all the rest of it.

Whether there is value in chiropractic care or not, I am not prepared to say. However, I would also agree, as will you, that *it has prospered through the years and it is a difficult thing to quarrel with success.*[245] (emphasis added)

Dr. Hendryson sent his report to Mr. Throckmorton of the AMA advising that while the report was preliminary, it was "the only study of its kind that has been made with any attempted objectivity in relation to manipulating techniques of chiropractic as evaluated against those ordinary methods that are commonly in use by our own [medical] profession."[246]

Unbelievably, the AMA buried his report for fear of its being "misconstrued" and consequently they ignored its conclusions.[247] This came despite the fact that Dr. Hendryson requested a follow-up report.[248] In fact, the Committee on Quackery actually received numerous reports from medical physicians favorable to chiropractic, and all were ignored.[249]

Another fortunate event occurred when a medical doctor testified in behalf of the chiropractors. Dr. Per Freitag, an orthopedic surgeon, professor of medicine with a PhD

---

245 Ibid. Letter by Dr. Irwin Hendryson to RB Throckmorton, PX-241, May 13, 1966.
246 PX-241, p. 1
247 PX-240, p. 2
248 PX-240, p. 2-8
249 PX 193,194, 241, 1876, 7005-57, 7059-76

in anatomy, and staff member at two Chicago hospitals, testified at the *Wilk* trial that doctors of chiropractic are remarkably useful in reducing by approximately fifty percent the average length of stay in a hospital for orthopedic patients.[250] Both hospitals in which he practiced had physiotherapists. *Only the hospital with the fifty percent average reduction in length of stay had doctors of chiropractic practicing in the hospital.* The record also indicated that no patient was harmed by chiropractic care.

Dr. Freitag's testimony confirmed his preference for chiropractic care:

> "... in my experience the chiropractors have been more accurate in their diagnosis as related to the general practitioner and the internist sending me patients...every patient that I have in the hospital with low back pain and sciatica, I usually ask the chiropractor to do spinal manipulations on them."[251]

He was asked by the medical attorney in cross examination why he referred patients to chiropractors: "For what purpose?"

Dr. Freitag answered, "To get them better."

Dr. Freitag also testified that he referred pregnant women for spinal manipulation and spoke of a woman with 50-60 pounds of water retention cured by chiropractic care after unsuccessful medical care:[252]

> During pregnancy, of course, back pain and sciatica is very common. And I don't remember even where I first heard about the idea of manipulating pregnant women, but I tried it on a few patients as an alternative to epidural steroid injections and it seemed to work, at least in the few that I came in contact with.[253]

After his testimony was given, one of the AMA's attorneys, Perry Fuller, made the mistake to ridicule this information, prompting a stern response from the court. Judge Getzendanner mentioned that she had had two babies, and if manipulation could have helped her avoid epidural shots to rid herself of the birthing pain and spasms, then she suggested that a chiropractor should always be in the labor room.[254] Only a female judge could have appreciated this testimony to help pregnant women with chiropractic care.

The AMA also ignored two important workmen's compensation studies on low back injuries, the most common on-the-job claim. "Study of Time Loss Back Claims" conducted by Dr. Rolland Martin, MD, of the Workmen's Compensation Board of the State of Oregon concluded that twice as many patients of chiropractic (82 percent) returned to work within one week of injury as did patients of physicians (41 percent) with comparable injury.[255]

---

250 Freitag testimony, *Wilk et al. v. AMA et al.* (May 20, 1987):812.

251 Ibid. p. 809.

252 Ibid. p. 814.

253 *Wilk v. AMA* trial transcript, (May 20, 1987):816.

254 G McAndrews via private communication with JC Smith, (September 16, 2009)

255 PX-193, p. 3.

The AMA moreover ignored another important study: a 1972 scientific study of more than six hundred employees entitled "Industrial Back Injury" by C. Richard Wolf, MD.[256] The study covered light to major injuries (some with more than 60 days of lost time) and concluded:

- Employee statement of lost time; 32 days average for MD-treated group versus 15.6 days average for the chiropractor-treated group.
- Percentage of employees reporting lost time in excess of 60 days, 13.2 percent of those treated by MDs versus 6.7 percent of those treated by doctors of chiropractic; and
- Percent of employees reporting no lost time, 21 percent of those treated by MDs versus 47 percent of those treated by doctors of chiropractic.

These scientific studies showed clearly that care provided by doctors of chiropractic was more than twice as effective as medical physicians, with an obvious corollary of enormous savings from a reduction in time off work. Thus, unlike optometrists who offer some of the same services offered by ophthalmologists; chiropractors were obviously offering a more effective service than offered by medical physicians.

George McAndrews noted the testimony at trial revealed patient care was never a legitimate concern for the AMA. Restricting chiropractors' use of public hospitals served to increase patient treatment time and costs with less effective medical treatments, thus increasing the incomes of AMA members.

McAndrews accused the AMA of boycotting of chiropractors from public hospitals solely to monopolize the public facilities and to keep its leading competitors out:

> They were going to appropriate to their own private use billions of dollars of bricks and mortar that they did not own and hundreds of millions of dollars worth of diagnostic equipment for which they paid not one cent.[257]

The boycott also effectively placed chiropractors outside of any medical discipline. This resulted in no referrals to chiropractors—ever. This suited the aim of the AMA to demean the *authority* of chiropractors, an issue it clearly feared:

> Once chiropractors can freely send their outpatients to our hospitals, they'll soon be able to admit inpatients. Once they can get all the scientific studies they order, it will be hard to refuse them medical staff privileges on the ground that their practice is unscientific.[258]

When one of the AMA's attorneys told the jury that patients go for "medical" care in "our" hospitals, Mr. McAndrews rebutted that "patients do not necessarily go to hospitals

---

256 PX-194.

257 G McAndrews closing argument, *Wilk v. AMA*, (December 9, 198):6751.

258 G Null, PhD, "Medical Genocide, Part Four: Painful Treatment," *Penthouse* (November 1985).

only for *medical* care, they go to *get well*," suggesting that a public hospital is not meant to be a low-overhead facility exclusively for medical physicians.[259]

Many hospitals today have been renamed "Medical Centers," again implying "medical" exclusivity and ownership of a public hospital. McAndrews also pointed out that only 0.2 percent of the 8,000 hospitals had chiropractors on staff, the boycotting parties controlled 94 percent of the hospital beds in the United States, the AMA alone included 50-60 percent of the medical doctors in the United States, and "enjoys a significant market power." And according to testimony of health care economists, "medical physicians earn monopoly profits."[260]

According to Mr. McAndrews:

> The purpose of this total ethics boycott was to isolate the profession of chiropractic, stifle demand for chiropractic services either from referrals or in a hospital setting, and cause the profession to "wither and die on the vine." Although the profession did not "wither and die," the defendants' ethical boycott met with substantial success. AMA members, including Doyl Taylor, admitted that the boycott succeeded in curtailing the growth of chiropractic. The record is replete with instances where medical doctors or hospitals who were otherwise willing to deal with doctors of chiropractic refrained from doing so due to the defendants' ethics ban.[261]

The AMA also ignored the 1972 "modest proposal" of a Dr. Healy, MD, editor of King County Medical Society in Seattle, Washington, to gather statistical evidence to determine whether chiropractic was detrimental to health care. The proposal stated:

> A thoughtful labor leader pointed out to me that most people don't care what the chiropractic theory is...they know that doctors of chiropractic help their backaches and muscle pains.
>
> *They offer something where we fail...maybe doctors of chiropractic help these folks.*[262]
> (emphasis added)

Some MDs were sympathetic to working with chiropractors for the benefit of their patients. Dr. David Stevens was a member of the Committee on Quackery who noted the cooperation and sympathy among many MDs who worked with chiropractors, "Many of us physicians are apathetic toward [the boycott campaign against] chiropractors and feel they have a place in the medical field."[263]

The Kentucky Medical Association, with Dr. Stevens assisting, conducted a survey to find negative public opinion to use against chiropractors. It backfired; the survey found

---

259 Historical summary taken from the *Wilk* appeal brief filed by attorney G McAndrews. The complete appeal brief is available online at www.chiroweb.com/trigon (last accessed 09/28/2009).

260 G McAndrews Aid to the Court, PX-7279, p. 89-91.

261 G McAndrews Aid t o the Court, p. 90.

262 G McAndrews, "Plaintiffs' Summary of Proofs as an Aid to the Court," Civil Action No. 76 C 3777, *Wilk*, (June 25, 1987):126.

263 G McAndrews closing argument, *Wilk v. AMA*, (December 9, 1980):6741

that at least one family member had used a chiropractor in 31 percent of the households polled, the highest rates being in the upper and middle class groups of the county. There was a feeling that a chiropractor had more specialized training than a medical doctor for musculoskeletal back and joint problems. Twenty-five percent indicated they would use a chiropractor if the need arose and stated they actually believed chiropractors provided an effective type of health service to certain patients.[264]

The survey concluded "Undoubtedly many patients with functional complaints feel better after the personal and manipulative treatments by a chiropractor." When asked of this survey in court, Dr. Stevens stood his ground as a member of the COQ and boasted:

> "We weren't out to be fair. We were advocates. Our job was to destroy chiropractic. We certainly weren't going to use anything that was favorable to them."[265]

The medical defendants treated all of these favorable studies and opinions with total silence. The list of examples goes on and on, showing that the medical defendants continued the boycott while ignoring the mounting evidence that chiropractic really was of extraordinary value and superior to medical care for the treatment of back pain.

Mr. McAndrews ridiculed this attitude of ignoring the evidence, testimony, and surveys that supported chiropractic care. "If it can't be surgically removed or written on a prescription pad, the medical physicians sorely ignore this part. But they couldn't ignore the results."[266]

Indeed, at trial many medical experts admitted that chiropractic had value as a health care modality. Many of the defendants' members testified to the same effect on cross-examination. In legal parlance, this "admission against interest" testimony by the medical witnesses to the benefits of chiropractic was considered the highest level of proof.

According to Mr. McAndrews, to be "objectively reasonable," the AMA defendants would have required a reasonable scientific body of information about chiropractic before deciding to "contain chiropractic and…eliminate it as a recognized healthcare service to the people."[267] It became clear that the defendants failed to obtain or even seek this proof. Not only were they biased to the extreme, they knowingly *suppressed* all evidence of benefits about chiropractic care including that from their own board member, Dr. Hendryson.

Mr. McAndrews showed that the majority of the Committee on Quackery members as well as the other defendants:

- had never been to a doctor of chiropractic
- had never read a chiropractic textbook
- had never been to a chiropractic school

---

264 Ibid. pp. 3049-50.

265 Ibid. p. 3055

266 Ibid. p. 3057

267 G McAndrews, "Plaintiffs' Summary of Proofs as an Aid to the Court," Civil Action No. 76 C 3777, *Wilk*, (June 25, 1987):126. PX-188.

- had never seen a chiropractic manipulation
- had never discussed chiropractic theory with a doctor of chiropractic
- had never conducted an unbiased test to determine the efficacy of chiropractic care
- had never polled any of the fifty state legislatures to determine why they had licensed chiropractic in the fifty states of this country
- had never conducted a meaningful survey of the many patients who reported successful treatment by a doctor of chiropractic

Doyl Taylor had only a "vague" notion as to what doctors of chiropractic do while his predecessor Youngerman admitted that there was "great value in manipulative therapy"[268] and that a medical physician (Dr. Thomas) had advised him that manipulative techniques used by medical physicians were identical to those used by doctors of chiropractic.[269]

AMA defendant Dr. Thomas Ballantine also admitted he was ignorant about chiropractic.[270] But that did not deter him in his message to his fellow AMA Committee On Quackery members to fight against chiropractors:

> "I would also like to point out that the AMA needs a cause to fight for on behalf of the public, the need to convince the public that we are really interested in the health and welfare of society…I can think of no better program to undertake than that of trying to eliminate quackery."[271]

Keep in mind that his definition of quackery included all healing arts that were non-allopathic medicine, not only those that were proven dangerous to the public. However, nowhere in the committee's literature was there any mention of other alternative methods or suspect experimental medical methods. The COQ dealt exclusively with chiropractic.

AMA defendant Dr. Sabatier revealed that the AMA never did any research into the efficacy of chiropractic.[272] He also admitted that he often treated patients with no proof of disease causation and using unscientific treatments based only on clinical proof of efficacy.[273] He further testified that he did everything he could to interfere with chiropractic practitioners' attempts to upgrade their education.[274]

Doyl Taylor stated that the "justification" for his efforts in the anti-chiropractic campaign was based on his alleged understanding that the fundamental principle of chiropractic is that all disease stems from one cause—spinal subluxations. This erroneous belief was derived from BJ Palmer's 1934 book, *The Subluxation Specific, The Adjustment*

---

268 Youngerman Dep. 42
269 Youngerman Dep. 204
270 Ballantine Dep. 33
271 Trever, p. 16.
272 Sabatier Dep. 32
273 Sabatier Dep. 37-38
274 Sabatier Dep. 57-63.

Specific: An Exposition Of The Cause Of All Dis-ease.[275] The historical record shows that this statement was rejected by mainstream chiropractors as soon as it was published. To suggest that modern chiropractors still strictly adhere to the tenets of DD Palmer from 1910 and BJ Palmer from 1934 is equivalent to accusing MDs of purporting to adhere to bloodletting, leeches, and lobotomies which were recognized medical treatments at one time.

Yet, Doyl Taylor and the AMA's Committee on Quackery should have known by the 1960's that this alleged perception of all disease being caused by spinal subluxation was rejected by the chiropractic profession. The chiropractors' national associations, both the American Chiropractic Association and the International Chiropractors' Association, published a White Paper in May, 1969, explaining that chiropractic was not premised on "one cause, one cure," and that it had not been for a "long, long time" according to James Winterstein, DC, then faculty member and today president of the National University of Health Sciences in Lombard, Illinois, near Chicago.[276] Moreover, by at least 1969, the AMA had clear, compelling reason to know that this "shibboleth was false," as attorney McAndrews mentioned.[277]

AMA Committee on Quackery simply ignored these published statements of two national chiropractic organizations. They purposely continued with their plan to contain and eliminate chiropractic using bogus reasons from yesteryear.[278]

Mr. McAndrews recognized the prejudicial mindset perpetuated by medical educators when he noted:

> This is the technocracy that the Marcus Welby phase has to be obeyed because they are the only ones fit to study healthcare in the United States.[279]

McAndrews also showed abundant evidence indicating that the medical boycott against chiropractic was established for two reasons, both unrelated to a genuine concern for patient care: (1) fear of competition from doctors of chiropractic[280]; and (2) as a rallying point to promote waning national physician unity and declining membership in the AMA ranks.[281] The medical army needed a cause for recruitment of new soldiers and chiropractic became the scapegoats to rally their troops.

Mr. McAndrews suggested in his closing argument that the Joint Commission on Hospital Accreditation had superseded the power of the state legislatures; in effect, the Joint Commission said, "You must first clear it with the Joint Commission before the

---

275 BJ Palmer, *The Subluxation Specific, The Adjustment Specific: An Exposition Of The Cause Of All Dis-ease,* Davenport, Iowa: Palmer School of Chiropractic, (1934)
276 Testimony of J Winterstein and plaintiffs. PX-344
277 Ibid.
278 Fineberg Dep. 296-297; Ballantine Dep. 251-252.
279 G McAndrews closing argument, ibid. p. 3389
280 PX-172, p. 8, Conclusion C: PX-241, p. 4; PX-1055
281 PX-466

representatives of the people can pass legislation favoring one of the health care professions licensed by that legislature."[282]

The boycott of chiropractors was spelled out clearly in an article entitled, "The Right and Duty of Hospitals to Exclude Chiropractors," written by the American College of Surgeons and published in the November 12, 1973, issue of the *Journal* of the AMA.[283] "The Commission looks on chiropractors as cultists. A hospital that encourages cultists to use its facilities in any way would very probably be severely criticized and lose its accreditation."[284]

MDs who were non-members of the AMA were also forced to comply with this edict or else lose their hospital privileges when the Joint Commission on Accreditation of Hospitals (JCAH) adopted the same restraints as the AMA.[285]

According to attorney McAndrews,

> The evidence showed that this was not just a simple, straight-forward wall erected, but *a series of concentric picket fences that no matter where the chiropractors went, they ran into another obstacle erected by these defendants.*[286]

> Defendants have failed to meet their burden of proof of objective reasonableness. In fact, their conduct was more than objectively unreasonable; it was, and remains, unconscionable. *Patients, indeed, patients who testified before this Court, have suffered because of defendants' boycott.* (emphasis added)

Mr. McAndrews characterized the AMA's attitude as "patient be damned":

> This might be a good time to mention and it is my duty as we are doing this traveling to stop and view some of the terrain. I want to make a point.

> This is not an effort by the chiropractors to become medical doctors and it is not an effort by the medical doctors to become chiropractors. That is a false issue in this case and when the defendants present it, it is not an issue presented by the plaintiffs.

> The plaintiffs are licensed chiropractors. They're experts in spinal adjusting and the non-drug care of some human ailments. They seek the help of superior knowledge, which is something that they should be credited for.

> The case attacks unreasonable restrictions placed by these professional societies on their members who wish to help chiropractors care for their patients.

> *In this day and age to suggest that there has to be an absolute dividing line between health care professionals, and the patient be damned, if one or the other has incomplete knowledge, seems bizarre.* (emphasis added)

> This is not an effort to have chiropractors practice brain surgery in hospitals or to administer medications beyond their state licenses. It is an effort for chiropractors to

---

282 G McAndrews, ibid.

283 Ibid. p. 6785

284 Ibid. p. 6787-90

285 MJ Pedigo, "Wilk vs. AMA: Was It Worth the Fight?" *Dynamic Chiropractic*, 16/15, (July 13, 1998)

286 Ibid. p. 6788.

chiropractically care for patients who need those services and to interrelate and inter-cooperate with any medical physicians that will willingly do so for the mutual benefit of the patient.

"Bizarre" was the apt term for the COQ's behavior and its defamation campaign that began to unravel during trial due to more peculiar events and strange bedfellows.

Wilk I Trial

During the discovery phase from 1976 to 1980, some of the medical defendants realized their conspiracy was indefensible and settled out of court with the chiropractors. By the time this case went to trial in 1980, the defendants remaining who had not settled were the American Medical Association (AMA), the Joint Commission on Accreditation of Hospitals (JCAH), the American College of Physicians (ACP), the American College of Surgeons (ACS), the American College of Radiology (ACR), the American Academy of Orthopaedic Surgeons (AAOS), and James H. Sammons, MD, an AMA official.

At the center of the chiropractic-plaintiff's contention of a boycott was Principle 3 of the AMA Principles of Medical Ethics. Before 1980 when it was changed, Principle 3 stated:

> A physician should practice a method of healing founded on a scientific basis; and he should not voluntarily professionally associate with anyone who violates this principle.

In an attempt to minimize the negative impact of its obvious discrimination, the AMA eliminated Principle 3 in 1980 during a major revision of ethical rules while the *Wilk* litigation was in progress. Its replacement stated that a physician *"shall be free to choose whom to serve, with whom to associate, and the environment in which to provide medical services."*

This change in policy came not from a sudden moral awakening by the AMA, but rather from a financial crisis. Aside from the *Wilk* trial in Chicago, the AMA was also involved with three other pending lawsuits in New Jersey, Pennsylvania, and New York. These lawsuits were costing the AMA more than $1 million annually to defend. To avoid bankruptcy and to aid its posture in the *Wilk* case, the AMA made a strategic policy change to avoid total collapse. In August of 1980, the AMA approved a new version of the Principles of Medical Ethics that allowed medical doctors to work with chiropractors.[287]

The case of *Wilk et al. v. AMA et al.* initially went to trial before U.S. District Court Judge Nicholas J. Bua in December, 1980. Aside from the evidence from the plaintiffs' witnesses concerning the antitrust action by the AMA, the judge allowed extraneous evidence and, in effect, he lost control of the antitrust focus of the trial.

A federal appeals court later would describe the trial as "free-for-all between chiropractors and medical doctors, in which the scientific legitimacy of chiropractic was hotly debated and the comparative avarice of the adversaries was explored."[288]

---

287 W Wardell, *Chiropractic: History and Evolution of a New Profession*, St. Louis, Mosby, (1992)
288 Wolinsky and Brune, ibid. p. 138.

Dr. Jerry McAndrews recounted conversation with his brother, George that typified the circus atmosphere during the *Wilk* trial:

> In the first morning of the *Wilk* case, George called me to ask, "What in the hell is the matter with you people? I just spent the worst morning of my professional life trying to defend the behavior of some of the chiropractors out there who make claims far beyond any objective evidence. I felt like I should get up from my chair and go over and sit with the attorneys for the other side."
>
> I apologized for the tough time "our" behavior had caused for him. "Don't get me wrong," George said, "the toughest part wasn't the trash so many chiropractors put out, it was that *I couldn't find any evidence of a single chiropractor speaking out against the atrocious behavior.*" [289] (emphasis added)

Despite a few dubious hyperbolic newspaper ads, the unethical instructions by some practice management firms, and the outlandish comments of chiropractic demagogues, the actual evidence did not support the AMA's claims that chiropractic care was unscientific. To the contrary, the more the AMA searched for evidence to support its allegations, the more it found evidence supporting chiropractic treatment as effective and, in some cases, more effective than medical care.

Among the many witnesses was John C. Wilson, Jr., MD, chairman of the American Medical Association's Section on Orthopedic Surgery (and subsequently president of the defendant AAOS). His testimony demonstrated that medical bias, not patient care, was at the center of this professional boycott.

The chiropractic treatment that the medical profession criticized most heavily was spinal manipulation therapy (SMT), a subject Dr. Wilson admitted he knew nothing about. Considering manipulation has existed since antiquity around the world, his ignorance of this ageless healing art was shocking although indicative of the medical boycott of chiropractic care.

The following excerpt, taken from the deposition of Dr. Wilson, shows the bias, contempt, and hostility that practitioners of chiropractic faced:

> Q: Is it possible to manually move a spinal joint through a range of motion?
>
> A: I simply cannot answer your question in that context.
>
> Q: Can you answer the question in any context including your own?
>
> A: No, because this is not a frame of reference in which medical doctors think, and we don't relate to turning spinal joints around through manipulation. That is the chiropractic concept, and we don't understand it. We don't relate to it. We don't know what you are talking about.
>
> Q: Have you ever done any research into that?
>
> A: No. And I don't have any desire to do any research into that or any other cult.

---

289 J McAndrews via personal communication to JC Smith. (May 8, 1998)

Q: I am not really talking about cults now. I am talking about the manual manipulation of spinal joints.

A: No. I have no interest in or desire to pursue the manipulation of spinal joints as a theory.

Q: Why?

A: Because I don't believe in this kind of thing. I don't know of any scientific basis that would cause me to pursue this as a way to help people.[290]

Wilson freely admitted he was ignorant of the concepts of joint play and manual manipulation of the spine, yet he had the audacity to condemn it as unworthy of his investigation. To make his testimony more ironic, in 1967, just a few years before his deposition, Wilson had written an article in *JAMA* admitting the deficiencies in medical education concerning treatment for low back pain and sciatica:

> Even the abundant and significant advances resulting from the medical profession's emphasis upon research have failed abysmally to relieve modern man of one of his most common and bothersome afflictions, low back pain…treatment of low back pain is inconsistent and less than minimal…MDs often displayed a disturbing ignorance of the cause and treatment of low back and sciatic pain, one of mankind's most common affliction.[291]

Although Dr. Wilson was painfully honest in his appraisal of traditional medicine's inability to diagnose and properly treat back pain, his gross condemnation of chiropractic concepts illustrated how his bias superseded his intellectual honesty on clinical issues. Recall this comes from a professional who prided himself on a so-called objective *scientific attitude*.

Not only did Dr. Wilson show his bias, so did Dr. Ernest K. Howard, the AMA president at the time of the medical attacks on chiropractic. Under oath, Dr. Howard admitted he had no proof or understanding of spinal manipulative therapy when asked by attorney McAndrews. Instead of any scientific knowledge of this healing art, Dr. Howard believed it was just psychosomatic:[292]

> Q: Did the AMA do any research into why those [chiropractic] patients were satisfied?
>
> A: I think the answer is no. I would have to add that it was clear from their public comments that we read, the usual comments of the patients, some of the letters, they were satisfied with the relationship. The psychotherapeutic approach which is part of the chiropractic service was practical.
>
> Q: Do you know if the AMA ever did any research to determine if spinal manipulation had any therapeutic value?

---

290 JC Keating, *Wilk et al. v. AMA et al.*, trial deposition, p. 57.

291 JC Wilson, "Low Back Pain and Sciatica: A Plea for Better Care of the Patient, Chairman's Address," *JAMA*, 200/8, (May 22, 1967):705-712.

292 Deposition of Ernest K. Howard by G McAndrews, (Dec. 15, 1980):1052.

A: I do not, no.

Q: In your time with the AMA did you, yourself, ever inquire as to whether or not spinal manipulative therapy had any therapeutic value?

A: The answer is no, I did not.

Q: Do you know of anyone that did?

A: No.

Q: Do you know whether spinal manipulative therapy has any health value?

A: Again there could be a psychotherapeutic value in the laying on of hands.

Q: Other than psychotherapeutic, mechanical value?

A: Not that I know of.

As president of the AMA that waged war on chiropractors, it is odd that Dr. Howard offered no proof of chiropractic's harm to patients, nor did he have any knowledge of chiropractic care whatsoever. Like a Storm Trooper, he simply followed his orders lock-step to the drum beat of the Committee on Quackery and AMA Board of Trustees.

Mr. McAndrews also asked Dr. Howard: "Was it your feeling that chiropractors should be eliminated?"

> It was my feeling then and it is my feeling today that the best way, one of the best ways to promote the public's health is to reduce the minimum possible quackery of all kinds including chiropractic, which I consider quackery.[293]

Howard's answer was shocking to reasonable people, but to the medical demagogues, his attitude typified their unrelenting mindset. Moreover, as an American living in a country built on equal rights, he failed to understand his wish to "to reduce the minimum possible quackery of all kinds including chiropractic" was antithetical to social justice and antitrust laws.

On the other hand, not all medical doctors fell for the anti-chiropractic dogma. Testimony by John McMillan Mennell, MD, enlightened the court as to the value of spinal manipulation during his testimony at the *Wilk* trial:

> Eight out of ten patients that come out of any doctor's office complain of a musculoskeletal system problem, regardless of what system the pain is coming from . . . I will say 100 percent of those complaints...are...due to joint dysfunction in the musculoskeletal [system]...*If you don't manipulate to relieve the symptoms from this condition of joint dysfunction, then you are depriving the patient of the one thing that is likely to relieve them of their suffering.*[294] (emphasis added)

Dr. Mennell also testified about the lack of education and training medical students receive in medical school on the musculoskeletal system:

> Q: At the medical schools with which you are familiar, do you know about the educational program in the musculoskeletal pain area for medical students?

---

293 Ibid. p. 1541.
294 Transcript of testimony of John McMillan Mennell, M.D., *Wilk v AMA* transcript pp. 2090-2093.

A: Usually it is anything between zero to four or five.

Q: Hours?

A: Yes, in four years. [295]

The court also heard incriminating testimony that the AMA committee was aware that:

- Some medical physicians believed chiropractic could be effective,
- Graduates from many medical schools failed to demonstrate basic competency on a validated examination of fundamental concepts of musculoskeletal care, and
- The court found that chiropractors were better trained to deal with musculoskeletal problems than most medical physicians.

According to Mr. McAndrews' closing argument to the court:

The American Medical Association has known since 1960 of a glaring deficiency in the musculoskeletal education of medical practitioners in the United States. There can be no doubt about that.

But there is something else that they knew. They knew and were placed on notice by an orthopedic surgeon, Dr. Hendryson, a member of the Board of Trustees and a professor of orthopedic surgery at the University of Colorado who had worked with a chiropractor on Guadalcanal. They knew the following, and I say they knew it because the document was suppressed. [296]

In his closing argument, Mr. McAndrews reminded the court of the testimony of Dr. John C. Wilson, one-time president of the American Academy of Orthopedic Surgeons, in his paper published in 1967 when he admitted to "prejudices and controversies":

At the postgraduate level, symposia and courses concerning the cause and treatment of low back and sciatic pain are often ineffective because of prejudices and controversies. Even the abundant and significant advances resulting from *the medical profession's emphasis upon research have failed abysmally to relieve modern man of one of his most common and bothersome afflictions, low back pain.* This situation could be very improved by correlation and dissemination of currently available knowledge of the etiology and treatment of low back pain and sciatic pain.[297] (emphasis added)

Of course, the "available knowledge of the etiology and treatment of low back pain and sciatica" failed to include any mention of manipulative therapy or chiropractic care. In essence, Dr. Wilson was a victim of his own deception.

McAndrews also presented a letter sent to Dr. Wilson in 1972 by Walter S. Wiggins, MD, Associate Secretary of the AMA, concerning the inclusion of chiropractic into California's workmen's comp program:

295 Ibid.
296 G McAndrews closing argument, *Wilk v. AMA*, (January 28, 1981): 6733.
297 JC Wilson, "Low Back Pain and Sciatica: A Plea for Better Care of the Patient, Chairman's Address," *JAMA*, 200/8 (May 22, 1967):705-712.

Dear Dr. Wilson:

> Governor Ronald Reagan of the State of California has recently signed a Senate
> bill directing insurance carriers in the State of California to provide the name of a
> chiropractor from a list of five names which must be given to an injured worker if he
> requests a change of physician and requests chiropractic care.

> At first glance the bill seems innocuous, but objective evaluation of the bill reveals
> it in effect legalizes the equality of chiropractic with medicine. I believe the orthopedic
> surgeons as a whole should be more concerned with the advances of chiropractic
> than perhaps any other specialty because of our knowledge of chiropractic activity in
> musculoskeletal disorders.

McAndrews also reminded the court of the many workmen's comp studies that
showed a 2:1 superiority rate for chiropractic care over medical care. He reminded the
court of the testimonies of Drs. Mennell and Freitag who also spoke of the superiority
of manipulation for low back pain cases. He emphasized the stirring testimony of Dr.
Hendryson, a member of the AMA's Board of Trustees who spoke highly of his report
observing chiropractic care at Guadalcanal during World War II.

McAndrews summarized the AMA's attitude about the abundance of evidence:

> What did the medical profession do about it? Nothing. They continued with a
> plan that was concocted back in the early '60s to contain and eliminate the profession.
> If nothing else, that type of report should have said, *"if we care one whit for the patient, we
> should investigate it."* There were hundreds of millions of dollars involved and untold pain
> and suffering coming from those types of industrial accidents.

> At no time do they talk about the patient. They talk about money. There is
> enormous—11 per cent of the entire gross national product of this nation—that means
> every dime, every cent spent for goods and services in the country, 11 percent of it goes
> to health care. The pot at the end of the rainbow was what was being protected by the
> monopoly we charge in this case.[298] (emphasis added)

No Medical Smoking Guns

Mr. McAndrews also pointed out the AMA attorneys did not bring in many witnesses.
They never brought to court one person from any of those commissions believed to be
"fixed" by Doyl Taylor (HEW, National Council of Senior Citizens) to testify that those
studies were honestly done. Taylor himself failed to testify when he fled to Arizona.
When the day of reckoning occurred, Taylor proved to be a coward.

According to Chester Wilk:

> Taylor was specifically named in our lawsuit and we had him scheduled to go to
> court. When it came time for him to appear in court he took an early retirement from
> the AMA and fled to Arizona and out of the jurisdiction of the Northern Illinois Federal

---

298 G McAndrews, ibid. p. 6739.

Court. He had devoted eleven years of his life and millions of dollars covertly trashing chiropractic behind the scenes and now when he was challenged to go to court to argue his case he ran like a coward.[299]

Taylor had his son come to court to testify that his dad had crippling arthritis and was unable to come to Chicago. The arthritis excuse was so outrageously phony that we hired a detective agency to watch Taylor in Arizona and study his activities and found that he was on the golf course golfing almost every day which is hardly a pastime for someone with crippling arthritis. Unfortunately the jury in our first trial was not allowed to hear this damning evidence which the jury should have heard.[300]

Also, none of the medical critics of chiropractic education testified despite their vehement objection when the New York Board of Regents accredited National College of Chiropractic and pronounced it "an outstanding educational institution."

Mr. McAndrews remarked at the lack of witnesses called by the attorneys for the medical defendants:

> *None of them have come through that door.* Dr. Sabatier, who called the chiropractors killers and rabid dogs, is a defendant in this action. Where is he? Dr. Tom Ballantine: they extolled his virtues, head of the Committee on Quackery, a defendant in this action, his name is on all of these letters going back and forth. Every one of the letters all in the web of combining and conspiring to destroy the profession of chiropractic, where is Dr. Tom Ballantine?
>
> They were not brought in so you [the jurors] could see them testify. Not one of them was brought in...none of these people that are central to this thing were brought in here. None of them.
>
> And they haven't brought in a patient. You'd think if all of these patients have been injured, some would come in here and say they were taken by a chiropractor. *Not one walked through the door.*[301] (emphasis added)

Mr. McAndrews addressed one of the main points of the defense–the issue of quackery. Again, no expert witnesses were provided to prove this point. Instead of bringing in experts in the field of spinal mechanics, neurophysiology, or orthopedic medicine to testify against the art or science of chiropractic, the best the medical attorneys could do was produce tacky and hyperbolic chiropractic ads. McAndrews showed by definition that many MDs are quacks when it came to spinal care:

> I have counted up the exhibits of the ads and there is no doubt that some of the ads were distasteful. I have seen one where the chiropractor has an ad that says "the only thing that can't be cured by spinal adjusting is rigor mortis itself."
>
> I do notice, though, that *for the AMA that claims it had a full-time committee for eleven years to produce approximately 50 ads from an entire profession, says something about the fact that*

---

299 CA Wilk, *Living a Prophesy: A Chiropractor's Incredible Story,* published by Chester A Wilk, (2008):31.

300 Ibid. pp. 31-32.

301 G McAndrews closing argument, ibid. p 7076-88.

they may not have found as many chiropractors behaving in an aberrant fashion as they would like the Court to believe.

The American Medical Association in their closing argument read three ads. The ads were clearly quackery, and the chiropractors know it. The ICA and ACA asked that their endorsement or background for any of those [Parker] charts be removed. You heard Dr. Rutherford [ICA president] state: "We're opposed to quackery. We're trying to clean it up." They were trying their darndest to help the chiropractors straighten out their act.

There were fringe practitioners and anyone that doesn't think that there are fringe lawyers, fringe medical doctors, fringe dentists, fringe podiatrists, psychologists and chiropractors just is ignoring common sense. There are charlatans wherever you go, and the chiropractors have tried to help themselves.

They use the definition of quackery: somebody who pretends to knowledge they do not have. Chiropractors that pretend to medical knowledge are quacks. And medical physicians who pretend to universal knowledge of human anatomy and biomechanics on this record should be called quacks if the definition is: somebody who pretends to knowledge they don't not have. That's quackery. We all agree on that. [302]

Mr. McAndrews also pointed out there was no effort by the AMA to incorporate the skills of chiropractors into the mainstream healthcare to help patients:

And what has happened here is that the might of a $60 million a year budget at the AMA was directed against eliminating the second largest health care profession in this country, not helping it, not joining hands, not sitting down and getting together and saying: you have certain skills, there's no doubt about that. Congress wouldn't include you in Medicare unless there is an over-whelming grass roots response from patients. They're getting some sort of help that they're not getting from the medical profession.

Indeed, the defendants' organizations responded to that. The way they responded was: we're not going to improve that health care group. We're not going to even talk to them. We won't debate with them. We won't help their colleges, we will oppose any effort they do to upgrade their educational base and then we'll call them stupid. What kind of concern and how does the name "physician" apply to someone that would do that? You can't do it. (emphasis added)

The trial evidence was clear the AMA *et al.* had based their war against chiropractors on falsehoods created by its own COQ. They presented no proof that chiropractic was a danger to the public, they refused to investigate chiropractic education or practice methods, and they refused to do research of their own despite the urging of one of its own board members, Dr. Hendryson. It became clear this was a war based on politics and greed, and certainly not on science, safety, or clinical effectiveness.

---

302 Ibid. p. 3051-52.

Judicial Malpractice

Despite the overwhelming evidence of the AMA's antitrust activities—the dirty tricks, the pilfered documents gleaned by Sore Throat, medical experts' "admissions against interest" testimonies in behalf of chiropractic care, as well as the New Zealand Report, the trial judge unhinged McAndrews' case with bad instructions to the jury.

Judge Bua told jurors they should not find the AMA guilty of wrongdoing *if its actions were merely designed to inform the public about defects in chiropractic,* adding that the AMA's advocacy was protected if it were aimed at lobbying for changes in law. This was clearly never stated by the AMA in evidence and served to mislead the jurors.

The AMA's attorneys used egregious emotional evidence to appeal to the jurors, including outlandish advertising claims by some chiropractors who claimed to cure most everything. This anecdotal evidence had nothing to do with the antitrust activities of the AMA, but was used to prejudice the jury that ultimately voted in favor of the defendants.

After an arduous eight-week trial, the jury concluded the AMA's anti-chiropractic campaign was within legal bounds.[303] Once again the downtrodden chiropractors had faced injustice, but this time it came from a federal judge who had misdirected the jury.

The jury had listened to the economic arguments presented by George McAndrews, but what they heard the loudest was the defendants' recitation of the fantastic and dubious clinical claims made by chiropractic technique peddlers and the greedy and unethical strategies recommended by the worst of those who instructed chiropractors on how to build their practices.[304] McAndrews in his closing argument proved that none of the plaintiffs used these methods and the defense attorneys never showed that any of the plaintiffs utilized them either.

When the two-month jury trial ended, one of the jurors phoned McAndrews' office and was clearly distraught and crying. The juror said, "What the AMA did was unethical and immoral, but some of those chiropractors [referring to the practice builders who made depositions] should be in jail."[305]

Afterwards, other distraught jurors contacted McAndrews office to say they believed the AMA was guilty, but based on the judge's instructions and the flagrant anecdotal evidence, they felt they had no choice but to judge the physicians' group innocent. McAndrews filed an appeal, arguing that Bua had erred in his handling of the case and instructions to the jury.

In his address to the Appellate Court on January 20, 1982, McAndrews presented the instructions from Judge Bua to the jurors that "best characterizes the incomprehensible and unsupportable position of the defendants." With respect to the Rule of Reason, the Trial Court actually told the jury, after having conducted the entire [eight-week] trial with this misunderstanding of the law, that:

303 Wolinsky, ibid. p. 138.
304 JC Keating, "The England Case and the Wilk Case: A Comparison, Part 2," *Dynamic Chiropractic* 25/20 (September 24, 2007)
305 Editorial Staff, "Wilk Plaintiffs Speak Out," *Dynamic Chiropractic* 11/08 (April 9, 1993)

If you find from the evidence that defendants engage in activities, meaning direct, private activities as distinguished from governmental activities, which have had substantial effect in preventing chiropractors from offering services which are reasonably interchangeable by consumers for the same purposes as the services offered by medical doctors, that would be <u>an element</u> weighing on the side of unreasonableness.

Mr. McAndrews noted the error of this judge's instruction to the jury in his address to the Appellate Court:

> *The Rule of Reason does not make a conspiracy to substantially prevent your competitors from offering their services a mere element in a violation. Substantially preventing your competitors from offering their services is a violation in and of itself."*

The American Medical Association and these defendants have no governmental authority whatsoever to restrain trade. Indeed, their conduct is diametrically opposed to the will of all 50 states. The AMA lost the battles to prevent licensure of chiropractors.

If chiropractors are incompetent, dangerous or dishonest it is the Illinois Department of Education and Registration which must act. Not these self appointed defendants... *the Supreme Court...made it clear that self-styled vigilantism in defense of public health, welfare and safety should not be placed on the scales.* Finally, in light of the evidence adduced by the defendants and permitted by the trial judge, plaintiffs were entitled to a plain and simple statement that good motives or a desire to protect the public health, safety and welfare is no defense to a Sherman Act claim.

We...ask that the Court remand the case for a new trial with instructions that will allow the plaintiffs to try the antitrust case they brought to Court, and not a malpractice or ethics case involving unscrupulous chiropractors not in court or an entrepreneur from Texas [Jim Parker] who conducts three or four day professional success seminars for chiropractors.[306] (emphasis added)

Wilk II Trial

On September 19, 1983, a forty-seven page decision from the Seventh Circuit Panel reversed in favor of the plaintiffs and remanded it for a new trial. The decision stated that errors had been made by the original trial judge in allowing inaccurate documents submitted by defendants into evidence and in the judge's instructions to the jurors.[307]

The court ruled there was a prejudicial error since the volume of material allowed as evidence was beyond the scope of the issues of the trial, that being the determination of whether the defendant medical groups had conspired to economically destroy the chiropractic profession.

In the second trial, the chiropractic-plaintiffs waived punitive damages in exchange for a trial by magistrate that required Federal Court Judge Susan Getzendanner to serve as the sole arbiter between the chiropractors and the AMA-defendants. After reviewing

---

306 G McAndrews appeal to the 7th Circuit court.
307 Wolinsky and Brune, ibid. p. 138.

all the evidence, she had to decide whether or not commerce had been illegally restrained, but she did not have to consider the financial magnitude of the economic loss to the plaintiffs.[308]

Chester Wilk commented on the selection of Judge Getzendanner:

> At that time one of the brightest judges in the Northern Illinois District Court, Susan Getzendanner, was looking for an exciting case to finish her career as a judge since she was planning to go into private practice. She came across our case and picked it out. I think God led her to our case and the judge did a flawless job which was upheld in the higher courts.[309]

During the proceedings, it was shown that the AMA attempted to:

- Undermine chiropractic schools; intimidate counselors to discourage prospective chiropractic students; threaten community colleges offering pre-chiropractic requirements.
- Undercut insurance programs for chiropractic patients; interfere with the initial Medicare legislation with a phony White Paper written by AMA operatives.
- Conceal evidence of the effectiveness of chiropractic care.
- Subvert government inquires into the effectiveness of chiropractic; block the inclusion of chiropractic into military health services and Department of Veterans Affairs.
- Promote other activities that would control the monopoly the AMA had on health care.

Much of the same evidence was presented, and in the closing arguments of the second *Wilk* trial, Mr. McAndrews commented on the low image cast upon chiropractors by the AMA propaganda:

> *This is the evil that is still permeating this country.* Every medical physician in this country has been exposed to that from the first day of medical school on. That's all we need, is the medical school students being told they are *rabid dogs* and *killers*, and not mentioning the fact that the medical students aren't getting the proper education in the musculoskeletal system.
>
> They have drummed into the medical physicians of this nation, not only their 260,000 members, but everyone down into the medical schools, that not only are you unethical, but *you are almost anti-human if you would dare entrust health care even in a cooperative setting to a chiropractor.*
>
> He {Dr. Sabatier} said he felt chiropractors were nice people, but they killed people. They couldn't possibly find evidence of that, and if they could have found it, it would have been here in

308 JC Keating, "The England Case and the Wilk Case: A Comparison, Part 2," *Dynamic Chiropractic* 25/20 (September 24, 2007)
309 CA Wilk, ibid. p.33.

court. After 25 years they haven't been able to find any evidence of that. They only evidence they had was that they helped people and they ran funny ads.[310] (emphasis added)

Mr. McAndrews also noted aside from the bad image cast upon medical propaganda of the cultural power the AMA took upon itself to damage chiropractic as a whole and how the medical society turned a blind eye to help patients.

These people were a fourth branch of government, self-subsumed title, and they were challenging both the Federal and State governments.

In this case we have got evidence that they play games with words: it's scientific if the MD does it. It's unscientific if the chiropractor does it. It's twice as effective if a chiropractor does it, but that just has therapeutic value, it's not scientific.

They want to set up at the gate not the owners of the hospital but their members that have been tainted and poisoned; that well has been poisoned by the AMA. These are your competitors. My God, they [chiropractors] are more effective than you are. The hospital is loaded with patients that could utilize chiropractic services…Forget how effective they are, but, remember, keep it within the hospital walls so we don't have antitrust implications.

They should have found out that medical physician studies were showing that it was twice as effective as medical care in certain orthopedic problems.

Mr. McAndrews summarized his closing remarks when he noted:

This is the first time anywhere in any trial where the Marcus Welby mask has been stripped away from them and they have been revealed for what they are. Their attitude was *'to heck with the patients'…* [311] (emphasis added)

In closing arguments, the AMA's trial lawyer Douglas R. Carlson inexplicably said the AMA acknowledged that chiropractic was becoming more scientific and even took partial credit for improvements in chiropractic: "We suggest that one reason that it changed was because of the criticism of its bizarre methods."[312] In fact, there was nothing bizarre about chiropractic clinical methods although there were some strange advertisements used by a very few chiropractors as McAndrews noted.

The courtroom "cracked up" when McAndrews, in his closing, retorted that Carlson's position was akin to a "German U-boat captain who took credit for the American Olympic swim team being so good because by sinking their ships, he taught them how to swim."[313]

McAndrews noted in his closing of *Wilk II* that by forcing Principles 3 and 4 upon its members, "the AMA has set the chiropractic profession back, has set the healthcare of this country back, and did it deliberately because it confused its trade union responsibilities with its responsibility to healthcare."[314]

---

310 G McAndrews closing arguments, *Wilk v. AMA*, (June 26, 1987):3093-97.

311 G McAndrews closing arguments, *Wilk v. AMA*, (June 26, 1987):3363-64

312 Transcript of Proceedings, *Wilk*, (May 26, 1987):3132.

313 Transcript of Proceedings, *Wilk*, (July 2, 1987):3396.

314 G McAndrews, *Wilk II*, ibid. p. 3090.

Lead plaintiff Chester Wilk summarized the personal impact of this medical war:

> As our daughters were growing up, I became deeply distressed with the dishonest
> propaganda and illegal conduct that was being used against chiropractic. Dishonesty is
> bad enough but when it exploits people in pain and suffering and even causes deaths it
> degenerates into the lowest form of contemptible human behavior. [315]

Due to the courage of Chester A. Wilk as well as the fortitude of the other remaining plaintiffs, James W. Bryden, Patricia A. Arthur, and Michael D. Pedigo, the case had been made that their constitutional rights had been violated. Their fate would be determined by a new judge after a two-month retrial that would become a landmark case and a step closer to social justice.

Legal Waterloo

After eleven years of legal wrangling after two trials in the District Court and one in the Appellate Court, the *Wilk et al. v. AMA et al.* antitrust lawsuit on September 25, 1987, Judge Susan Getzendanner issued a 101-page opinion that affirmed the AMA had violated Section 1 of the Sherman Act.[316]

Also convicted with the AMA were the American College of Surgeons and the American College of Radiologists. The presiding judge found these medical allies guilty of a "lengthy, systematic, successful, and unlawful boycott"[317] designed by the AMA to eliminate the profession of chiropractic as a competitor in the American healthcare system.

The judge dismissed charges against the American College of Physicians, the Joint Commission on Accreditation of Hospitals and the American Academy of Orthopedic Surgeons. Charges were also dismissed against James H. Sammons of Chicago, an AMA trustee who had served as head of the Committee on Quackery, which was disbanded in 1974. Defendants Taylor, Sabatier, and Ballantine were dismissed by the court over plaintiffs' objection. When asked why these three leading culprits in the medical war were dismissed, attorney McAndrews replied, "They were tiny fish and the judge knew we were going after the giants. They had retired long before the trial. Their employers were responsible for their activities."[318]

Five defendants settled earlier after affirming the rights of chiropractors. Defendant American Osteopathic Association settled and agreed to consent injunction on October 29, 1980. Defendant American Academy of Physical and Medical Rehabilitation settled and entered into consent injunction on December 8, 1980. Defendant Illinois State

---

315 CA Wilk, *Living a Prophesy: A Chiropractor's Incredible Story*, published by Chester A. Wilk, (2008):21.
316 *Wilk v. AMA*, 671 F. Supp. 1465, N.D. Ill. 1987.
317 *Chester A. Wilk, James W. Bryden, Patricia A. Arthur, Michael D. Pedigo v. American Medical Association, Joint Commission on Accreditation of Hospitals, American College of Physicians, American Academy of Orthopaedic Surgeons,* United States District Court Northern District of Illinois, No. 76C3777, Susan Getzendanner, Judge, Judgment dated August 27, 1987.
318 G McAndrews via private communication to JC Smith, (May 3, 2010)

Medical Society settled after first trial. Defendant American Hospital Association settled during the second trial.[319]

The judge summarized the situation that the AMA and its officials had:

> "...instituted a boycott of chiropractors in the mid-1960s by informing AMA members that chiropractors were unscientific practitioners and that it was unethical for a medical physician to associate with chiropractors. *The purpose of the boycott was to contain and eliminate the chiropractic profession.* This conduct constituted a conspiracy among the AMA and its members and an unreasonable restraint of trade in violation of Section 1 of the Sherman Act."[320] (emphasis added)

The court noted the AMA had offered a "patient safety" defense which it failed to prove. On the other hand, data from workers' compensation studies served to validate chiropractic care. Specifically, evidence before the Committee on Quackery proved conclusively that chiropractic treatment was more effective than traditional medicine in treating certain kinds of back injuries. The COQ was also aware that some medical physicians believed chiropractic to be effective and that chiropractors were better trained to deal with musculoskeletal problems than most medical physicians. [321]

In regard to the "patient safety" defense, Judge Getzendanner opined that "most of the defense witnesses, surprisingly, appeared to be testifying for the plaintiffs" [aka, *admissions against interest*]:

> The plaintiffs...point out that the anecdotal evidence in the record favors chiropractors. The patients who testified were [treated] by chiropractors and not by medical physicians. Dr. Per Freitag, a medical physician who associates [professionally] with chiropractors, has observed that patients in one hospital who receive chiropractic treatment are released sooner than patients in another hospital...which does not allow chiropractors. Dr. John McMillan Mennell, MD, testified in favor of chiropractic. Even the defendants' economic witness, Mr. Lynk, assumed that chiropractors outperformed medical physicians in the treatment of certain conditions and he believed that was a reasonable assumption. The defendants have offered some evidence as to the unscientific nature of chiropractic...*but most of the defense witnesses, surprisingly, appeared to be testifying for the plaintiffs.* Taking into account all of the evidence, I conclude only that the AMA has failed to meet its burden on the issue of whether its concern for the scientific method in support of the boycott of the entire chiropractic profession was objectively reasonable throughout the entire period of the boycott.[322] (emphasis added)

"These admissions were not mere puffery," she said. Although the AMA never disciplined any members for associating with chiropractors, the judge said the existence of

---

319 Ibid.

320 Getzendanner, Memorandum Opinion and Order, 5.

321 Ibid. p. 7

322 Ibid. p. 7.

the ethical stricture against such relations "is inherently a forceful mandator of conduct... Enforcement was not necessary to obtain compliance with the boycott."[323]

Judge Getzendanner accepted the Committee on Quackery's acknowledgement that it had succeeded in containing chiropractic:

> The AMA believed that the boycott worked—that chiropractic would have achieved greater gains in the absence of the boycott. Since no medical physician would want to be considered unethical by his peers, the success of the boycott is not surprising. However, chiropractic achieved licensing in all 50 states during the existence of the Committee on Quackery.[324]

She mentioned in her Opinion:

> The activities of the AMA undoubtedly have injured the reputation of chiropractors generally...In my judgment, this injury continues to the present time and likely continues to adversely affect the plaintiffs. The AMA has never made any attempt to publicly repair the damage the boycott did to chiropractors' reputations.[325]

"There has never been an affirmative statement by the AMA that it is ethical to associate with chiropractors,'" the judge said, and she described the conspiracy "systematic, long-term wrongdoing, and the long-term intent to destroy a licensed profession."[326]

> The AMA's purpose was to prevent medical physicians from referring patients to chiropractors and accepting referrals of patients from chiropractors, to prevent chiropractors from obtaining access to hospital diagnostic services and membership on hospital medical staffs, to prevent medical physicians from teaching at chiropractic colleges or engaging in any joint research, and to prevent any cooperation between the two groups in the delivery of health care services.[327]

To combat the continuing effects of the conspiracy, she ordered the AMA to admit to the "lawlessness of its past conduct" and to alter its official policy on chiropractic.[328] As a result, the injunction was published in the AMA *Journal* on January 1, 1988, with an editorial by AMA general counsel Kirk B. Johnson explaining why such an unusual document appeared in the scientific publication.[329]

The Court's *Permanent Injunction Order Against the AMA* found that the "AMA was unable to establish that during the entire period of the conspiracy its position was objectively reasonable":

---

323 Getzendanner, Memorandum Opinion and Order, pp. 23.

324 Ibid. p. 1

325 Opinion p. 10

326 *Associated Press*, "U.S. Judge Finds Medical Group Conspired Against Chiropractors," *New York Times* (1987)

327 S Getzendanner, US District Judge, *Permanent Injunction Order Against the AMA* (Sept. 25, 1987), published *in JAMA*, 259/1 (January 1, 1988):81

328 *Associated Press*, "U.S. Judge Finds Medical Group Conspired Against Chiropractors," *New York Times*, (August 29, 1987)

329 S Getzendanner, ibid. 140.

The court concluded that the AMA had a genuine concern for scientific methods in patient care, and that this concern was the dominant factor in motivating the AMA's conduct. However, *the AMA failed to establish that throughout the entire period of the boycott, from 1966 to 1980, this concern was objectively reasonable.* The court reached that conclusion on the basis of extensive testimony from both witnesses for the plaintiffs and the AMA that some forms of chiropractic treatment are effective and the fact that the AMA recognized that chiropractic began to change in the early 1970s. Since the boycott was not formally over until Principle 3 was eliminated in 1980, *the court found that the AMA was unable to establish that during the entire period of the conspiracy its position was objectively reasonable.* Finally, the court ruled that the AMA's concern for scientific method in patient care could have been adequately satisfied in a manner less restrictive of competition and that a nationwide conspiracy to eliminate a licensed profession was not justified by the concern for scientific method. *On the basis of these findings, the court concluded that the AMA had failed to establish the patient care defense.*[330]

Judge Getzendanner wrote in the AMA *Journal* of her decision:[331]

As part of the injunctive relief to be ordered by the court against the AMA, the AMA shall be required to send a copy of this Permanent Injunction Order to each of its current members. The members of the AMA are bound by the terms of the Permanent Injunction Order if they act in concert with the AMA to violate the terms of the order.

In addition to the AMA being ordered to notify its 275,000 members of the court's injunction, the American Hospital Association (AHA) sent out 440,000 separate notices to inform hospitals across the United States that the AHA had no objection to allowing chiropractic care in hospitals.

Although the judge may have unlocked the doors to the nation's public hospitals, her decision did little to open these medical fortresses to chiropractors. To obtain hospital privileges still required approval by the controlling medical staff. Just having a state license does not entitle anyone to practice in a public hospital without approval of the local medical society.

Indeed, just as desegregation laws did not lessen racial bigotry in society for many years, neither did the *Wilk* decision sway *"Jim Crow, MD,"* to embrace the ostracized chiropractors with open arms into their medical fortresses.

Dr. Alan Nelson, chairman of the AMA board of trustees, told the *Associated Press*, "We don't think there was ever a boycott or a conspiracy."[332] Considering the volume of evidence in these two trials, it is unfathomable how Nelson came to that conclusion, but typical of one who cannot see his own bigotry.

---

330 S Getzendanner, US District Judge, *Permanent Injunction Order Against the AMA* (Sept. 25, 1987), published in *JAMA*, 259/1 (January 1, 1988):81

331 Ibid. pp. 81-82.

332 *Associated Press*, ibid.

AMA attorney Kirk B. Johnson inexplicably touted this defeat as a victory:

> We still believe that the lower courts erred in their decision. However, their decision did not call for the AMA to change any policies. The lower court found that AMA's policy for the past 10 years regarding professional interaction between physicians and chiropractors was lawful. The court's decision did not endorse chiropractic. No damages were awarded. Therefore, the decision will have little or no impact on patients and their physicians.[333]

Regrettably, both the comments by Johnson and Nelson illustrated the same biased attitude that denied chiropractors social justice and denied patients the best treatment for the pandemic of back pain. Like the Southerners after the Civil War, their defiance led to resentment and belligerence rather than an ethical reawakening to equality and justice for all. This attitude was not lost on the Court.

The evidence at the trial prompted Judge Getzendanner to comment:

> Although the conspiracy ended in 1980, there are lingering effects of the illegal boycott and conspiracy which require an injunction. Some medical physicians' individual decisions on whether or not to professionally associate with chiropractors are still affected by the boycott. The injury to chiropractors' reputations which resulted from the boycott has not been repaired. Chiropractors suffer current economic injury as a result of the boycott. The AMA has never affirmatively acknowledged that there are and should be no collective impediments to professional association and cooperation between chiropractors and medical physicians, except as provided by low. Instead, the AMA has consistently argued that its conduct has not violated the antitrust laws...*An injunction is necessary to assure that the AMA does not interfere with the right of a physician, hospital, or other institution to make an individual decision on the question of professional association...*[334] (emphasis added)

Hopefully, Mr. Johnson is wrong when he writes this "opinion will have little or no impact on patients and their physicians." It seems he missed the point that chiropractic care would improve patient care, but it is obvious the AMA continues to delude itself. Apparently, he failed to hear the Court's opinion of the effectiveness of chiropractic care when she wrote in her injunction:

> The court did not reach the question of whether chiropractic theory was, in fact, scientific. However, the evidence in the case was that some forms of chiropractic manipulation of the spine and joints were therapeutic. AMA witnesses, including the present Chairman of the Board of Trustees of the AMA, testified that some forms of treatment by chiropractors, including manipulation, can be therapeutic in the treatment of conditions such as back pain syndrome.[335]

Fortunately, a saner mindset prevailed in court than in the leadership of the AMA. "Labeling all chiropractors unscientific cultists and depriving chiropractors of association

---

333 Editorial Staff, "Looking Back: 1988," *Dynamic Chiropractic* 26/06 (March 11, 2008)
334 S Getzendanner, US District Judge, *Permanent Injunction Order Against the AMA* (Sept. 25, 1987), published in *JAMA*, 259/1 (January 1, 1988):82
335 Ibid.

with medical physicians, injury to reputation was assured by the AMA's name-calling practice," Judge Getzendanner said. [336] The court stressed, however, that her ruling should not be construed as an endorsement of chiropractic, nor would she preside over a shotgun wedding between the professions. "Certainly no judge should perform that ceremony."[337]

Getzendanner found the behavior by both the AMA and chiropractic to be a mixed bag of contradictory issues. She said the AMA acted in the blind belief that it was protecting patient welfare by combating chiropractic. Meanwhile, she noted "alarming practices by some chiropractors" that were potentially harmful to patients:

> The defendants have offered some evidence as to the unscientific nature of chiropractic. The study of how the five original named plaintiffs diagnosed and actually treated patients with common symptoms was particularly impressive.[338]
>
> This study demonstrated that the plaintiffs do not use common methods in treating common symptoms and that the treatment of patients appears to be undertaken on an *ad hoc* rather than on a scientific basis. And there was evidence of the use of cranial adjustments to cure cerebral palsy and other equally alarming practices by some chiropractors.[339]
>
> I do not minimize the negative evidence, but *most of the defense witnesses appeared to be testifying for the plaintiffs.*[340] (emphasis added)

George McAndrews later mentioned, "The judge read with interest and had a knee-slapping outburst" to the defendant's interrogatory response that cited the positive medical studies about chiropractic care. "Their own documents condemn themselves and praised chiropractors," he noted of these admissions. [341]

The AMA's present position on chiropractic is that it is ethical for a medical physician to professionally associate with chiropractors provided the physician believes that such association is in the best interest of his patient. A physician now may, without fear of discipline or sanction by the AMA, refer a patient to a duly licensed chiropractor when he believes that referral may benefit the patient. The AMA confirmed that a physician may also choose to accept or to decline patients sent to him by a chiropractor. Also, the AMA confirmed that a physician may teach at a chiropractic college or seminar.[342]

Supreme Decisions

After the *Wilk* trial, the AMA experienced more legal setbacks. The district court's decision was affirmed by the Court of Appeals on February 7, 1990.[343] The AMA

---

336 *Associated Press*, ibid.

337 Ibid. p. 49.

338 Tr. 2208-319.

339 Tr. 917.

340 S Getzendanner, ibid, 35.

341 Speech before the National Chiropractic Legislative Conference, March 2002, Washington D.C.

342 Ibid.

343 *Wilk v. AMA*, 895 F.2d 352, 7th Cir. 1990

petitioned the Supreme Court three times, but each time the Court denied *certiorari*. The Court grants *certiorari* only when a case presents a novel question of law and the *Wilk* case was a straightforward application of the Sherman Act.

Attorney McAndrews commented on this appeal:

> This makes the third time that the AMA has lost in the Supreme Court. In fact, it has never won at that level. Time has been running out on the AMA's ability to bully other health care providers in the increasingly competitive health care market. The studies, from reputable medical and governmental sources, have been increasingly pointing to the fact that members of the AMA have been deprived of access to more effective health care procedures by a boycott that denied them and their patients access to the documented skills of doctors of chiropractic. *The AMA has been tripped up by the very scientific studies that it demanded and which now have been used in court to confirm the finding of guilty in the antitrust case.* It is certainly hoped that medical and chiropractic physicians, recognizing the scientific proof of the efficacy of chiropractic care, will now cooperate for the benefit of patients everywhere.[344]

After negotiating for more than a year, the AMA in December, 1991, agreed to make a $3.5 million payment for the chiropractors' legal costs and to publish a new position on its ethical opinions explicitly stating that medical doctors and chiropractors could associate professionally.[345]

Not only did the chiropractors cry foul against the AMA's antitrust activity to eliminate competitors, but in 1981, the Federal Trade Commission also brought suit against the AMA when it had discovered that their monopolistic actions had created problems in the treatments for patients, and called it "a formidable impediment to competition in the delivery of health care services by physicians in this country":

> That barrier has served to deprive consumers of the free flow of information about the availability of health care services, to deter the offering of innovative forms of health care and to stifle the rise of almost every type of health care delivery that could potentially pose a threat to the income of fee-for-service physicians in private practice. *The costs to the public in terms of less expensive or even, perhaps more improved forms of medical services are great.*[346] (emphasis added)

In support of the FTC, the Justice Department argued that the AMA had ignored the law in the past:

> In fact, [AMA's] long history of illegal behavior strongly supports the need for a remedy to reverse the effects of the restraints of trade they have imposed. *And although*

---

344 Editorial Staff, "Chiropractors Strike American Medical Association Out in Supreme Court," *Dynamic Chiropractic* 08/26 (December 19, 1990)

345 Wolinsky, "After 15-Year Fight, AMA Gives OK to Chiropractors," *Chicago Sun-Times*, (January 9, 1992):3.

346 Organized Medicine on Trial: The Federal Trade Commission vs. the American Medical Association - *Journal of Policy History* 12/4 (2000):445-472.

petitioners are now quick to admit that their past conduct was unlawful, they have not been so quick to mitigate the effects of their past violations. The Commission's remedial order does what petitioners themselves have been unwilling to do. It dissipates the effects of past violations and protects the public against their repetition.[347] (emphasis added)

Post *Wilk II*

Under Section 16 of the Clayton Act (which was established to prevent such future behavior), Judge Getzendanner issued a permanent injunction order against the AMA; it has, however, had little impact on the continuing covert boycott. Despite the legal victory by the chiropractors in the *Wilk* antitrust lawsuit, the boycott of chiropractors continued underground like the KKK to thwart chiropractic's inclusion in hospitals,

The chiropractic profession believed the *Wilk* antitrust case would be a defining moment for its professional image and cooperation. Not true. Sadly this landmark decision went without much fanfare and, in effect, actually stiffened medical opposition. Few hospitals allow chiropractors on staff, few medical doctors regularly refer patients for chiropractic treatment, and medically-controlled organizations like workers' compensation still marginalize chiropractic care despite the fact that low back pain is a leading on-the-job injury.

Mr. McAndrews blamed the AMA for what he termed a "bastardization of ethics" in its attitude toward chiropractic. He said that some ethical problems in the chiropractic profession, such as spurious advertisements, were caused by the AMA driving chiropractic into a "ghetto," isolated from the health care mainstream where it remains.[348]

> *"There are a lot of faults attributed to people that have been ghettoized. But you don't look to the person that has been placed in that position for the blame.* You look to the medical societies with all of their resources and all of their so-called education for the blame. When you put someone in that condition you can't argue then that the outgrowth of that condition is something that they can use to destroy them." [349]

Dr. Michael Pedigo, one of the chiropractic-plaintiffs, said he and other chiropractors wanted "to be allowed to compete freely in the marketplace."[350] Sadly, his hope is unfulfilled and chiropractors remain in the medical ghetto considering only six percent of chiropractors today have hospital privileges according to the American Chiropractic Association.[351]

In commenting on the permanent injunction, Chester Wilk stated:

> The AMA is not a charitable organization. It is a trade association that exists to protect the financial needs of its members even when the goal runs counter to the

---

347 Ibid.

348 Ibid.

349 G McAndrews, closing arguments, *Wilk v. AMA*, (June 26, 1987):3093-97.

350 Ibid.

351 N Schetchikova, "For the Good of the Patient: The Integrative Chiropractor," *ACA News* 5/3 (March 2009):12-15.

health, welfare, and safety of the American people, and even when it is directly contrary to the will of all 50 state legislatures and the Congress of the United States.

The AMA obviously did not learn a lesson from its prior convictions for violating the antitrust laws. I and the nation's chiropractors can only hope that the third finding of guilty will convince the AMA leadership that the AMA is not above the law. I look forward to commencing usual dialogue and cooperation with medical physicians for the benefit of all our patients.[352]

This federal antitrust trial revealed the shocking tactics, language, and attitude of the AMA. As Judge Susan Getzendanner admitted, "The AMA has never made any attempt to publicly repair the damage the boycott did to chiropractors' reputations." Indeed, the damage was done, a small price was paid in reparation, and the offenders went unpunished. This despicable conduct of the AMA remains a dark chapter in medical history. This is the untold story in the paradox of chiropractic, one that clearly needs more light shed upon it so people will understand the true basis of today's skepticism of chiropractors comes from a rival association and not from the government or public.

In commenting on the decision, Dr. Jerry McAndrews stated:

The AMA took both arrogance and ignorance to new levels of foolishness. Between those characteristics the AMA crushed all common sense. As an educator and administrator, I spent almost twenty-five years combating the despicable actions of the AMA now declared to be illegal by the Court. How many students, patients and professionals have had to suffer from the AMA's folly? Perhaps now the government will listen when we point out the corrupt power exercised by the AMA. Perhaps now the people of the United States can get cooperative care from all segments of the health care spectrum.[353]

This case was not simply an antitrust case where one competitor tried to corner the market; it was a blitzkrieg of cultural, economic, and political might by the AMA to destroy the chiropractic profession completely. George McAndrews in his speech at the 1983 ACA Annual Convention in Atlanta, Georgia, commented that "Antitrust law is the window through which the clean air of competition has entered the healthcare world."

McAndrews recommended that to "get the message out...let the public and medical doctors read [the positive medical studies] where medical doctors are praising chiropractors."[354] Indeed, this is the untold story of chiropractic–the research that shows the superiority of hands-on care to drugs, shots, and surgery for most back pain cases.

"The AMA has been tripped up by the very scientific studies that it demanded and which now have been used in court to confirm the finding of guilty in the antitrust case. It is certainly hoped that medical and chiropractic physicians, recognizing the scientific

---

352 Editorial Staff, "Looking Back," *Dynamic Chiro* 27/10 (1987).
353 Ibid.
354 G McAndrews, speech before the National Chiropractic Legislative Conference, March 2002, Washington D.C.

proof of the efficacy of chiropractic care, will now cooperate for the benefit of patients everywhere," said McAndrews. [355]

He further stated that, "the world doesn't know these studies proving chiropractic superiority exist," and that chiropractors can stop "begging for the right to exist. Now [the medical doctors] have to beg for the right to exist" in this area of care, and they should "not be allowed to masquerade their position to harm patients."[356]

Mr. McAndrews noted that the evidence and testimonies indicated the AMA continues to lag behind both in clinical methods and training for the epidemic of musculoskeletal disorders:

> ...the medical physician community represented by defendants is years away from being able to duplicate the superior services of chiropractic. Slander of the profession and continuation of the boycott is therefore necessary to cover the interim while medical physicians try to adopt chiropractic methods in this area. That cannot be done overnight. The New Zealand Commission quoted Dr. Haldeman's testimony that "12 months full-time training in spinal manipulative therapy following a medical degree would be appropriate."[357]

Mr. McAndrews is adamant that "medical doctors are no longer gatekeepers to chiropractors," stating that "somewhere people of goodwill will wake up to the abilities of chiropractors that are un-matched for the twenty percent of patients in all physicians' offices who complain of neuromusculoskeletal problems."[358]

Medical Admissions

The impact of the *Wilk* trials transcends a simple legal victory over the medical cartel. For the first time publicly, George McAndrews and his staff compiled the known proof of chiropractic care as well as evidence of the inferior medical education in this area and ineffective medical treatments by the medical witnesses' own admissions. He leveled the playing field from a shouting match of epithets to a war of science and evidence.

Indeed, Mr. McAndrews shifted the focus from unproven allegations and slander against chiropractors by placing the burden of proof on the medical profession to admit its own failings and illegality:

- Never before had anyone heard a renowned medical man like John C. Wilson, Jr., MD, Chairman of the American Medical Association's Section on Orthopedic Surgery, admit to the inadequate medical education and treatments in the field of musculoskeletal disorders: "At the postgraduate level, symposia and courses concerning the cause and treatment of low back and sciatica pain are often ineffective because of prejudices and controversy."

---

355 Editorial Staff, "Looking Back: 1988," *Dynamic Chiropractic* 26/06 (March 11, 2008)
356 Ibid.
357 G McAndrews, "Plaintiffs' Summary of Proofs as an Aid to the Court," Civil Action No. 76 C 3777, *Wilk*, (June 25, 1987):80. (PX-1829).
358 Ibid.

- Never before had the public heard any medical professional like Dr. John Mennell say, "If you don't manipulate to relieve the symptoms from this condition of joint dysfunction, then you are depriving the patient of the one thing that is likely to relieve them of their suffering."
- Never before had the public known how unqualified MDs are for back problems as Drs. Mennell and Stevens admitted.
- Little did the public know that the AMA's prime mission was, first, the containment of chiropractic and, ultimately, the elimination of chiropractic.
- Little did the public know of the Oregon and California state workmen's compensation studies show the 2:1 effectiveness rate of chiropractic over medical care for back pain.
- Never had the public known of Dr. Per Freitag's testimony confirming this 2:1 ratio of superiority for in-hospital care.
- Never had the public heard about the New Zealand Royal Commission's endorsement of chiropractors as experts over MDs in this field.
- Never had anyone known that the AMA's own trustee, Dr. Irwin Hendryson, had said "I must say quite honestly that there are still aspects of the manipulative therapy itself which impress me and which I feel practicing clinicians should be using in the management of low back pain."

Instead of these facts for at least three generations since the days of Morris Fishbein, the public and media were constantly fed lies about chiropractic care. The more research the plaintiff's attorneys uncovered, the more they established that the AMA was not only guilty of an illegal boycott, the record makes clear that most everything the Committee on Quackery had disseminated to the public and media were boldface Big Lies that, furthermore, hid their own incompetence in this area of back pain care. Indeed, if any doctors were quacks, it is clear that medical doctors were, at least when it came to the management of musculoskeletal disorders.

Not unexpectedly, very little was mentioned by the media about the landmark legal ruling of the *Wilk* case. Few in the public or press knew the extent of dirty tricks done to undermine the chiropractic profession. Moreover, no one knew of the burglary of the plaintiffs' attorney's office, wiretapping, and illegal surveillance. Considering that George McAndrews had to meet with his brother secretly in a cornfield for fear of surveillance, it is understandable why the facts revealed in the *Wilk* antitrust trial made the Watergate burglary look amateurish.

Although the judge found "injury to chiropractors' reputations which resulted from the boycott have not been repaired," the AMA was not required to compensate the thousands of chiropractors who went to jail for practicing chiropractic. The judge also admitted, "Chiropractors suffer current economic injury as a result of the boycott,"[359] but

---

359 *Wilk et al v AMA et al.,* US District Court Northern District of Illinois, No. 76C3777, Susan Getzendanner, presiding judge; Judgment dated August 27, 1987.

no reparations were given to the thousands of chiropractic stalwarts who suffered from this boycott for nearly a century of conflict.

The court gave the AMA a verbal reprimand and ordered them to pay court costs, but this trial was just a small bump in the road for this Goliath. No one went to jail, no public apology was made to the chiropractors, and no admission of guilt was offered. The AMA simply issued an explanation to its own members that was published in its *Journal* of the AMA, stating it was now ethical to associate with practitioners of chiropractics, and made a nominal $300,000 donation to the Kentuckiana Children's Center founded by Lorraine Golden, DC, in 1957, that offers integrated medical and chiropractic care for kids.

No act of contrition was ever offered by the AMA, no *tabula rasa* to reconstruct the damaged chiropractic image, and no *mea culpa* to apologize for its past transgressions. It is the same as when the Civil War ended slavery, but racism continued with *Jim Crow* laws and segregation. Indeed, while the AMA was beaten by the chiropractic foe in a defining legal moment, an underground medical apartheid continued in American healthcare just as racism continued after slavery was abolished.

Regrettably, most consumers are unaware that for many years–in spite of the good work it performed—the image of chiropractic as an "unscientific cult" was purposefully, illegally, and without merit crafted and promoted by a well funded AMA under the leadership of Morris Fishbein, Roger Throckmorton, and H. Doyl Taylor. That public image continues in large measure to this day—evident each time someone says, *"I don't believe in chiropractors."*

George McAndrews noted years later in his speech before the National Chiropractic Legislative Conference in March, 2002:

> Thirty years ago our goal was getting rid of the quack label, now it's about equality and fairness. If we go hat-in-hand, they'll give us nothing. They're still launching salvos because we're taking their money. I don't care if they get angry, that passed a long time ago. We don't need to apologize. It's all about money now.[360]

Though it has always been about power and money for the AMA; for the chiropractors, it was always about survival. The struggle for social justice continues for chiropractors seeking free enterprise and for patients seeking their freedom of choice in healthcare.

From the steps of the Lincoln Memorial on August 28, 1963, Martin Luther King, Jr, in his "I Have a Dream" speech called for racial equality and an end to discrimination. He urged Americans to judge a person not by the color of his skin, but by the content of his character. This is good advice that is applicable in many areas, including health care.

Rev. King also once said, "Of all forms of inequality, injustice in health care is the most shocking and inhumane." Certainly denying health care to the poor or elderly is inhumane, but just as shocking was to learn the injustice to those chiropractors who struggled to bring their brand of health care to all.

---

360 G McAndrews speech before the American Chiropractic Association at the National Chiropractic Legislative Conference in Washington, DC, (March 2002)

King's sentiment of injustice were revealed throughout this *Wilk* trial when we heard two words that the medical men used repeatedly—"contain" and "eliminate." Their intent, however, was not to contain disease and eliminate pain, as one might think. Their real goal was to contain the reach of chiropractic care and to eliminate chiropractors by any means possible.

It is past time for the medical profession and the public to do as Rev. King urged—to judge chiropractors not by the medical propaganda, but by their good clinical results. Indeed, it is past time for the good actions of chiropractors to speak louder than biased words from medical bigots. It is time to end the injustice in healthcare for patients and practitioners alike.

Masters of Deception

Two attacks by political medicine exemplified the use of propaganda as a weapon to contain or eliminate chiropractic: one attack on Congress and another attack at Florida State University. Both revealed the power of the medical monarchy to thwart the will of the people and to see chiropractic "wither on the vine."

Spin Doctors

"Propaganda is a truly terrible weapon in the hands of an expert."
Adolf Hitler, 1924 [361]

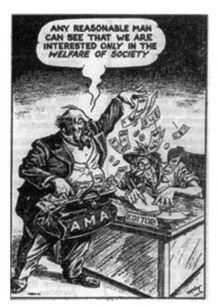

S. Levin, "America's Biggest Lobby, the A.M.A.,"
*Journal of the National Chiropractic
Association* 19/12 (Dec 1949): 27-28, 64, 66.

Morris Fishbein's use of viral journalism to attack chiropractic set the standard for others to purposely misrepresent the value of manipulative therapy and mischaracterized chiropractors by branding them as dangerous and unscientific cultists.

Between 1910 when the medical war began and 1950 after Fishbein retired, there was the notable lack of transparency of the medical association by the free press. There were no investigative reporters like *The Washington Post's* Bob Woodward and Carl Bernstein of Watergate fame[362] to expose the AMA's underbelly—the illegal tactics, unbridled political power, illicit funding from tobacco and drug companies to wage war, and the defamation it did to chiropractors.

361   S Luckert and S Bachrach, "State of Deception: the Power of Nazi Propaganda," United States Holocaust Memorial Museum handout.
362   The Watergate scandal resulted from the break-in to the Democratic National Committee headquarters at the Watergate office complex in Washington, D.C. Effects of the scandal ultimately led to the resignation of the President of the United States Richard Nixon on August 9, 1974.

When a few newsmen did speak out against the obvious propaganda, they too felt the wrath of the medical establishment. After all, *"everybody* knows chiropractic is an unscientific cult" was the prevailing mindset the AMA sold to the media, and if you did not buy into this Big Lie, then the inference was something was wrong with you, too.

An editorial in the *Valley Morning Star* from Harlingen, Texas, in 1966, provided a reasonable and insightful response to the AMA's accusation of quackery thrown at chiropractors. "As long as there are human beings there will be 'quacks,' persons who make false claims," wrote the editor. "And," he recognized, "some of them may even belong to that sacrosanct American Medical Association." Perhaps it takes a strong-willed Texan to write such bold truths with such dry humor:

AMA Tries To Discredit Nation's Chiropractors

The American Medical Association, one of the strongest unions of 'em all, has made another attempt to discredit chiropractors, a rival group engaged in the healing arts.

It's too bad the practitioners of medicine and chiropractic can't get along and may be they could if the AMA would tend to its business and let the chiropractors alone. It looks like there should be room for both groups.

The AMA recently staged its third "Congress on Medical Quackery," in which an effort was made to show that chiropractors are making false claims about their ability to help the sick, the generally accepted meaning of quackery.

We also know that medical doctors have been known to seek help from chiropractors, on occasions. However, they probably enter the chiropractor's office through the back door. But no matter.

On the other hand there is a definition of the verb "quack" which is "to talk pretentiously without sound knowledge of the subject discussed." In that case, one might say that a spokesman for the AMA was doing a bit of quacking.

"The confrontation between medicine and chiropractic is not a struggle between two professions," said the spokesman, Dr. Thomas M. Ballantine, Jr. of the Harvard Medical School. "Rather it is more in the nature of an effort by an informed group of individuals to protect the public from fraudulent health claims and practices." Among other things, Ballantine accused chiropractors of treating cancer patients, and he said patients suffering from serious illness risk death when treated by a chiropractor.

We suppose there are chiropractors who do claim to be able to help patients suffering from cancer. But we have been told of medical doctors who are treating cancer patients without benefit.

We do not know whether chiropractic is of aid to cancer patients, just as we do not know whether there are benefits to some other products the AMA and American Cancer Society and their partners in the state and federal health bureaucracy claim are quackery. *We do know there are people who claim to have been helped by unorthodox methods of treatment. And we contend the AMA has no right to deny those persons their right to choose a method of treatment.*

As long as there are human beings there will be "quacks," persons who make false claims. *And some of them may even belong to that sacrosanct American Medical Association.*

The AMA is doing no service to humanity to use every trick to attempt to show that its members have the only answer to healing the sick. Some people still want to choose their own means of treatment, regardless of what the medical men say. To devote a public forum to attacking others the AMA members disapprove, smacks something of quackery itself.[363] (emphasis added)

It is refreshing to see that one journalist during the height of this medical war could see through the AMA's smokescreen. Since there never was a *public* outcry against chiropractic care, the state government officials, licensing board members, and district attorneys had no significant cause to act against chiropractors without provocation from the medical societies. Despite the lack of evidence of harm, the AMA continued to use propaganda to twist and distort the truth about chiropractic in the court of public opinion.

To clarify what constitutes propaganda, which is a very serious accusation to levy at the medical profession, let me quote directly from the book, *State of Deception: The Power of Nazi Propaganda,* by Steven Luckert and Susan Bachrach written in conjunction with the current exhibition at the United States Holocaust Memorial Museum in Washington, DC. [364]

"Propaganda," Adolf Hitler wrote in 1924, "is a truly terrible weapon in the hands of an expert." The word itself conjures up images of lies, distortions, and brainwashing. Even in democratic societies that guarantee freedom of expression, fears about mass manipulation by government, extremists in the media, and "spin doctors" with a political agenda appear on occasion, such as in America during the 1940s and 1950s when the Red Scare of "McCarthyism" used reckless and unsubstantiated accusations of communism and demagogic attacks on the character of political adversaries.

According to the United States Holocaust Memorial Museum, propaganda is biased information spread to shape public opinion and behavior. It is characterized as such:

- Uses truths, half-truth, or lies ("chiropractic is an unscientific cult")
- Omits information selectively (ignores studies, guidelines, or medical experts that endorsed chiropractic care)
- Simplifies complex issues or ideas ("chiropractic is quackery")
- Plays on emotions ("chiropractors are dangerous")
- Advertises a cause ("to protect public safety")
- Attacks opponents (chiropractors are "killers" and "rabid dogs")
- Targets desired audiences (physicians, students, politicians, media, and just about anyone)

---

363 Editorial, "AMA Tries to Discredit Nation's Chiropractors," *Valley Morning Star* (Harlingen, TX) (November 1966)

364 S Luckert and S Bachrach, United States Holocaust Memorial Museum, "State of Deception: the Power of Nazi Propaganda." WW Norton & Company, Inc. New York, NY. (January 2009)

Propaganda is not only an historical issue as we have seen with the Medical Mussolini, but one that continues to this day in the medical war against chiropractic with misleading journalism that ignores the research supporting chiropractic care and omits chiropractic from discussion on the epidemic of back pain. Despite the obvious social injustice toward chiropractors, this issue has been virtually ignored by the media.

Unquestionably Morris Fishbein, Robert Throckmorton, and H. Doyl Taylor were experts at medical propaganda—the epitome of medical "spin doctors." For nearly a century, the AMA spent millions of man hours and millions of dollars as it worked tirelessly to persuade public opinion against chiropractors with distortions, denigration, and demonization of chiropractic in general.

"Nazism," Victor Klemperer wrote in 1946, had "permeated the flesh and blood of the people through single words, idioms, and sentence structures which were imposed on them in a million repetitions and taken on board mechanically and unconsciously."[365]

Just as the Nazis used the Big Lie to undermine the image of Jews, so did the AMA use its own versions of the Big Lie to defame chiropractors. In the same vein, the medical misinformers repeated their lies about chiropractic so often and for so long they actually believed them despite having no proof. In fact, when the *Wilk* trial and New Zealand Inquiry revealed evidence to the contrary, it still did not change the biased attitudes of the unrepentant medical professionals.

There are many journalists and medical personnel who still deny the devastating impact of the medical war upon the chiropractic profession or the pandemic of pain it has caused millions of Americans. The media has also developed a bad case of "professional amnesia" as Dr. Anthony Rosner described those who forget the ascendancy of chiropractic in this back pain epidemic as the researchers have shown. [366]

For example, on April 6, 2010, National Public Radio reported in an enlightening article on *All Things Considered*, "Surgery May Not Be the Answer to an Aching Back." On June 7, 2010, the *Associated Press* began a six-part series on overtreatment in the United States. The second installment on June 8 was titled "Back Pain Widely Overtreated in the U.S."[367] A similar article appeared October 14, 2010, with the lead headline on MSNBC.com that read, "Back Surgery May Backfire on Patients in Pain."[368]

Of course, chiropractors were in total agreement with these articles and expected a balanced analysis of this epidemic of back pain and unnecessary surgery. To our dismay, none of these articles mentioned chiropractic care in any depth as the recommended treatment of choice. They did, however, properly cite some of the extensive research of the excessive spine surgery and the high costs, but once again the writers failed to mention the primary alternative to spine surgery, which is chiropractic care. Alas, the medical

---

365 Luckert and Bachrach, ibid. p.141

366 A Rosner, "Evidence or Eminence-Based Medicine? Leveling the Playing Field Instead of the Patient," *Dynamic Chiropractic*, 20/25 (November 30, 2002)

367 L Neergaard, "Back Pain Widely Overtreated in the U.S." *Associated Press* (June 8, 2010)

368 L Carroll, "Back Surgery May Backfire On Patients In Pain," MSNBC.com (10/14/2010)

propaganda about chiropractic care continues as evident by this professional amnesia in the mass media.

This is no small oversight when you keep in mind that chiropractors constitute the third-largest physician-level health profession in the world, yet it somehow remains virtually ignored. Indeed, when was the last time a chiropractor was featured on national TV as a spokesperson on health concerns like Dr. Sanjay Gupta on CNN or Dr. Isadore Rosenfeld on FOX News?

When has a chiropractor ever been questioned on healthcare reform or as an expert speaking on spinal health care matters? Considering the $100 billion back pain business, undoubtedly the full implementation of chiropractic care in every hospital, every workers' compensation program, and in the military health services could drastically reduce this bill. This remains the untold benefit of chiropractic care.

Few times, if ever, has there been a chiropractor TV character hero like the original medical sitcom, *Marcus Welby, MD*, played by Robert Young, or a character on the TV comedy shows like *M*A*S*H** or *Scrubs*. At best, the chiropractor role portrayed in the TV sitcom *"Two and a Half Men"* by actor John Cryer is that of the neurotic boob compared to his cousin, a handsome playboy played by Charlie Sheen. This portrayal is not too distant from the chiropractor role of a loser played by Burt Lancaster in the 1952 movie, *"Come Back, Little Sheba."*

Apparently this emasculated image has been the standard in Hollywood for chiropractors, an image Morris Fishbein created when he characterized chiropractors in his book, *Medical Follies*: "The one who comes through the cellar is besmirched with dust and grime; he carries a crowbar and he may wear a mask."[369] Indeed, the leap of this lowly image from medical propaganda to the silver screen was an intentional misrepresentation of chiropractors, not merely a coincidence.

Not only has the image of chiropractors been distorted, the important historical events like the *Wilk* trial, AHCPR guideline, Manga Reports, and the New Zealand Inquiry have been ignored by the media. In effect, the media has been active medical misinformers as they continue in their role as invaluable spin doctors for the medical profession, but they played by one important rule to always stay behind the scenes.

The Committee on Quackery headed by H. Doyl Taylor fully understood the power of the press to spread misinformation about its chiropractic rivals when he created "Quack Packs" that included defamatory articles written by hired hands that were given to the public, press, politicians, and educators as proof of the evils of chiropractic from supposedly objective third parties. As the *Wilk* trial proved, this was a total ruse, but the public to this day still has no idea of the COQ's Big Lies.

In 1962, General Counsel Robert B. Throckmorton spelled out in his Iowa Plan the deceptive nature of the Committee On Quackery: "Action taken by the medical profession should be firm, persistent, and in good taste [and] *behind the scenes* whenever

---

369 M Fishbein, *Medical Follies*, New York, Boni & Liveright (1925):98

possible."[370] As if he had taken a lesson from Joseph Goebbels, this clandestine tactic mirrored the Nazi's effort to keep its Final Solution out of the public eye.

Certainly, *"behind the scenes"* meant instructing, enabling, and using the mass media, celebrities, columnists, and freelance writers as co-conspirators with the AMA's plan to contain, besmirch, and defame chiropractic. No detail was left to doubt in this anti-chiropractic campaign.

The media has been the purveyor of Fishbein's and Taylor's Big Lies to deceive anyone about the value of chiropractic. The AMA has repeated for decades, *"everybody* knows chiropractic is an unscientific cult,"* and, for the most part, it was the media who taught this to the public, especially through the use of one of the most famous journalists in the nation, Ann Landers.

Assault on the Medical Bastille

Another huge battle that stunned the medical world occurred when an agency of the U.S. Public Health Service, the Agency on Health Care Policy and Research (AHCPR), endorsed spinal manipulation as a "proven treatment" for adults with acute low back pain. This recommendation was issued on December 8, 1994, after a federal appeals court ended an injunction to prevent its release that was issued in the summer of 1994 sought by the North American Spine Society (NASS) and the manufacturers of spinal fusion surgery hardware like pedicle screws.

This recommendation was the first and largest (albeit circuitous) endorsement of chiropractic care by a U.S. federal agency; the ramifications of this study were huge and the medical society knew it, which is why they worked so hard to kill it. Once the injunction failed, the medical insurgents resorted to more notorious methods in its propaganda battle against this federal agency.

The history of this event began when the U.S. Public Health Service was designed to be an ongoing partner with the health professions in an effort to improve medical care in America. During the first Bush administration in 1989, they were charged by Congress to be a federal arbiter of evidence-based, clinical-practice guidelines for many common treatments and tests; the AHCPR was to study and make recommendations.

The AHCPR's responsibility was to choose conditions, focusing on high-cost, high-use procedures like back surgery for low back pain. The AHCPR convened multi-disciplinary panels consisting of 18 to 25 highly-regarded researchers to create guidelines that were to be updated as new evidence was discovered. The goal was to improve the quality and cost-effectiveness of care.

Democrats and Republicans alike hoped that the AHCPR's research would help rein in costs by giving doctors better direction and offering payers—especially Medicare—the ammunition they needed to make evidence-based coverage decisions. More significantly, the agency promised to improve the quality of health care by helping to ensure that doctors would give patients the treatments they really needed and refrain from giving them care that could harm them. Under the leadership of Newt Gingrich (R-GA) in

---

370 Ibid. p. 127.

the House, this goal came to a screeching halt when the AMA went ballistics over the fourteenth guideline on acute low back pain.[371]

In 1994, AHCPR issued a 170-page study entitled "Acute Low Back Pain in Adults," along with an accompanying 30-page "Quick Reference Guide for Clinicians" entitled "Acute Low Back Problems in Adults: Assessment and Treatment."[372] A Patient Guide was also disseminated to the public with the same recommendations in laymen terms.

The low back pain study was conducted by a multidisciplinary panel comprised of twelve medical physician experts, other healthcare professionals, and consumer representatives, who were brought together by the AHCPR to perform an evidence-based analysis of all research trials on all treatment approaches to acute low back pain in adults. Abstracts of over 10,000 research papers were reviewed, almost 4,000 articles were retrieved, and the study took nearly two years to complete. It was the most thorough investigation of low back pain ever conducted in the United States, only rivaled by the New Zealand Inquiry into Chiropractic in 1978-79.

This study also showed the enormity of the low back pain (LBP) epidemic in America.[373] Although back pain is not a killer like cancer or heart disease, it does afflict more people during their lifetime:

- 80-90 percent of all adults will suffer with acute low back pain sometime in their life;
- BP is the leading workers' compensation injury;
- LBP is the leading cause of disability for people under the age of 45;
- LBP is the second-leading cause of visits to doctors' offices;
- LBP is the third-leading cause for hospital admissions;
- LBP the second-leading cause of surgery other than heart surgeries.

The chiropractic and medical professions waited with bated breath for the results, and when the results were announced, the medical profession was livid. After this two-year investigation, the AHCPR concluded that spinal manipulation was a "proven treatment" for acute low back pain in adults and was the preferred initial professional treatment for acute low back pain. This recommendation was, in effect, an endorsement of chiropractic care.[374]

This Patient Guide stated:

> This treatment (using the hands to apply force to the back to 'adjust' the spine) can be helpful for some people in the first month of low back symptoms. It should only be done by a professional with experience in manipulation.[375]

---

371 S Brownlee, "Newtered," Overtreated: Why Too Much Medicine Is Making Us Sicker and Poorer, http://overtreated.com/extras01.html

372 Bigos *et al.* US Dept. of Health and Human Services, Public Health Service, Agency for Health Care Policy and Research, Clinical Practice Guideline, Number 14: Acute Low Back Problems in Adults AHCPR Publication No. 95-0642, (December 1994)

373 Ibid. p. 90.

374 PG Shekelle, *et al*, RAND Corporation Report, *The Appropriateness of Spinal Manipulation for Low-Back Pain*

375 S Bigos, ibid, Patient Guide, (1992):7.

The most shocking recommendation focused on back surgery. The panel of experts found back surgeries were costly, were sometimes based on misleading tests such as MRIs, and were generally deemed ineffective. This information, when released to the media and public, would have been a dagger in the pocketbooks of many spine surgeons and hospitals.

This conclusion came as no surprise to MDs since similar findings were published in the *Journal of the American Medical Association* in 1992 by J. Turner, *et al.*, "Patient Outcomes after Lumbar Spinal Fusions."[376] Since the public media rarely reports on such scientific articles, this critical analysis, among many others, was kept secret. But when the AHCPR entered this fray, it also found the research on low back pain concluded there was no evidence to support spinal fusion surgery and that such surgery commonly had complications.

The section on Spinal Fusion from the AHCPR's Clinical Practice Guideline clearly summarized the research:

> There appears to be no good evidence from controlled trials that spinal fusion alone is effective for treatment of any type of acute low back problems in the absence of spinal fractures or dislocation....*Moreover, there is no good evidence that patients who undergo fusion will return to their prior functional level.* (emphasis added)[377]

What angered traditional medicine the most about the AHCPR study was its finding that confirmed the rare need for surgery except in the most severe cases that did not respond to conservative care. The following was stated in its Patient Guide, *Understanding Acute Low Back Problems*:

> Even having a lot of back pain does not by itself mean you need surgery. *Surgery has been found to be helpful in only 1 in 100 cases of low back problems.* In some people, surgery can even cause more problems. This is especially true if your only symptom is back pain.
>
> People with certain nerve problems or conditions such as fractures of dislocations have the best chance of being helped by surgery. In most cases, however, decisions about surgery do not have to be made right away. Most back surgery can wait for several weeks without making the condition worse.
>
> If your health care provider recommends surgery, be sure to ask about the reason for the surgery and about the risks and benefits you might expect. You may also want to get a second opinion.[378]

Shannon Brownlee, author of *Overtreated: Why Too Much Medicine Is Making Us Sicker and Poorer*, described the reaction in the medical community:

> But when the AHCPR's panel concluded that there was little evidence to support surgery as a first-line treatment for low back pain, and that doctors and patients would be wise to try nonsurgical interventions first, back surgeons went wild.[379]

---

376 J Turner, *et al.*, "Patient Outcomes after Lumbar Spinal Fusions," *Journal of the American Medical Association* 287/7 (August 19, 1992):907–11.
377 S Bigos, ibid. p. 90.
378 S Bigos, ibid. p. 8.
379 Ibid.

The surgeons in the North American Spine Society (NASS) could not accept the fact that their spine surgeries were being touted as ineffective, supposedly based on a suspect abnormal disc premise, and the shocking recommendation by a federal agency for spinal manipulation over traditional medical treatments was too much to bear. To rub salt in this NASS wound, the AHCPR panel was headed by an orthopedic surgeon, Stanley Bigos, MD, so they could not vilify him as they might have any other type of doctor.

The recommendations also upset the physical therapists. Standard forms of passive care by physical therapists were also not recommended for lower back pain. The Patient Guide published by the U.S. Public Health Service also states:

> A number of other treatments are sometimes used for low back symptoms. While these treatments may give relief for a short time, none have been found to speed recovery or keep acute back problems from returning. They may also be expensive. Such treatments include: Traction, TENS, massage, biofeedback, acupuncture, injections into the back, back corsets, ultrasound.[380]

The AHCPR guideline stated spinal manipulation was the preferred initial treatment of choice. The Patient Guide lists three "Proven Treatments":

- Over-the-counter NSAIDs, which "have fewer side effects than prescription medicines."
- Heat or cold applied to the back.
- Spinal manipulation. This treatment (using the hands to apply force to the back to 'adjust' the spine) can be helpful for some people in the first month of low back symptoms. It should only be done by a professional with experience in manipulation.[381]

Of course, this recommendation implies chiropractic care, but the panel was forced to state "spinal manipulation" since some other practitioners also employ this healing art. RAND earlier had reported that 94 percent of all manipulative care was delivered by chiropractors, with osteopathic physicians delivering 4 percent, and general practitioners, physical therapists, and orthopedic surgeons accounting for the remainder.[382]

Considering chiropractors have carried the banner of manipulative therapy since 1895 while, for the most part, the osteopaths relinquished this art in the early 1960s, physical therapists have ignored this treatment, and medical physicians have chosen to vilify this form of care, it is obvious that chiropractors are the professionals who lay claim by far to the most experience in manipulation, and rightfully so.[383]

---

380 Ibid.
381 Ibid. p. 7.
382 PG Shekelle, AH Adams, MR Chassin, E Hurwitz, RE Park, RB Phillips, RH Brook, "The Appropriateness of Spinal Manipulation for Low-Back Pain: Project Overview and Literature Review," RAND (1991):3. Santa Monica, Calif.
383 Ibid.

More importantly, the AHCPR study specifically defined spinal manipulation as the type of manipulation used by all chiropractors as opposed to mobilization methods used by physical therapists:

> Spinal manipulation includes many different techniques. For this guideline, manipulation is defined as manual therapy in which loads are applied to the spine using short and long lever methods. The selected joint is moved to its end range of voluntary motion, followed by application of an impulse loading. The therapeutic objectives of manipulation include symptomatic relief and functional improvement.[384]

Perhaps most significantly, the guidelines stated that unlike non-surgical interventions, spinal manipulation offered both pain relief and functional improvement. This "functional improvement" is what gets patients back to work faster and at less expense, whereas drugs, shots, and spine surgery are primarily interested in pain control.

But the resounding conclusion of the AHCPR guideline for acute low back pain not caused by fracture, tumor, infection, or cauda equina syndrome, was clear: the treatment of choice was spinal manipulation through chiropractic care.

Because acute low back pain is the most prevalent ailment and most frequent cause of disability for persons younger than 45 years of age in the United States, adherence to these practice guidelines would have substantially decreased medical costs and significantly increased the numbers of patients referred to chiropractors for spinal manipulation. As Louis Sportelli, DC, noted: "If the doctors of chiropractic only cornered the market on one condition, back pain, there would not be enough [chiropractors] now to handle the volume."[385]

While the chiropractic profession took great pride in this guideline's recommendation for spinal manipulation as a federal endorsement, the medical profession was not about to take it so lightly. After years of condemning chiropractic as an "unscientific cult" and manipulation as "dangerous," they simply detested the fact that this newfound guideline refuted the AMA's propaganda to the public. Although the AHCPR panel was comprised of the most knowledgeable medical researchers ever convened and was convinced of chiropractic's effectiveness, the medical profession chose to fight the new guideline and initiated a counter offensive.

Counter Attack on Capitol Hill

Furious at the release of the AHCPR guidelines, political medicine fought back by launching a propaganda scheme to destroy an act of Congress signed by President George H.W. Bush to improve our nation's health. This multi-faceted assault on Capitol Hill illustrated the wrath of special interests as never before seen, and by using the strategy of the Committee on Quackery to stay behind the scenes, the assault remained hidden from

---

384 Bigos, ibid.
385 L Sportelli, "AHCPR: It Did Not Happen By Accident," *Dynamic Chiropractic* 13/2 (January 16, 1995).

the public view. It may be one thing to attack a rival profession, but when the medical corps attacked Congress, it reinforced its reputation as the *"most terrifying trade association on earth."*

First, the NASS sounded its battle cry:

> We, the North American Spine Society, feel that this document should not be published in its present form. Instead, a new consensus should be sought, with appointed input from all relevant medical specialties dealing with low back pain issues, and with AHCPR staff that is responsive to the criticisms of the methodology raised in this letter. [386]

Inexplicably, *the consensus the NASS sought is exactly what AHCPR had done.* The panel members were selected from nominees of all medical, osteopathic, physical therapy, and chiropractic professions. The AHCPR itself came as no surprise to the NASS; what surprised them were its conclusions. The true objection by NASS was the panel's recommendation about unnecessary spine surgery.

Unable to accept the experts' criticisms of spinal surgery, NASS claimed the research team was biased and inept, despite the fact that the team was headed by Stanley Bigos, MD, an orthopedic surgeon, along with 22 other spine experts. It was also interesting to note that the NASS criticized only this one guideline and only one of the preferred forms of therapy: spinal manipulation.

An historical review of the battle between AHCPR and NASS, *Health Affairs: The Policy Journal of the Health Sphere,* summarized how and why AHCPR was attacked and lost a sizeable amount of its budget after this firestorm over low back treatments. [387] Unlike the first thirteen guidelines produced by AHCPR that received little condemnation by the medical profession, the fourteenth guideline on acute low back pain in adults and its criticism of back surgery posed a much more serious threat to the spine surgeons.

Opponents to the report attempted to shut down the agency by eliminating its funding. NASS argued that AHCPR was redundant, inefficient, and wasteful. They noted that medical societies and HMOs had already turned out 1,500 guidelines. They told the Republican Congress that came into power in 1995 that AHCPR was inappropriately meddling in what doctors should do and was inefficiently turning out guidelines, only fifteen in five years.[388]

AHCPR was also confronted with a bogus third-party advocacy group, the Center for Patient Advocacy, whose main goal was to get it de-funded. In reality, this was not

---

386 Ibid.

387 BH Gray, MK Gusmano, and SR Collins, "AHCPR and the Changing Politics of Health Services Research: Lessons From the Falling and Rising Political Fortunes of the Nation's Leading Health Services Research Agency," *Health Affairs: The Policy Journal of the Health Sphere* (June 25, 2003) http://content. healthaffairs.org/cgi/content/full/hlthaff.w3.283v1/DC1?maxtoshow=&HITS=10&hits=10&RESULTFO RMAT=&author1=bradford+gray&fulltext=politics&andorexactfulltext=and&searchid=1&FIRSTINDE X=0&resourcetype=HWCIT

388 J Weeks, "Back Surgeons, Chiropractic, and the Murder of a Federal Agency on Evidence-Based Medicine," theintegratorblog.com (June 11, 2006).

an actual "patient" group, but were members of NASS formed by Neil Kahanovitz, MD, a back surgeon from Arlington, Virginia. They organized a letter-writing campaign to gain congressional support for its attack on AHCPR.

NASS created an ad hoc committee which attacked the literature review and the subsequent AHCPR practice guideline on acute care of low back pain. In a letter published in 1994 in their journal *Spine*, the committee not only criticized the methods used in the literature review, they also expressed concern that the conclusions might be used by payers or regulators to limit the number and types of spinal fusion procedures. This was its real agenda—to keep its cash cow alive and protected from regulation.

On January 9, 1995, Eric J. Muehlbauer, executive director for NASS, sent out a memorandum to NASS members regarding the release of the clinical practice guideline from AHCPR on acute low back problems in adults. The front page of the 1995 summer edition of *NASS News* proclaimed, "AHCPR Guidelines Disputed," suggesting that "this has become a political, and not a scientific document."[389] Ironically, the NASS made it a political issue since the AHCPR panelists were diverse, apolitical, and scientific in their approach.

The article made many statements to rationalize its objection to the guideline, such as:

- Patients should not have treatment selected or denied based on the guidelines *(the point of the guideline was to determine evidenced-based treatments rather than the whimsy of individual practitioners)*;
- The guidelines relied upon limited scientific information *(how can 10,000 published articles be considered "limited"?)*
- The consensus method did not necessarily identify the best forms of treatment or diagnosis *(it certainly did)* and,
- Clinical judgments made by the AHCPR panel should have been balanced with those of relevant medical societies *[every spine profession was represented on the panel; in other words, what the NASS really meant was the panel should consider the vested interests of NASS before making recommendations]*. [390]

Congress created AHCPR to establish goals to help improve healthcare outcomes and reduce costs in America. The multidisciplinary panel accomplished all four goals stated by NASS. The evidence clearly showed the surgeon's methods were criticized by medical researchers on the best available research.

Most inconsistent was the NASS response letter that criticized reliance on randomized control trials (RCTs), the gold standard for research. It seems odd for NASS and the medical society to protest the strict reliance on RCTs, given its history of demanding such trials as evidence, a demand put upon chiropractic for decades. Now the table was turned, and the NASS did not like it at all.

---

389 Ibid.
390 Ibid.

The letter also charged that AHCPR had wasted taxpayer dollars on the study.[391] Republican Congressman Sam Johnson (R-TX) proposed elimination of the agency and mocking referred to it as the "Agency for High Cost Publications and Research."[392] The point was lost that by avoiding unnecessary back surgeries, billions of taxpayer dollars would be saved and millions of patients would be saved from suffering failed back surgery syndrome.

The surgeons found sympathetic ears among House Republicans, led by Speaker Newt Gingrich, who were prepared to believe the worst about the agency after the failed Clinton Health Care Reform Act in 1993-1994. They were also very beholding to the donations made by the medical special interests such as AMPAC and surgical hardware vendors to their campaigns. Obviously money speaks louder than science.

The AHCPR found more supporters in the Senate than in the House. A letter by Edward Kennedy (D-MA), Jay Rockefeller (D-WV), James Jeffords (R-VT) and Orrin Hatch (R-UT) called for the maintenance of FY 1995 funding for the agency. It observed that "there has been some misunderstanding about the role, purpose, and mission of AHCPR," and argued that "it is essential to have a federal agency that works with the private sector to provide consumers with information to make informed choices, measure, and improve the quality of care, and improve the cost and effectiveness of our health care system." [393]

The Senate Appropriations Committee and the Senate itself approved a reduced budget figure for the agency ($127,310,000) that was similar to the amount that had been approved by the House Appropriations Committee. In the conference committee, the House leadership, as promised during the floor battle months before, supported the Senate's figure. On April 26, 1996, almost seven months into the fiscal year, President Clinton signed the appropriations bill that, after a final small across-the-board reduction, was only slightly less than the amount approved by the Senate. The agency had survived with a 21 percent budget cut, but *it had been stripped of the ability to make treatment recommendations.*[394]

The AMA used its political punch to gut the AHCPR, which today is out of the guideline business and reauthorized with a new mandate and name—the Agency for Healthcare Research and Quality (AHRQ). The AHRQ is charged with "improving the quality, safety, efficiency, and effectiveness of healthcare," but it can no longer make recommendations for treatment even though it was originally ordered to develop guidelines by a 1989 congressional mandate. It would seem the wishes of special interest

---

391 A White, *et al.*, Letter to the Editor, *Spine* 19/1 (1994):109–10.

392 Congressional Record, (August 3, 1995)

393 BH Gray, *et al.*, "AHCPR and the Changing Politics of Health Services Research: Lessons From the Falling and Rising Political Fortunes of the Nation's Leading Health Services Research Agency," *Health Affairs: The Policy Journal of the Health Sphere* (June 25, 2003) http://content.healthaffairs.org/cgi/content/full/hlthaff.w3.283v1/DC1?maxtoshow=&HITS=10&hits=10&RESULTFORMAT=&author1=bradford+gray&fulltext=politics&andorexactfulltext=and&searchid=1&FIRSTINDEX=0&resourcetype=HWCIT

394 BH Gray, ibid.

groups like AMA's political action committee or NASS superseded Congress' wish to determine the best treatments for common ailments. Indeed, the AHCPR had been castrated by the spine surgeons.

Flip-Flopping Guideline

When the AHCPR panel's guideline was published in 1994, the reaction of American spine surgeons was certainly heated; many surgeons ignored the guideline, especially those who were emboldened by the Republican smack-down of the AHCPR.

However, reaction was also mixed among the rational elements in healthcare. On one hand, they were incensed that their biggest money-maker, spine fusion, was criticized and they were afraid insurance might stop paying for the procedure. The endorsement of spinal manipulation also infuriated many surgeons. On the other hand, some of their own reviewers admitted that they agreed with the AHCPR guideline.[395]

"Perhaps the NASS experience typifies the evolution most groups undergo as they wrestle with practice guidelines," the editorial staff of *Dynamic Chiropractic* journal opined. "Could it be that rage, denial, review, and grudging acceptance are all part of the guidelines experience for most health care providers?"[396]

The AMA also feared the next AHCPR publication (#15) on cervicogenic and tension headaches that reportedly was prepared to endorse spinal manipulation. Political medicine also killed this headache study after thwarting the implementation of guideline #14 on acute low back pain. However, it must be repeated that the AMA never complained about the first thirteen guidelines issued by AHCPR. Only when it might hurt the pocketbooks of the spine surgeons did the AMA propagandists use their devious political tricks to kill this federally-mandated program.

The Headache Report was later continued by Duke University in 2001, with the sponsorship of the Foundation for Chiropractic Education and Research (FCER), and became the most notable publication that endorsed manipulative therapy for headaches.[397] This might create a new bag of worms for the medical profession.

Imagine if the public were told by the federal government and the media that according to the AHCPR experts and the office of the U.S. Public Health Service–the best medical and scientific minds in America–that "*if you have low back pain or headaches, you should go see your chiropractor first.*" Certainly the AMA would never allow this to happen without a fight despite the facts.

---

395 Editorial Staff, "North American Spine Society: Flip-Flopping on AHCPR Low Back Guidelines?" *Dynamic Chiropractic* 13/23 (November 6, 1995)

396 Ibid.

397 D McCrory, *et al.*, *Behavioral and Physical Treatments for Tension-type and Cervicogenic Headache* (Duke University Evidence-based Practice Center, Center for Clinical Health Policy Research; Durham, NC (2001).

The lawsuit to stop the release of the AHCPR guideline on acute low back pain by the Center for Patient Advocacy (the bogus NASS advocacy group) has also had the effect of intimidating present and future critics by eliminating the messengers who may report the many ineffective and costly medical procedures that have driven up the direct and indirect costs of back pain to $100 billion annually in America according to RAND.[398] Research also suggests of the 300,000+ disc surgeries done in the U.S. annually, as many as 90 percent are unnecessary and ineffective.[399]

A member of the AHCPR panel, Richard Deyo, MD, MPH, co-authored an article in *The New England Journal of Medicine*, "The Messenger Under Attack: Intimidation of Researchers by Special Interest Groups."[400] In it, he commented of this heavy-handiness to thwart progressive researchers:

> Attacks on health researchers are not new. Pierre Louis, for example, was vilified nearly two centuries ago for suggesting that bloodletting was an ineffectual therapy.[1] In an open society such as ours, controversy is common and often socially useful. The fact that scientists are sometimes challenged by special-interest groups should be no surprise. However, with widening media coverage of health research, growing public interest in health hazards, and expanding research on the outcomes of clinical care, such attacks may become more frequent and acrimonious. *The huge financial implications of many research studies invite vigorous attack...*Intimidation of investigators and funding agencies by powerful constituencies may inhibit important research on health risks and rational approaches to cost-effective health care.

For decades political medicine has called chiropractic unscientific and demanded research from the chiropractic profession to prove itself. Yet, when a comparative effectiveness study was finally done by the most universally accepted and acclaimed expert group of researchers ever assembled (AHCPR), the same proof of the standard medical methods fell short.

"Even if you take all of the research at face value, you have to conclude that spinal fusion is only modestly effective," said Deyo. "It's not a slam dunk."[401]

The medical mob was emboldened by victory on Capitol Hill, and it was a green light to do more spine surgeries, not fewer. Between 1997—just three years after the AHCPR's guidelines were published—and 2006, the number of spinal fusions went up 200 percent, from a little more than 100,000 a year to 303,000 annually.[402]

---

398 Paul G., Shekelle, *et al*, RAND Corporation Report, *The Appropriateness of Spinal Manipulation for Low-Back Pain*, 1992.

399 BF Finneson, "A Lumbar Disk Surgery Predictive Score Card: A Retrospective Evaluation," *Spine* (1979): 141-144.

400 RA Deyo, BM Psaty, *et al.*, "The Messenger Under Attack: Intimidation of Researchers by Special Interest Groups," *NEJM* 336/16 (April 17,1997):1176-79.

401 J Silberner, "Surgery May Not Be The Answer To An Aching Back," *All Things Considered*, NPR, (April 6, 2010)

402 S Brownlee, "Newtered," Overtreated: Why Too Much Medicine Is Making Us Sicker and Poorer, http://overtreated.com/extras01.html

Once again the political power of the AMA fought any reform effort to improve healthcare in America. According to Shannon Brownlee, "We've been set back a decade in reforming this system, thanks in part to the handiwork of Gingrich's House."[403]

NBC *Today Show's* Spin Doctor

The AHCPR recommendations had been the most significant recognition to date in the U.S. of the many unnecessary spine surgeries and the importance of manipulative therapy for the epidemic of low back pain. Instead of being heralded as champions helping this epidemic of pain and suffering, chiropractors got short shrift by the spokesmen in the media who virtually ignored or distorted this landmark study.

Media misinformation occurred on several occasions after the AHCPR report was released in December of 1994. Every news organization ignored the NASS backlash against Congress, all ignored the distorted findings in the AMA's "Pocket Guide to Back Pain," and many conservatives fostered the spin doctor's attitude that "Congress cannot tell doctors how to practice medicine."

However, some in the media initially acknowledged the endorsement of chiropractic manipulation. The *Associated Press* and major newspapers throughout the country immediately recognized that the AHCPR study was a boon to chiropractors and a setback for medical doctors. Announcements in the *Chicago Sun-Times*, *Washington Post*, and *Chicago Tribune*, were typical of media reports around the nation that touted chiropractic care over medical care:

- *Chicago Sun-Times*, December 8, 1994

   "When it comes to lower back pain, think twice before resorting to the usual remedies and bed rest. Try a chiropractor instead."

- *Washington Post*, December 9, 1994

   "A panel of medical experts yesterday threw out bed rest and endorsed exercises and spinal manipulation as treatments with proven effectiveness for episodes of acute lower back pain…it found that spinal manipulation, a treatment often performed by chiropractors and osteopaths was safe and effective…many doctors have long discouraged their patients from trying such treatments."

- *Chicago Tribune*, December 9, 1994

   "Chiropractors get a boost in new government-backed guidelines on how to treat low back pain."

By the time the AHCPR recommendations on acute low back pain had reached the news talk programs and magazines, many elite media reporters twisted the conclusions of this thorough study to misrepresent the findings about chiropractic care. *Consumer*

---

403 Ibid.

Reports, Parade magazine, ABC's *Good Morning America*, and NBC's *Today Show*, to name but a few of the more prominent sources, all belied the actual thrust of the AHCPR report.

Undoubtedly the most glaring example of media misrepresentation of the AHCPR's findings occurred on NBC's *Today Show* when the in-house medical spokesman, Art Ulene, MD, presented the results of this impressive two-year study on back pain. In a week-long series on back pain, Ulene mentioned the startling results of this study: Only one in 100 back surgeries is helpful; physio-therapeutics such as ultrasound, TENS, hot packs, and other standard treatments by physical therapists were also short term at best and considered ineffective to change the underlying causes; and spinal manipulation was the preferred initial professional treatment.

To his credit, Dr. Ulene detailed the findings accurately, but he could not contain his medical bias after *Today Show* host Matt Lauer concluded, "So, if you have a back problem, then you should see a chiropractor first."

"Oh, no," said Ulene, "I would *never* recommend a chiropractor. Go see an osteopath instead." Sadly, the Big Lie remains alive.

There was an immediate pause on the show; Matt Lauer looked stunned and confused. You could have heard a pin drop on the stage since his condemnation stood in direct opposition of the AHCPR findings, and everyone knew it.

In one fell swoop, Ulene thwarted the possible upsurge of interest in chiropractic in the minds of millions of viewers. He should have known that most osteopaths today do not do spinal manipulation as a routine treatment and that chiropractors do the vast majority (94 percent) of all spinal manipulation according to RAND.[404] Indeed, if not for the courage and stamina of the chiropractic profession for over 100 years, the healing art of spinal manipulation therapy could have been lost due to the likes of Fishbein and Taylor, but these facts were lost to Ulene altogether.

In the long line of medical misinformers, Ulene's bias was obvious. He still conveyed his message that the public should boycott chiropractors even when recommended by the U.S. Public Health Service. Ulene's misrepresentation of the guideline was a great disservice to both the suffering public and to the chiropractic profession; this was exactly his goal.

It is one thing to win an antitrust trial in the courtroom or to convince fair-minded investigators of the New Zealand Inquiry and the AHCPR of the effectiveness of chiropractic, but until the media acknowledges the new paradigm shift to hands-on therapy, the jury will still be out in the court of public opinion. After decades of misinformation, the media's skepticism remains a powerful problem that hinders the public from learning the truth of the benefits of chiropractic spinal care. The longer we wait, the more people continue to suffer.

---

404 PG Shekelle, *et al*, RAND Corporation Report, *The Appropriateness of Spinal Manipulation for Low-Back Pain* (1992)

According to author Shannon Brownlee,

> Back pain patients would probably do well to think about that, because the surgery they're about to undergo poses real risks, including infection, continuing pain, pseudoarthrosis, a condition called "failed back syndrome," and occasionally even death.
>
> One day medical historians will look back at many current medical practices and see 21ˢᵗ century equivalents of bloodletting and leeches....Spinal fusion surgery serves as the poster child for much of what's wrong with the current debate over what to do about health care costs; it may, according to Dr. Jerome Groopman, be "the radical mastectomy of our time."[405]

Headaches & Strokes

The fifteenth guideline from AHCPR on headaches would have been another windfall for chiropractors. After the NASS attack and the AHCPR was relinquished from the guideline business, the headache project was moved to the Duke University Evidence-Based Practice Center in Durham, NC, that released in 2001 a systematic review by McCrory and Penzion *et al.* which found that spinal manipulation was safe, effective, and appropriate for patients with common forms of primary headache and offered a valuable alternative to patients concerned about the side effects of medications.[406]

Instead of the media reporting on this elimination of the important headache guideline or the supportive research from Duke University that would have helped both millions of headache sufferers and the chiropractic profession, it fell on deaf ears once again.

In its place, the medical media waited with bated breath for another controversial issue to reload its propaganda guns. A malpractice case in Canada got international attention when a chiropractic patient, Lana Lewis, died from a stroke two weeks after getting a neck adjustment. The Canadian media, with encouragement from the medical society, jumped on this case to frighten the public and even demanded that chiropractors not be allowed to do cervical adjustments.

Despite the supportive research concerning the safety of spinal manipulation, this lone incident resurrected the fear that chiropractors may cause strokes or paralysis. The evidence in this case was spurious and unsupported, but the medical propagandists did not let the facts get in their way and used the event to tarnish the professional image of chiropractic once again as dangerous.

Lewis' chiropractor was eventually found not negligent in this case. At trial researchers brought to light many interesting facts about spinal manipulative therapy (SMT) and stroke that never made it past the headlines or subsequent newspaper articles to rebuild chiropractic's reputation after the initial headlines had already convicted it in the court of public opinion.

---

405 S Brownlee, "Newtered," Overtreated: Why Too Much Medicine Is Making Us Sicker and Poorer, http://overtreated.com/extras01.html
406 DC McCrory, DB Penzien, *et al.* "Evidence Report: Behavioral and Physical Treatments for Tension-Type and Cervicogenic Headache," Des Moines, IA: Foundation for Chiropractic, (2001)

Dr. Adrian Upton, head of the Department of Neurology at McMaster Health Sciences Centre testified at the inquest that, based on all of the evidence he had reviewed, Ms. Lewis died of a stroke caused by advanced atherosclerosis. During examination, he stated that a chiropractic neck adjustment she received not long before her stroke was at best "a remote possibility at the bottom of the list of probabilities" for causation. Ms. Lewis was extremely hypertensive, off her meds, and a heavy tobacco smoker at the time of her death—as Dr. Upton put it, "she was a time bomb ready to explode."

The expert testimony that concluded Lewis' death was due to intra-cranial atherosclerosis causing 100 percent and 70 percent stenosis of her basilar arteries rather than one cervical adjustment two weeks before. Nonetheless, the amount of bad press has had its ripple effect on all chiropractors despite the expert testimony. Chiropractors were, in effect, guilty by inference after the press had done a "tremendous over-simplification of this issue."[407]

According to research by Alan Terret *et al.,* the rate of iatrogenic problems associated with spinal manipulative therapy as rendered by doctors of chiropractic is only 1 in 5.85 million cases, which is less than the chance of stroke in a hair salon or being hit by lightning (one in 600,000). It equated to one occurrence in 48 chiropractic careers.[408]

"We didn't see any increased association between chiropractic care and usual family physician care, and the stroke," said Frank Silver, one of the researchers and also a professor of medicine at the University of Toronto and director of the University Health Network stroke program.

> The association occurs because patients tend to seek care when they're having neck pain or headache, and sometimes they go to a chiropractor, sometimes they go to a physician. But we didn't see an increased likelihood of them having this type of stroke after seeing a chiropractor.[409]

A recent Canadian study by The Bone and Joint Decade 2000-2010 Task Force on Neck Pain and Its Associated Disorders indicated there was no increased risk related to chiropractic treatment in the debate about whether neck adjustments can trigger a rare type of stroke. *Researchers found patients are no more likely to suffer a stroke following a visit to a chiropractor than they would after stepping into their family doctor's office.*

The findings, which were published in the journal *Spine,*[410] helped to shed light on earlier studies that had cast a cloud on the chiropractic profession and suggested that their

---

407 2002 ICSM Proceedings. The Proceedings is available on CD-ROM or as a book through www.fcer. org or by calling 800-622-6309

408 AGJ Terret, "Current Concepts in Vertebrobasilar Complications Following Spinal Manipulation," NCMIC Group Inc, West Des Moines, Iowa, (2001)

409 G Bronfort, M Haas, R Evans, G Kawchuk, and S Dagenais, "Evidence-informed Management of Chronic Low Back Pain with Spinal Manipulation and Mobilization," *Spine* 8/1 (January-February 2008):213-25.

410 JD Cassidy, E Boyle, P Cote, Y He, S Hogg-Johnson, FL Silver, and SJ Bondy, "Risk of Vertebrobasilar Stroke and Chiropractic Care Results of a Population-Based Case-Control and Case-Crossover Study," *Spine* 33/4S, (Feb. 2009): S176–S183.

actions resulted in some patients suffering a stroke after treatment. In fact, the findings support the chiropractic position of its extreme safety when compared with drugs and surgery.

If we were to take a look at the rates of iatrogenic deaths from medical care, the numbers are staggering. Barbara Starfield, MD, MPH, of the Johns Hopkins School of Hygiene and Public Health, reported that medical care is now the third-leading cause of death in the U.S., causing 225,000 preventable deaths every year. She also stated, "The fact is the US population does not have anything near the best healthcare system in the world."[411]

In 2006, Jay Triano, DC, PhD, wrote about the stroke issue in his publication, *Current Concepts in Spinal Manipulation and Cervical Arterial Incidents,* that included 675 references and a comprehensive discussion of cervical artery injury and manipulation. He also came to the sobering conclusion that chiropractic is very safe:

- The increased risk of death resulting from NSAID use is 1,500 times greater than the risk of tetraplegia following cervical SMT.
- On analysis, SMT as delivered by chiropractors is one of the most conservative, least invasive and safest of procedures in the provision of health care services.
- The risks of SMT pale when compared to known medical risks. Chiropractors, by their training and skill in SMT and special emphasis on the spine, are the best positioned to deliver this mode of health care to the public.
- Conclusion: VBA stroke is a very rare event in the population. The increased risks of VBA stroke associated with chiropractic and PCP visits is likely due to patients with headache and neck pain from VBA dissection seeking care before their stroke. We found no evidence of excess risk of VBA stroke associated chiropractic care compared to primary care. [412]

The fact is malpractice insurance companies know which doctors are hurting patients, and the actuaries show that chiropractors have the lowest malpractice rates among all spine practitioners. Chiropractors pay approximately $1,600 annually[413] compared to spine surgeons, who typically derive as much as 62 percent of all of their professional income from performing surgical procedures on the lumbar spine, will pay approximately $71,000 to over $200,000,[414] which clearly suggests the safety of care provided by chiropractors.

---

411 B Starfield, "Is US Health Really the Best in the World?" *JAMA* 284/4 (July 26, 2000):483-485.
412 Ibid.
413 National Chiropractic Mutual Insurance Company rate (2009)
414 The Burton Report, "Why Spine Care is at High Risk for Medical-Legal Suits," www.burtonreport. com/infforensic/MedMalSpCommonCause.htm

A study by Anthony Rosner, PhD, comparing medical procedures to chiropractic care concerning strokes flipped this coin to mention patients need to be warned of the dangers of *medical* procedures rather than *chiropractic* care. As he suggests, "The statistics really begin to spin one's head."[415]

Using a baseline figure of one per one million as an estimate of stroke incidence attributed to cervical manipulations, one finds a:

- two times greater risk of dying from transfusing one unit of blood;[416]
- 100 times greater risk of dying from general anesthesia;[417]
- 160-400 times greater risk of dying from use of NSAIDs;[418]
- 700 times greater risk of dying from lumbar spinal surgery;[419]
- 1000-10,000 times greater risk of dying from traditional gall bladder surgery;[420]
- 10,000 times greater risk of serious harm from medical mistakes in hospitals.[421]

Obviously these medical risks are unknown by the public and untold by the medical propagandists to the media, yet the same MDs who criticized chiropractors forget to mention these facts (the "professional amnesia" Dr. Rosner suggests) of the remote danger of manipulation or the fact that patients who seek medical care are equally susceptible, if not more so, to medical mistakes and iatrogenic problems.

Despite the overwhelming support for chiropractic manipulation for neck problems, the medical misinformers have again raised unwarranted concern for strokes caused by manipulation. A 2010 study from England, "Deaths After Chiropractic: A Review Of Published Cases," by Edzard Ernst of the Medical School at the University of Exeter, once again raised the level of fear over chiropractic care when he noted that "Twenty-six fatalities were published since 1934 in 23 articles."[422]

Considering this covers 76 years and equates to 0.34 deaths per year, instead of sounding an alarm to scare people as Ernst attempted, he should have praised chiropractic care for its obvious safety since this is an extremely low rate in comparison with equivalent medical methods for the same diagnostic condition.

---

415 A Rosner, "Evidence or Eminence-Based Medicine? Leveling the Playing Field Instead of the Patient," *Dynamic Chiropractic* 20/25 (November 30, 2002)

416 J Paling www.healthcare speaker.com, 2000.

417 Paling, ibid.

418 V Dabbs, W Lauretti. "A Risk Assessment Of Cervical Manipulation Vs NSAIDs For The Treatment Of Neck Pain," *Journal of Manipulative and Physiological Therapeutics* 18/8 (1995):530-536.

419 RA Deyo, DC Cherkin, JD Loesser, SJ Bigos, MA Ciol, "Morbidity and Mortality In Association With Operations On The Lumbar Spine: The Influence Of Age, Diagnosis, And Procedure," *Journal of Bone and Joint Surgery Am* 74/4 (1992):536-543.

420 Paling, ibid.

421 Paling, ibid.

422 E Ernst "Deaths After Chiropractic: A Review Of Published Cases," *Int J Clin Pract*, 64/8 (July 2010):1162–1165

Ernst's paper drew quick criticism from leading medical and chiropractic scholars. According to SM Perle, S French, and M Haas:

> Ernst ignored the evidence against a causal relation between spinal manipulation and death. Instead, he went boldly along a path of fear mongering and propaganda that we expect was predetermined to establish the dangers of CSM (cervical spinal manipulation).[423]

Another review from The Dartmouth Institute for Health Policy and Clinical Practice was equally critical:

> Three deaths were reported during the last 10 years of the study, so for that most recent time period, the absolute risk could be estimated to be 3/10 per 100 million, or three deaths for every billion chiropractic encounters...This rate is so low that it cannot possibly be considered significant...An interesting flip side to the research question might be: by undergoing a course of chiropractic spinal manipulation, *how many patients were able to avoid death by avoiding complications of surgical intervention?*[424] (emphasis added)

Although chiropractic scored a big victory in the legal court room with the *Wilk v. AMA* trial, however, in the court of public opinion chiropractic remains obscured behind medical propaganda. Until chiropractic has equal access to the media with spokesmen on every news program, the medical spin doctors like Ulene and Ernst will continue to spew one-sided and biased information to the public.

Unfortunately, medical bigotry still permeates political medicine today. This was clearly evident during the Obama healthcare reform effort in 2010 when the AMA suggested in news releases that alternative therapies, including chiropractic, were not scientific. Considering the plethora of evidence against spine surgery, drugs, and shots, this claim is ridiculous, but the naïve public and compliant press were unaware of this irony that was, in effect, the pot calling the kettle black.

"Much of the information currently known about these [CAM] therapies makes it clear that many have not been shown to be efficacious," the AMA said in a July, 2009 policy statement.[425] Again, the AMA had turned a blind eye to the public popularity and recent research supporting chiropractic care that threatens its income stream and willingly misled the media and governmental bodies.

When comparative effectiveness trials were done to discern which treatments were best, the AMA again objected to them. For example, just in the past few years, comparative

---

423 SM Perle, S French, and M Haas, "Critique of Review of Deaths after Chiropractic, 4" Letters to editor, *The International Journal of Clinical Practice*, 65/1 (January 2011):102-106.

424 JM Whedon, GM Bove, MA Davis, "Critique of review of deaths after chiropractic, 5" Letter to editor, *The International Journal of Clinical Practice*, 65/1 (January 2011):102-106.

425 M Kranish, "Senators Seek Coverage For Alternative Therapies," *Boston Globe*, (July 24, 2009)

effectiveness studies have shown that most back surgeries[426], heart procedures[427], and knee surgeries[428] were no better than non-invasive conservative care, yet in each case, the AMA cried out "junk science" and screamed, "we're not going to let bureaucrats tell us how to practice." Apparently what the AMA really said was, "Don't confuse us with the facts," just as we saw with the AHCPR study on acute low back pain.

Certainly for the medical profession to levy criticism at chiropractic care is simply crying wolf and is now seen as a shameless attack on competition. The AMA denied trying to stifle competition and said it was only trying to ensure that medicine was based on science, according to an article in the *Boston Globe,* "Senators Seek Coverage for Alternative Therapies."[429] This alibi was similar to the smokescreen excuse of "public safety" used by the AMA in the *Wilk* trial.

Undeterred, Senator Tom Harkin (D-Iowa) came to the defense of CAM when he said at a congressional hearing that "It's time to end the discrimination against alternative healthcare practices."[430]

Of course, this met with strong criticism from medical chauvinists like Dr. Harriet Hall, a retired Air Force flight surgeon, who said she worried that "ill-informed members of Congress will elevate practitioners of alternative medicine to the same level as medical doctors." [431] As chairman of the Office of Alternative Medicine for the past 16 years, undoubtedly Sen. Harkin must have been rather offended at her remark that he is "ill-informed."

Obviously Dr. Hall seemed more concerned about keeping the medical monarchy when she appeared annoyed that "Congress will elevate practitioners to the same level as medical doctors." Her arrogance was clear that there is no room on the medical throne for anyone other than MDs.

Dr. Hall continued to show her bias when she said, "If it were shown to be truly effective, it would be part of regular medicine." Once again we hear Morris Fishbein speaking from his grave when he said, *"Scientific medicine absorbs from them that which is*

---

426 JN Weinstein, JD Lurie, TD Tosteson, JS Skinner, B Hanscom, ANA Tosteson, H Herkowitz, J Fischgrund, FP Cammisa, T Albert, RA Deyo, "Surgical vs. Non-Operative Treatment For Lumbar Disk Herniation: The Spine Patient Outcomes Research Trial (SPORT) Observational Cohort," *JAMA,* 296 (2006):2451–9.

427 WE Boden, RA O'Rourke, KK Teo, PM Hartigan, DJ Maron, M Knudtson, M Dada, P Casperson, CL Harris, BR Chaitman, L Shaw, G Gosselin, S Nawaz, LM Title, G Gau, AS Blaustein, DC Booth, ER Bates, JA Spertus, DS Berman, GBJ Mancini, WS Weintraub, for the COURAGE Trial Research Group, "Optimal Medical Therapy with or without PCI for Stable Coronary Disease," *NEJM,* 15/356 (April 12, 2007):1503-1516.

428 A Kirkley, TB Birmingham, RB Litchfield, JR Giffin, KR Willits, CJ Wong, BG Feagan, A Donner, S H Griffin, L D'Ascanio,, JE Pope, and PJ Fowler, "A Randomized Trial of Arthroscopic Surgery for Osteoarthritis of the Knee," *NEJM* 359/11 (Sept. 11, 2008):1097-1107

429 Kranish ibid.

430 Ibid.

431 Ibid.

good, if there is any good, and then they die."[432] Considering the evidence from the *Wilk* trial and AHCPR as well as the many international studies that support manipulative therapy for back pain, it is obvious Dr. Hall is spewing propaganda.

Ironically, if medicine were "truly effective" as Dr. Hall suggests, we would not be in the present healthcare crisis. If this is not proof of the medical prejudice that still prevails in healthcare, what would better illustrate this lingering discrimination against CAM health providers? Obviously the medical monarchists like Hall have no wish to see their medical Bastille toppled by equality among the ranks of non-allopathic providers. Indeed, it must be foggy to see the truth from the rarified air atop the medical pedestal.

Until a true healthcare reform ends the medical monarchy and its prevailing prejudice that fuels this medical war; until comparative effectiveness studies assure that patients will be given the best of evidence-based guidelines such as non-invasive, non-drug, hands-on spinal care first; and until insurance companies stop throwing good money after bad at the surgeons, patients need to remember one bit of advice: Buyer Beware.

It is time for the media to stop ignoring chiropractic's benefits and stop parroting the medical propaganda. It is time to tell the whole truth about the benefits of chiropractic care rather than repeating the medical propaganda we have heard for nearly a century. It is time to restore sanity in healthcare.

---

432 M Fishbein, *Medical Follies*, New York, Boni & Liveright, (1925):43.

Wither on the Vine

"The chiropractic profession as a whole...
is ready to step up to the plate and to let its belief systems
be tested scientifically.
Let the chips fall where they may." [433]

J. Jay Triano, DC, PhD

The medical war against chiropractors has been fought on many battlefields in the courtrooms, hospitals, the media, and, most repugnantly, in the sanctity of our nation's classrooms and universities. Although most Americans cherish the freedom of thought in our educational institutions to debate issues in a fair-minded fashion, political medicine realized shaping negative public opinion about chiropractic meant controlling academia.

In 1962, General Counsel Robert B. Throckmorton clearly spelled out in his Iowa Plan, "What Medicine Should Do about the Chiropractic Menace"[434] that included a section to "contain chiropractic schools":

f. Contain chiropractic schools.

> ...Any successful policy of 'containment' of chiropractic must necessarily be directed at the schools. To the extent that these financial problems continue to multiply, and to the extent that the schools are unsuccessful in their recruiting programs, the chiropractic menace of the future will be reduced and possibly eliminated.

---

433 K Miller, "FSU Faculty Members Debate Chiropractic School," *Palm Beach Post* (January 14, 2005)
434 Ibid. PX-172 (November 11, 1962)

Action taken by the medical profession should be persistent and behind the scenes whenever possible.

If chiropractic was to "wither on the vine" in the court of public opinion, it had to start early by influencing children through their teachers and counselors. When the AMA investigated the attitudes of youngsters, it was mortified to learn from its own survey that 70 percent of high school seniors in the 1960s thought that chiropractors were best for neck and back pain.[435] In response, the Committee on Quackery (COQ) under the direction of H. Doyl Taylor produced "The Quack Pack" to disseminate misinformation to high school counselors to distribute to prospective chiropractic students.[436]

As well, in order to demean chiropractic's academic legitimacy, the COQ had to smear chiropractic's image and "contain" its expansion in the ranks of higher education with intimidation and censorship. Indeed, no leaf was left unturned by the AMA in its effort to contain its competitors, and it began by warping the minds of educators and their students with propaganda.

The Iowa Plan sought to prevent the government from granting chiropractic student loans and to prevent any government research grants at chiropractic colleges. While the AMA worked to starve chiropractic education, it also complained loudly that the caliber of chiropractic education was poor and that chiropractors did not do enough research to prove its scope of treatment, illustrating the duplicity of political medicine.

As well, the Committee on Quackery developed a plan to resist any federal recognition of and financial assistance for chiropractic education. As long as the education of chiropractors appeared inadequate compared to medical schooling, the AMA could use this as leverage against chiropractors gaining equal status.

The Iowa Plan also addressed the issue to contain the improvement of chiropractic education by prohibiting medical professionals from consulting with chiropractors about patients or teaching. According to attorney George McAndrews in his closing remarks in the *Wilk* trial, "The plan encompassed keeping them from having adequate teachers in their schools. So then you could turn around and condemn the schools for being inferior."[437] The Iowa Plan also prohibited MDs from attending seminars where chiropractors lectured or allowing MDs to lecture at chiropractic colleges or seminars.

This was the tactic used in the late 1950s and early 1960s in the medical war in the state of Louisiana, which was the last state to legislate a separate scope of practice law for chiropractors in 1974. The *England* case, as it became known, was filed by Dr. Jerry England and other Louisiana chiropractors who sought the right to practice chiropractic without hindrance from the medical establishment. This lengthy legal process that began

---

435 G McAndrews closing argument, *Wilk II* (June 26, 1987):3057
436 Ibid. p. 3082.
437 G McAndrews, closing remarks before the Honorable Nicholas J. Bua, *Wilk et al. v. AMA et al.*, (December 9, 1980):66.

in 1957 and ended in 1966 was appealed all the way to the US Supreme Court, which in 1964 remanded it back to the District Court.[438]

J. Minos Simon, chief counsel in the *England* case, spoke to the Louisiana Chiropractors' Association in May, 1960, to buoy their spirits after decades of discrimination and despair in their battle for equality:

> There was a time not long ago when the Chiropractors of Louisiana were spent of all reasonable hope...They were fined and imprisoned and deprived of their constitutional right to practice their profession as swiftly as the criminal and civil machinery of the Louisiana judiciary permitted...
>
> The allopaths embarked on a concerted program of vilification and slander, scurrilously maligning the Chiropractor, and irresponsibly assailing the undeniable principles of Chiropractic. So consummate was the effort, so vicious was the unrelenting attack, that the Chiropractor and his family soon became the object of obloquy and boorish derision. The dark clouds of gloom came crowding about them. The weight of oppression was unbearable. Life itself held little for them...
>
> With nimbleness of brawn and brain they now contend that while chiropractic is good for some things, it is not good for all things, and, therefore, Chiropractors should not be permitted to attend the sick for anything. Such chameleonic versatility is destined to doom...
>
> We see, therefore, that the struggle between the Chiropractor and the medical doctor is a struggle between truth and the avarice of man...the opposition to chiropractic, when it comes from the medical doctor, from one who should be learned in the sciences, necessarily must be based entirely on a fear of economic competition.
>
> Look to the future, therefore, not with rancor... not with a sense of vengeance, but with a sense of righteous determination that chiropractic as chiropractic will be established and vindicated, and that it peaceful residence, side by side, with the other healing arts will endure forever, to the end finally that the sick will have the benefits of all healing sciences in an atmosphere of absolute freedom of choice.[439]

Despite Mr. Simon's eloquent speech, the medical war in Louisiana was the last stand by the Committee on Quackery. It was not by coincidence that Louisiana was also the home state of Dr. Joseph Sabatier, better known in the medical profession as the chairman of the Committee on Quackery and a co-defendant in the *Wilk* trial that began in 1976. The Pelican State was the last ditch effort by Sabatier to thwart chiropractic's legal recognition that had previously occurred in all other states.

Similar to the tactics in the first *Wilk* trial, the unethical practices and advertisements of some chiropractors were exposed to the three-judge tribunal. The medical attorney

---

438 RB Phillips, "Joseph Janse: the Apostle of Chiropractic Education," (2006):164-181.
439 J. Minos Simon, chief counsel, *England* case, convention of the Louisiana Chiropractors' Association, New Orleans, May, 1960.

also emphasized the lack of federally-recognized accreditation for chiropractic schools. In 1965, the judges ruled in favor of the medical board. The tribunal ruled that the proper venue for seeking change in the laws governing licensure was not the responsibility of the judiciary but should come from the legislature.[440]

Once the tribunal had ruled in favor of the medical board, arrests of chiropractors commenced again after the nine-year legal battle. In 1967, Dr. England and his wife left Louisiana in the middle of the night to avoid going to jail, relocating in Alabama for the next 27 years.[441]

Renowned chiropractic educator Joseph Janse, DC, ND, president of National College of Chiropractic (NCC) in Chicago, was embarrassed as a witness during the *England* trial when he was forced to admit to the lack of federal accreditation of chiropractic by the U. S. Office of Education (USOE), unlike all other health professions that had this recognition.

According to the historian of National College of Chiropractic, Ronald P. Beideman, DC, ND, "He vowed he 'would correct this fault…or leave the profession.'"[442] Being a "scrapper" that Janse was known to be all his life, this ridicule motivated him to seek accreditation for NCC, which he accomplished six years later when his college received regional accreditation.[443]

He did not leave the profession and his efforts led to federal recognition in 1974 when the Council on Chiropractic Education (CCE-USA) was finally recognized by the USOE as the professional accrediting body for chiropractic colleges. In the same year, Louisiana chiropractors were finally granted recognized status by statute.

The fear of incarceration was not that long ago when EJ Nosser was the last chiropractor in the United States to go to jail in 1975 in Shreveport, Louisiana. He was charged with practicing medicine without a license before the 1974 chiropractic scope law was passed, but his original conviction was appealed by J. Minos Simon to the U.S. Supreme Court where it was remanded back in 1975 to the lower court to the same judge who had convicted him.[444]

Despite the fact that the law had changed by then, the judge sentenced Dr. Nosser to fifteen days in jail with a $500 fine and, as luck would have it, the bailiffs who led him away to jail were also patients of his. To illustrate how times have changed in Louisiana, years later the mayor of Shreveport would proclaim "Dr. EJ Nosser Day" on May 24, 2007, in recognition of his 50 years of service since graduating from Palmer School of Chiropractic in 1957.[445] Dr. EJ Nosser exemplified the ordeal from persecution to vindication that too many chiropractors endured to safeguard this healing art.

---

440 JC Keating, "The England Case and the Wilk Case: A Comparison, Part 1, *Dynamic Chiropractic*, 25/19 (September 10, 2007)

441 Ibid. p.180.

442 R Beideman, *In the Making of a Profession: The National College of Chiropractic 1906-1981.* National College, Lombard, Ill. (1995): 260.

443 Phillips, ibid. p.161.

444 Tom Nosser via private communication with JC Smith on January 14, 2011.

445 I Hunter, "Rubbing Patients the Right Way," *Shreveport Times* (May 29, 2007)

Recall the arrest of Dr. Nosser came just one year before the *Wilk* lawsuit was filed, and due to the initial failure of the *England* case, the American Chiropractic Association and many chiropractors were initially hesitant to support Chester Wilk and return to a legal battle in another courtroom with a much stronger opponent.

Both the *England* and *Wilk* legal battles had to be fought and, despite initial defeats in the courtroom, the subsequent appeals proved positive. The *England* case that led to improving educational standards was essential for chiropractic's survival as well as important in the *Wilk* trial by removing a legitimate criticism of chiropractic—its lack of federally-recognized educational standards.

Sabatier and the Committee on Quackery (COQ) had no wish to see chiropractic improve on the educational front. Two of the stated goals of the Sabatier's COQ were the distribution of propaganda to the nation's teachers and guidance counselors to discourage students from seeking careers in chiropractic and punishing community colleges that offered pre-chiropractic programs. Of course, this extended to the established universities' medical schools to resist the implementation of any chiropractic academic programs, which remains in effect yet today.

Both Morehead College in Kentucky and the College of St. Thomas in Minneapolis attempted to begin a two-year pre-professional course for students seeking to attend a chiropractic college. In both instances, the local medical society put pressure on the college president to stop the affiliation or else lose their accreditation.[446] Certainly, losing face among the medical peer group was another huge inducement to follow the boycott of chiropractic curriculum.

For example, in 1971, the C.W. Post College, a division of Long Island University in New York State, was asked by Lincoln College of Chiropractic to cooperate in setting up a Chair of Chiropractic and to teach the pre-professional basic sciences. C.W. Post indicated a desire to have this chiropractic college work with them.[447]

However, this program was scuttled when the college capitulated to the threat of the AMA to cut funds and withdraw accreditation. The New York medical society sent newsletters throughout the state to its member physicians stating "the lights of the Empire State have gone out." In July, 1972, issue of the Medical Society of the State of New York, an article, "Long Island University says it will not teach pre-chiropractic students," reported that "the proposal was protested vigorously by the Medical Society..."[448]

Ernest R. Jaffe, Acting Dean of the Albert Einstein College of Medicine of Yeshiva University, sent a letter to Long Island University that said, "I urge you to take all appropriate measures to terminate any relationship with Lincoln College of Chiropractic. It can only bring discredit to your university."[449]

---

446 Ibid. p. 7078-79
447 Minutes of "Meeting of the Logan College Board of Trustees" in St. Louis (Logan Archives) (June 17, 1971)
448 Null, ibid.
449 Ibid.

George McAndrews commented on the "objective reasonableness of any men or women of science saying that they are going to benefit patient care by undercutting the educational base of a licensed healthcare profession. But that is what they did, I might say, probably to their everlasting shame."[450]

Henry I. Feinberg, then chairman of the Committee on Quackery, reported that the medical staff at C.W. Post had threatened to resign if the chiropractic proposal was implemented:

> It is reprehensible that a number of intellectuals of an accredited institution of higher education would even consider participation in this chicanery. Our purpose is to alert everyone engaged in the legitimate practice of medicine to the tremendous danger of setting up a program for those who wish to *practice medicine through the back door.*[451]

Once again we hear the echoes of Morris Fishbein speaking.

George McAndrews summarized the intent of the AMA to thwart chiropractic education was to "have the appearance of lack of education":

> That's equivalent of book burning. You can't give a lecture to these people because we want to accuse them of being stupid so we can eliminate them. You can't teach in their schools because we're going to maintain the appearance they don't have any knowledge. And they never know when to send anyone to an MD, so we're going to make it unethical for them to refer a patient to us. And since all they do well is biomechanical things, we are going to make it unethical for an MD to ever refer a patient to a chiropractor under any circumstances even when the MD intimately knows the chiropractor. They left no room.[452]

Indeed, chiropractic had become a taboo subject for many colleges due to this intimidation. To this day, not one major American university has a chiropractic program. Author Gary Null, PhD, summarized this twisted sense of medical ethics that had no bearing to improve patient welfare, but did improve the AMA's own economic welfare to thwart the progress of a rival profession:

> Placing this kind of pressure on academic institutions was central to the strategy of the AMA and the other medical organizations involved. If chiropractors had access to the same university privileges that the medical profession enjoyed—including internships and residencies in university medical school hospitals—it would undercut the medical profession's arguments that chiropractors lack the education necessary to diagnose or treat human ailments.[453]

The Illinois State Medical Society (ISMS) drew its own line in the sand when it published a sarcastic article, "Snap, Crackle and Pop," written by William Lees, MD,

---

450 Ibid. p. 3082-83.
451 Ibid. p. 3085-86.
452 G McAndrews, (December 9, 1980):7086.
453 Null, ibid.

Chairman of the ISMS Board of Trustees. This article was immediately sent around the United States by Doyl Taylor.

Among many incriminating statements, Dr. Lees wrote:

> Physicians must become fully knowledgeable, must educate their patients, and must help ISMS to concentrate activity to eliminate chiropractic.
>
> It is also recommended that physicians not compete with chiropractic practitioners since this lends status and credence to them and implies a certain equality.[454]

When Lees learned that a chiropractor had been allowed in the door of a tax supported public state university, he wrote to the Illinois College of Medicine:

> It might be wise to prohibit any contact of any kind at any time by persons at the medical center with any chiropractor.[455]

One might think the chiropractor had the bubonic plague that would contaminate the college staff. Instead, in the opinion of Lees, he had something more dangerous—a chiropractic degree.

A good example of this academic discrimination occurred to J. Jay Triano when he submitted his first peer-reviewed article accepted by *SPINE* magazine that refused in 1981 to acknowledge his DC degree:

> "Please be advised that it is the policy of *SPINE* to print only designations indicting University degrees or equivalents to or extensions upon such degrees following an author's name. Therefore, we would propose to acknowledge your M.A. degree only. If you find this a suitable arrangement, please indicate. *SPINE* will then be prepared to finalize publication."[456]

Mr. McAndrews addressed this attitude at trial when he said, "This is what you call total absolute ostracism, segregation, isolation, and humiliation."[457]

Despite the medical criticism of the poor standards of chiropractic education, when the USOE began the process to establish a federal accrediting agency to improve chiropractic education, the Council on Chiropractic Education (CCE), the AMA adamantly complained again with any effort to improve chiropractic education.

> On March 1, 1974, Dr. Ernest B. Howard, Executive Vice-President of the American Medical Association, made a second attempt, following a similar attempt in 1972, to get the U.S. Commissioner of Education to discontinue its consideration of recognition of an accrediting agency for chiropractic education. *The thrust of his argument was that chiropractic had no scientific validity or social usefulness.* [458]

---

454 G McAndrews closing argument, p. 6800

455 Ibid.

456 JJ Triano via personal communication with JC Smith, 6-2-10

457 Ibid, p. 6800-01

458 JC Keating, *"Wilk et al. vs. AMA et al."* National Institute of Chiropractic Research (05/11/08):45.

Howard presented no facts or research to prove his allegations. The AMA would not stop in its relentless pursuit to obstruct federal accreditation of chiropractic colleges by the USOE because along with federal accreditation came guaranteed student loans, the lifeblood of any college.

At the May 23-24, 1974, hearing of the USOE Advisory Committee on the CCE Application for Recognition in Washington, D.C., the AMA sent its new chairman of the Committee on Quackery, Boston neurosurgeon, Dr. H. Thomas Ballantine. He made a vicious attack on the chiropractic profession, the CCE, and its Commission on Accreditation. He characterized the chiropractic profession as a cult and stated that "medical authorities agree that chiropractic has no validity... and represents a significant hazard to the public."[459]

Once again, Ballantine presented no facts or research to prove his allegations. The AMA would do anything to have chiropractic colleges wither on the vine, including lying to the courts. The alibi that chiropractic is an "unscientific cult" was later reiterated at the *Wilk* trial in 1976 and the New Zealand Inquiry on Chiropractic in 1978 and shown to be an unproven allegation without merit, but that did not stop these medical generals from stating such propaganda.

Despite the notion of academic freedom in higher education, the AMA and its Committee on Quackery made a mockery of this enclave of learning. The Iowa Plan undermined chiropractic education and illustrated the power of one special interest group to impose self-serving policies on public institutions—scholastic, hospitals, and health programs in general—that affects millions of Americans. In effect, the AMA's plan to ban chiropractic was an egregious attack on academic freedom and an affront to every civil minded person. This mindset did not end when the CCE was accredited by the USOE making student loans available for chiropractic students. It may have lost this one battle, but the medical war to thwart chiropractic education and research was far from over.

As shocking as this lack of academic freedom may seem today, it was typical of the bigotry many Americans experienced before the Civil Rights era in the early 1960s. Racial de-segregation in schools created strong resentment often leading to deadly attacks. Sadly, the chiropractic profession would experience a similar academic injustice decades later at Florida State University.

The Imperfect Storm in Florida

The thrust to expand chiropractic education from small private colleges operating on shoe-string budgets to a major university level became the goal of the Florida Chiropractic Association. They lobbied five years to convince the state legislature and Governor Jeb Bush to implement a chiropractic program at Florida State University (FSU) and to make available the research capabilities at its Tallahassee campus Medical School.

---

459 Ibid.

The fact that not one major public state university in the United States and Canada offers a chiropractic graduate level program speaks volumes about the influence of the medical profession considering chiropractic is the third-largest physician-level profession in the world, only behind allopathy and dentistry. Academia remains a bastion of allopathic dominance and the attempt to upend this academic monarchy became an imperfect storm in Florida that blew in like a hurricane to destroy a heroic effort to implement a chiropractic program at FSU.

In 2004, the Florida state legislature, led by Senate President Senator Dennis Jones, a chiropractor, and FSU alum Jim King gave FSU the authority to offer a chiropractic degree and provided the university $9 million a year for a School of Chiropractic Medicine. This legislation was hugely supported by the legislators. SB 2002 was the first bill sent to Gov. Bush during the 2004 legislative session after being approved 38-1 by the Florida Senate on March 4, and approved by the House unanimously, 113-0, the following day.[460] Needless to say, a *total vote of 151 to 1 against should indicate the strong public support* for this program, but that did not stop the medical society from interfering.

"Throughout this long effort, the Florida Chiropractic Association (FCA), its lobby team, and legislative leadership never lost sight of the goal to have a public option for a chiropractic education," said the FCA's CEO Debra Brown. "We have a long list of legislators, chiropractic leaders, educators and others to thank for helping to achieve this success."

"We look forward to sharing the great news with the chiropractic world that this program is funded and that future chiropractic students at last have an option of a public education," said Florida State Association CEO Emeritus Ed Williams, DC.

A public chiropractic school at FSU was the longtime goal of Senate Majority Leader Dennis Jones, a 1963 graduate of Lincoln College of Chiropractic and former president of the FCA. While serving in the House of Representatives, he argued for decades that Florida had no chiropractic school to call its own, causing hundreds of people who were interested in studying chiropractic to move out of state to obtain a degree.[461]

FSU proposed a joint Masters degree program that would be five years in length, as opposed to the usual four years of study in other chiropractic programs. In addition to the doctor of chiropractic degree, students would be required to obtain a collateral masters degree in microbiology, nutrition, health policy or biomechanics, depending on their course of study.[462]

Rand S. Swenson, DC, MD, PhD, and Associate Professor of Anatomy and Medicine at Dartmouth Medical School was retained by the Board of Governors as a consultant to review the proposal. Dr. Swenson indicated in his report that the proposed chiropractic program would benefit from its relationship with the integrated master's programs, and

---

460 Editorial Staff, "Florida Legislature Approves Funding for Chiropractic College at FSU," *Dynamic Chiropractic* 22/8 (April 8, 2004)

461 Ibid.

462 M Yeager, "Question of Science," Tallahassee *Democrat*, (12/12/2004)

he also suggested that those programs (and others at FSU) might be enhanced by the addition of chiropractic education.

The University also responded to the call both within and external to the profession for more scientific research related to chiropractic health care and a more evidence-based approach to professional practice. [463]

The integrated MS program emphasized the following themes:

- Science-based educational curriculum
- Evidence-based care and research
- Prevention, health promotion and wellness
- Complementary and integrative health care
- Health care information and quality improvement
- Patient-centered care with focus on special populations

Dr. Swenson indicated in his consultant's report that a chiropractic program at a public institution may be more effective in attracting minorities because of the decreased cost of attendance.

The FSU program would have been a turning point in chiropractic research and education, according to J. Jay Triano, DC, PhD, a leading chiropractic researcher who had by then obtained his PhD and was instrumental in the development of this program. "The transition is from the stereotypical impression of chiropractic as a bunch of people running around claiming they can treat everything, to a very evidence-based but open-minded practice approach."[464]

The goal of the evidence-based chiropractic program was to do research at a major university that had the facilities, faculty, and funding to determine the scope of chiropractic care, but this noble cause was killed after it was conceived in the legislature when medical demagogues and political subterfuge crushed the proposed chiropractic program before it was implemented.

The monumental task of a small cadre of chiropractic researchers addressing these clinical questions has always been a problem in the privately owned chiropractic colleges working without the financial help of federal funding for this research so necessary to the advancement of chiropractic clinical science. The FSU program would have opened a big door to research never permissible before, but this hope was dashed by the actions of a medical mob.

In a combination of events never seen before in the ranks of American higher education, this became a imperfect storm consisting of a power struggle among the state legislature, the Board of Governors, the Board of Trustees, and the FSU administration; an objectionable medical faculty; a divided chiropractic camp; and a gullible media that narrated without question the path of this storm to the public.

---

463 Florida Board Of Governors Minutes, Subject: Implementation Authorization for a Doctor of Chiropractic at FSU, (January 27, 2005)

464 G Fineout, "Chiropractors, Doctors Feud Over FSU Plan," *Miami Herald*, (January 13, 2005)

According to newspaper reports, the FSU Provost Abele had done a "commendable job" in putting together a chiropractic plan that attempted to bridge the gaps in chiropractic science and establish loftier academic standards. Despite his support, he felt compelled to distance this program from the poor image of chiropractic education emanating from Life Chiropractic College (LCC) in nearby Georgia that was supplying chiropractic graduates to many of the Southeastern states.

The role of LCC in the FSU proposal was a big factor in this imperfect storm. Not only as a direct competitor for students, LCC stirred controversy with its unfounded position on the scope of chiropractic care as noted by the FSU Provost when he referred to the *Journal of Vertebral Subluxation Research (JVSR),* an upstart chiropractic publication from LCC that had met mixed reviews, some often harsh, from within chiropractic itself for pushing the envelope of research with questionable case studies.

This controversial journal drew the attention of the FSU Provost:

> Our first commitment is to a rigorous scientific educational program, one that would explicitly reject some current chiropractic activities, such as many of the articles published in the *Journal of Vertebral Subluxation Research,"* he wrote. The *Journal* includes such "peer-reviewed science" as the benefits of spinal manipulation to promote fertility in infertile women, or to reverse multiple sclerosis and Parkinson's disease.[465]

The Provost's decision to cite the *JVSR* was also problematic. The original scientific mainstay of chiropractic indexed research is the *Journal of Manipulative & Physical Therapeutics (JMPT).* Indeed, the decision by the provost to reference any articles from the *JVSR* was unusual—the equivalent to quoting the *National Enquirer* instead of the *National Review* on political matters.

The image of LCC and its controversial president, Sid E. Williams, was a well-known problem within the chiropractic profession, as others testified:

> Chiropractors, who traveled from Canada and New York, acknowledged there were fringe elements that damaged the legitimacy of spinal manipulation. But, they said, with FSU's help, chiropractic medicine could trim the fringe and become a respected practice.[466]

Nonetheless, the FSU program was to research the scope of chiropractic care, which would in itself be a huge undertaking considering there are different levels of treatments within the chiropractic field as the New Zealand Inquiry noted. Foremost are the musculoskeletal disorders (Type M) like neck pain, low back pain, and headaches, the most common reasons why patients seek chiropractic care. These Type M disorders include neuromusculoskeletal disorders (NMS) that include radiating pain like sciatica.

On the other hand, some organic health problems (Type O) have also known to respond to chiropractic care as the New Zealand Inquiry had reported. Of course, this

---

465 Ibid.
466 K Miller, "Confused FSU Trustees OK Chiropractic Plan," *Palm Beach Post,* (January 15, 2005)

was a source of contention despite the emerging, albeit scant, supportive research on the neurophysiologic aspect of spine care. This explains why such research at a well-funded university was important to implement.

Most controversial, and also noted by the New Zealand Inquiry, was the vitalistic component of chiropractic philosophy extolling the body's ability to heal itself. This philosophical tenet of chiropractic had become the Achilles heel that was attacked by the medical opponents as "pseudoscience." This alluded to the cure-all notion of chiropractic care emanating from the traditional "straight" chiropractic branch—the metaphysical aspect of the Palmer tenets that are faith-based rather than science-based.

Certainly any philosophy by definition is pseudoscience, but medical critics use this to mischaracterize all of chiropractic as such. To mainstream chiropractic proponents, this philosophical issue was nothing more than a red herring issue that became a stumbling block rather than a stepping stone to better understanding the dynamics of the healing process.

This aversion to vitalism may also stem from an unnerving admission by Francis R. Collins, MD, director of the National Institutes of Health. From his personal experience, he admits as many as sixty percent of doctors and scientists are atheists.[467] Dr. Collins spoke of his experience in medical school when the prevailing academic dogma to be strictly scientific ridiculed any supernatural belief in the God factor in the healing process.

Undoubtedly this attitude made it easy for atheistic MDs to attack chiropractors who did believe in the God factor—in chiropractic parlance, the Innate Intelligence in the body that DD and BJ Palmer wrote about profusely and was attacked as quackery by the medical profession. Apparently American medicine has become so cynical that a simple belief in God is now a professional sin that should be shunned in academia. On the other hand, it may explain the callous attitude they have toward chiropractors and the feeling of superiority they have about themselves.

This became the trump card for the medical critics who fought to stop the chiropractic program at FSU. Rather than seeing the value of the main goals to explore the clinical scope of chiropractic and conduct research in an academic setting with the staff, facilities, and funding available only at a major university, this vitalistic philosophy of chiropractic became the source of ridicule for the medical opponents at FSU. What should have been an academic debate would take on the fervor of a religious war to keep the heretics out of the medical den of iniquity.

Academic Demagogues

The goal of the FSU chiropractic program was supported overwhelmingly by the Florida state legislators by the combined vote of 151-1, but that did not persuade the medical opponents who did not like the idea of any chiropractic presence on campus, no

467 Interviewed by David Hirschman, Recorded September 13, 2010, BigThink.com

matter the lofty academic goals, research objectives, or the popular support for chiropractic in the state legislature. Although all other major universities have boycotted a chiropractic curriculum, never before had medical interference with chiropractic education taken on such an open display of academic demagoguery that quickly became another huge factor in this imperfect storm in Florida.

Raymond Bellamy, MD, orthopedist and adjunct professor at FSU, became the lightning rod who led an academic revolt against this proposed chiropractic college that would have highlighted the profession's struggle to move from broad unscientific claims to evidence-based treatments.

In effect, Bellamy's effort was not a studious argument as much as it quickly digressed into a tirade of propaganda and slanderous accusations that reflected the ranting of Morris Fishbein in the 1930s rather than an informed college professor in the 2000s.

Bellamy told the media he was fearful that establishing a chiropractic school would "devalue his FSU degree, the university's reputation, and its medical school." In effect, his argument sounded eerily familiar to "race defilement" to avoid contamination by chiropractors. He was unconcerned about the quest for academic inquiry as one might expect at an institution of higher learning.

"I'm trying to avoid embarrassing FSU or threatening their funding, but it may not be possible," Bellamy said. "My sense is the only way we have of stopping this chiropractic school is getting the public educated."[468]

He also admitted to "tapping into national experts who work against chiropractic education."[469] It was shocking admission to discover that the AMA still had "national experts" whose goal was to "contain and eliminate" any presence of chiropractic on any campus as the Iowa Plan called for nearly forty years ago in 1963.

The following excerpt from the *Palm Beach Post*, "Question of Science" by Melanie Yeager, clearly illustrated the academic demagoguery espoused by Bellamy:

> A frenzy of e-mail exchanges...Conference calls and closed-door meetings, petitions circulating through the Internet...
>
> Criticism against Florida State University's planned chiropractic program has gained momentum in the last few weeks as Dr. Ray Bellamy, a longtime Tallahassee orthopedic surgeon, has quickly become the loudest naysayer in town.
>
> Calling chiropractic medicine 'pseudoscience,' Bellamy is telling all who will listen - FSU administrators, trustees, state officials - that the program needs to be stopped.
>
> "There are quacks. There is no question," Provost Larry Abele said of the chiropractic profession. "But it's incorrect to say all chiropractic is non-science and non-evidence based." And he said FSU wants to bring better scientific practices to a health service used annually by 15 million Americans.

---

468 M Yeager, "Question of Science," Tallahassee *Democrat*, (12/12/2004)
469 K Miller, ibid.

But Bellamy still thinks *most chiropractic care is based on "gobbledygook... not one shred of science."* He said it degrades FSU's entire scientific effort.

"It looks to me like the university's for sale here," Bellamy said. Bellamy's primary beef is academic and personal, not financial. He's fearful that *establishing a chiropractic school would devalue his FSU degree, the university's reputation and its medical school, where he teaches as an adjunct faculty member.*

"I'm trying to avoid embarrassing FSU or threatening their funding, but it may not be possible," Bellamy said. *"My sense is the only way we have of stopping this chiropractic school is getting the public educated."*

"Not one single major scientific contribution has been made by chiropractic in 100 years, about *the dangers of high neck manipulation* and so on, but all I ask is that the facts be given a chance," Bellamy said. [470] (emphasis added)

"... all I ask is that the facts be given a chance," Bellamy pleaded. Too bad the readers had no idea his facts were skewed, he was ignorant of the recent research endorsing chiropractic, or that he would not give the chiropractic program the same fair chance he asked for himself.

Ironically, on one hand Bellamy wants to educate the public against the proposed chiropractic school, but on the other hand, he resists educating the public (students) about chiropractic in an academic setting in a scholarly fashion at FSU. Instead, he literally took to the streets to incite a medical mob to attack chiropractic on malicious pretensions.

Bellamy's claim that chiropractic "has not one shred of science" reeks of the same unproven bias heard for years from the medical propagandists: *"everyone* knows chiropractic is an *unscientific* cult." Once again we hear Fishbein speaking.

The fact that Bellamy failed to appeal to the Florida legislature revealed his strategy was not to stage his battle until he had surrounded himself with his medical allies on the FSU campus rather than at the state capital where he would have faced 151 legislative proponents who voted for the chiropractic program.

The avoidance of a confrontation with the legislators on their turf in the capital was reminiscent of the AMA's battle in the 1960's when the Illinois State Medical Society executive director, a Mr. White, who was not an MD, challenged Doyl Taylor of the COQ when Taylor recommended the ISMS adopt the COQ's policy against chiropractors. White wrote the following response to Taylor on November 25, 1966:

> The current AMA campaign to brand all chiropractors as cultists poses a problem for us in our dealings with the general assembly. Insofar as Illinois is concerned, you should know that many members of the legislature are not convinced that most chiropractors are quacks, many have told me personally that they have been to a chiropractor or some member of their family has been to a chiropractor and they have found relief.[471]

---

470 M Yeager, ibid.

471 G McAndrews, *Wilk I* closing argument (December 9, 1980):6798

Undoubtedly the Florida legislators felt the same support for chiropractors considering they passed the bill by a vote of 151-1. Instead, the medical mob chose to fight its battle on its home turf at FSU and in the media where it could avoid any critical feedback as it would have gotten on the legislature floor.

Although Bellamy's accusations were unsubstantiated, the public and press were unaware that his own brand of academic gobbledygook and confounding accusations were derived from historic Fishbein and Committee on Quackery propaganda deeply embedded into the medical consciousness and not in scientific proof.

In retrospect, it can be seen that Bellamy's strategy was to make the proposal of a chiropractic program into a propaganda exercise instead of an academic debate by using the classical tactics of demagoguery.

Humorist H. L. Mencken once defined a demagogue as "one who will preach doctrines he knows to be untrue to men he knows to be idiots." Throughout history many demagogues have followed this doctrine which also aptly describes both Morris Fishbein and Raymond Bellamy in this medical war.

The following characterize the tactics of demagoguery specifically in this FSU fiasco:

- to misrepresent chiropractic as a "pseudoscience," "an unscientific cult," and "gobbledygook,"
- to mischaracterize chiropractic care as "dangerous" with "not one shred of evidence,"
- by not allowing any academic or public debate for chiropractors to refute these allegations with research studies,
- predicting a doomsday outcome for the university's image by suggesting "the university's for sale here," and
- to stir action among his biased supporters, mainly other medical professors on faculty, by pushing the buttons of passion, fear, and prejudice by suggesting the mere presence on campus of a chiropractic program "devalues the FSU degree."

Despite his assertion that his concern was not financial, the truth belied his claim since Bellamy had an obvious conflict of interest in this matter as "a longtime Tallahassee orthopedic surgeon" which may explain why he "has quickly become the loudest naysayer in town" according to the article in the Tallahassee *Democrat*. [472]

As Upton Sinclair once said, "It is difficult to get a man to understand something when his salary depends on his not understanding it." This truism described Bellamy perfectly—he had no interest in understanding chiropractic, just defaming it.

In the face of his obvious conflict of interest as an orthopedist and his use of blatant demagoguery, still no one in the media challenged Bellamy's lack of objectivity. Nor did any reporter do any homework that would have revealed the many research studies and guidelines that supported chiropractic and refute his claims of gobbledygook and pseudoscience.

---

472 M Yeager, "Question of Science," Tallahassee *Democrat*, (12/12/2004)

By the time this FSU fiasco took place, many research studies had already occurred, such as AHCPR, Manga, RAND, UK BEAM, to name but a few, as well as the *Wilk* trial evidence and the findings of the New Zealand Commission. Bellamy failed to mention any of these positive studies in his condemnation of chiropractic and the media failed to confront his ignorance.

Instead, the media seemed content to quote his exaggerations and pejoratives; it appeared the more sensational he became, the more copy the newspapers gave Bellamy. Undoubtedly, just as Fishbein swayed the mainstream media for decades with yellow journalism, Bellamy did the same on this battlefront to "getting the public educated"— "educated" to his Big Lie, that is.

Obviously Bellamy ignored the point of the FSU chiropractic program advocated by Jay Triano, DC, PhD, who served on the advisory committee for the FSU School. "The chiropractic profession as a whole…is ready to step up to the plate and to let its belief systems be tested scientifically," said Dr. Triano. "Let the chips fall where they may."[473]

Bellamy did admit to the *Palm Beach Post* that many patients do feel better after visiting a chiropractor, and confessed he had seen studies that showed some improvement to low-back pain, although he believed it was minimal. He also acknowledged research showing patients were more satisfied with chiropractors than with doctors.[474] Most notably, he failed to mention the call for restraint in spine surgery.

"Other than for low-back pain, in very specific instances of recent back pain, almost everything they do is bedside manner and placebo effect…Patients like to be fussed over," Bellamy said. "I think doctors need to learn to listen to patients more and be more hands-on and more caring."[475]

It was obvious Bellamy was clueless about spinal mechanics and the benefit of manipulative therapy. Instead of "fussing over" patients as he suggested, chiropractors did something more impactful when they adjusted their patients' spines to correct joint dysfunction, a physiological benefit ignored by Bellamy as an effective treatment.

Not only did he not step up to the plate for a fair fight, Bellamy rigged the game before it started with his intimidation of officials, "I'm trying to avoid embarrassing FSU or threatening their funding, but it may not be possible." He also misconstrued his support for this warfare when he told the press, "Everybody wants somebody else to kill it."[476] Considering this proposal passed the state legislature by a combined vote of 151-1, it does not appear "everybody" else wanted to see it killed, just he and his medical mob.

Indeed, the press never took Bellamy to task over his conflict of interest as an orthopedist and member of a rival trade association. Certainly, it was academic demagoguery at its worst–a medical lynch mob that fought to eliminate a rival on spurious grounds using inflammatory rhetoric with gross misrepresentation of the truth and mischaracterization

---

473 K Miller, "FSU Faculty Members Debate Chiropractic School," *Palm Beach Post*, (January 14, 2005)

474 Ibid.

475 Ibid.

476 R Matus, "Chiropractic School Angers FSU Professors," *St. Petersburg Times* (December 29, 2004)

of their opponents. This FSU mob became the driving force behind this imperfect storm with Bellamy as its ringleader.

Perhaps the most shocking question *not* asked was *how* this demagoguery happened on a public university campus where diversity of thought, scholarly debate, and intellectual inquiry are cornerstones of higher education. With emotions running on high and the strong presence of Bellamy and his medical mob, opposition to Bellamy by other academicians must have been impossible for fear of being branded as traitors, too reminiscent of Principle 3.

Did rational academicians really believe, as Bellamy claimed, that "FSU is for sale" or their degrees would be "devalued" if there were a chiropractic graduate program on campus? Did the public actually believe Bellamy when he touted chiropractic was a "pseudoscience" all the while making chiropractic services the third-most sought health care behind medical and dental care? Did the medical staff believe Bellamy when he said there was "not one shred of science" behind chiropractic after the landmark AHCPR study and numerous other studies proved otherwise? Indeed, just how gullible was the media, the faculty, and the public to his lies in light of these obvious revelations?

This alludes to a larger question: where were the stalwart defenders for academic freedom at FSU? Where was the Board of Trustees or the Provost of the University or the Board of Governors when this academic assault began? Were they also afraid of the public display of political power by the medical monarchy and, rather than confronting this medical bully, they capitulated to his whim?

Apparently George McAndrews was prophetic during the *Wilk* trial when he likened the AMA's resistance to improving chiropractic education to Southern bigotry. McAndrews noted this appalling academic apartheid created by the AMA:

> Any medical physician that tried to teach in a chiropractic college was banned. He was anathema. He was unethical...you haven't had anything like that in modern history except down in the South where they used to say you can't educate blacks. There aren't many instances of anything like that in the history of the United States, that you can't educate someone and you can exercise sufficient power to bully a university system supported by taxpayers into not giving education to someone.[477]

Instead of demeaning black Americans as unworthy of a college education alongside white students, Bellamy and his mob debased chiropractors as unworthy of a university presence alongside them. Once again there is not enough room on the medical pedestal at FSU for anyone other than MDs.

What is so shocking is the fact that this demagoguery would never have happened in any other academic discipline. For example, imagine the uproar if Democrats were able to block the study of conservative Republican politics from the FSU poli-sci program. What if faith-based Creationists were allowed to ban Darwinism and the study of evolution from the biology program? Imagine the outcry if peaceniks were able to bar the ROTC program from campus as war-mongerers.

---

477 G McAndrews, ibid. p. 3087-88.

Of course, none of this would be tolerated, but when the medical society harangues and attacks chiropractic on bogus propaganda left over from the Fishbein era, the FSU administration and media kowtowed to their demands as the medical faculty led by Bellamy goose-stepped to display their hatred of the medical heretics. This is a sad indictment of higher education at FSU, but typical of the mindset fomented by the Iowa Plan.

As Bellamy told the press, "I've got hundreds of petitions saying that this school is not wanted. It's a stupid idea."[478] On the other hand, there were probably just as many if not more fair-minded people in a silent majority who disagreed with him but where intimidated by his outlandish rhetoric. As well, where were these petitions when the state legislature voted on this issue? The time to be heard was before the vote in the legislature, not afterwards on campus by mob rule during a rebellion.

Certainly non-discriminatory and fair-minded academicians had to exist at FSU, but Bellamy and his medical mob made it impossible for them to express their opposition to his academic demagoguery, just as fair-minded Americans were voiceless when *Jim Crow* protestors were spraying Civil Rights activists with fire hoses in Selma, Alabama, not too far literally and figuratively from the mindset on the FSU campus.

Moreover, the whole idea of this program would be to separate fact from fiction as well as to do credible research into the arena of neuroscience and spinal mechanics, the subject of Dr. Triano's doctoral expertise. This field is virtually ignored due to the prevailing medical bias toward manual medicine and, particularly, chiropractic care.

Sadly, once this effort had been christened by the legislature, Bellamy as the lightning rod struck it down before it could find a safe harbor in the sanctity of the university. This imperfect storm was a disaster for both chiropractic and for academic freedom in Florida.

Unquestionably the most outlandish, if not the most childish, stunt by the medical lynch mob occurred with the distribution of the infamous "FSU Science Map." Bellamy further mocked the proposal by circulating to the press a map of the campus, placing a "Bigfoot Institute" and a "Crop Circle Simulation Laboratory" next to the proposed Chiropractic Medicine School. This map included other such whimsical landmarks like the School of Astrology, Yeti Foundation, Institute of Telekinesis, Department of ESP, Faith Healing, School of UFO Abduction Studies, School of Channeling and Remote Sensing, Foundation of Prayer Healing Studies, Creationism Foundation, Past Life Studies, College of Dowsing, Palmistry, Tarot Studies, School of Acupuncture, Institute of Tea Leaf Reading, School of Parapsychology, Pyramid Power Studies, and Alien Autopsy Laboratory.

This mockery illustrated another sad indictment of higher education at FSU. This childish stunt fanned the flames of ridicule and prejudice among the faculty and student body in a symbolic act of hanging a chiropractor in effigy.

---

478 R Matus, "Chiropractic School Angers FSU Professors," *St. Petersburg Times*, (December 29, 2004)

FSU Science Map

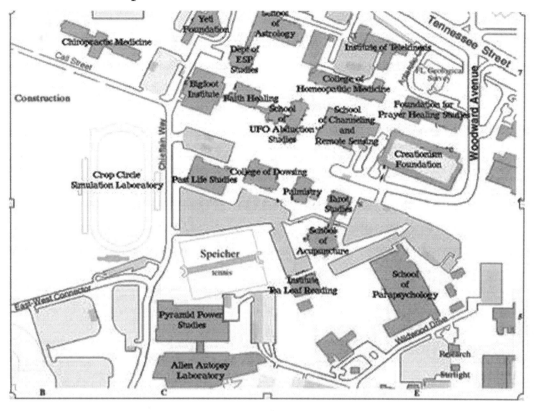

Bellamy was unapologetic when he admitted his role in this mob's behavior, "I did not design the FSU Science Map, but did forward it to others, including the press. It was sent to me by a biochemistry professor."[479] Enabling bigotry seems fine to Bellamy.

Since turnabout is fair play, let me recommend a few additions to this FSU Science Map to include:

- an Infirmary for Victims of Failed Back Surgery Syndrome,
- a Rehab Clinic for Medicinal Drug Abuse and Addiction,
- an Institute for the Study of Super Germ Infections,
- a Hospice for Late Term Abortions,
- a Rescue Shelter for People Bankrupted by Medical Bills,
- a Medical Museum of Bloodletting, Leeches, and Lobotomies.

All of these buildings could be sponsored by the Tobacco Institute that has already paid millions to the AMA to endorse its cancer-causing products in medical journals. Indeed, two can play at this game if Bellamy wants to throw mud and cast aspersions, but in this case, these are realistic and not ridiculous claims.

---

479 R Bellamy via private communication with JC Smith, Sat 6/20/2009 12:10 PM, RE: response to FSU chiropractic school commentary.

Rather than being apologetic for this childish display, Bellamy was proud of the reaction it fomented among the FSU faculty:

> There were nearly 500 email responses from the FSU science faculty opposing the chiropractic school. About 93 from the FSU College of Medicine, with about 12 clinical faculty declaring their intent to quit the teaching faculty if the chiropractic school came to FSU. I did forward to the press some of these emails opposing the chiropractic school if given permission by the sender.[480]

"I would no longer wish to volunteer my teaching energies to FSU medical school, should it encompass a school of chiropractic," said Dr. Ian Rogers, an assistant professor at FSU's Pensacola campus told the *St. Petersburg Times*. "This is plainly ludicrous!"[481]

"If they resign, so be it," said state Senator Dennis Jones, a chiropractor himself. "The instructors don't deserve to teach at FSU if they're putting their credentials with people known for promoting professional bigotry."[482]

The medical mob at FSU was, in reality, members of one trade association that politicked to have its rival association barred from campus. Once again, the medical profession lived up to its reputation as the *most terrifying trade association on earth* that extended into our university classrooms as the Iowa Plan intended.

The FSU administration also played an interesting under-handed role to sabotage the chiropractic program when it was discovered that they had already spent the $9 million allocated to the chiropractic program by the Florida legislature.[483] According to the *Palm Beach Post* newspaper, allegations swirled that the FSU president and its board conspired with the press by allowing the medical critics to impugn chiropractic in the minds of the public, faculty, and Board of Governors to justify their rejection, knowing all the time the money was already spent.

This may explain why the media was so one-sided in its account of this situation and, if a covert conspiracy did occur, it would explain why this program was blindsided so suddenly by the media and the FSU mobsters after five years of work in the Florida legislature that voted to fund $9 million for its implementation. Indeed, where were these opponents during the legislative battle when they would have met a stronger and more objective resistance from the 151 legislators who supported this bill? Apparently the medical mob was waiting in the wings to ambush the effort on the FSU campus rather than on the open battlefield of the state legislature.

The Enemy of Your Enemy is Your Friend

Another twist in this imperfect storm of the defeat of this chiropractic proposal was the fact that not all chiropractors were pleased to see the proposed public chiropractic

---

480 Ibid.
481 R Matus, "Chiropractic School Angers FSU Professors," *St. Petersburg Times* (December 29, 2004)
482 Ibid.
483 K Miller, "President Says FSU Can't Return Chiropractic School Money To State," *Palm Beach Post* (February 23, 2005)

program at FSU. Regrettably, this storm also brought together chiropractic demagogues who joined forces with the medical opposition to destroy this effort, illustrating the idiom that the enemy of your enemy is your friend.

First of all, Life Chiropractic College (LCC) in Marietta, Georgia, located only a few hundred miles north of Tallahassee, Florida, where FSU resides, opposed this proposal adamantly. LCC enjoyed a virtual monopoly in the Southeast United States as the biggest chiropractic college in the world and had no wish to see its market in Florida cut into by a state university that reportedly would have charged less in tuition, offered better funded graduate programs, and, most of all, emphasized science rather than the Palmer philosophy as its core.

It must be strongly emphasized that the majority of accredited chiropractic colleges do not subscribed to the old time BJ Palmer chiropractic tenets or the LCC style of curriculum to only "detect and correct subluxations," eschewing responsibility of primary care physicians such as differential diagnosis, the use of other treatment modalities, or the obligation to refer when necessary to medical doctors.

LCC was an easy target for Bellamy to exemplify all that was wrong with chiropractic education. The loss of accreditation at Life Chiropractic College only two years beforehand in 2002 fueled the imperfect storm of these medical critics at FSU as proof of the spurious chiropractic curriculum and academic leadership. Indeed, when the antics of LCC and Williams were called out by regional and federal accrediting bodies, it proved the need but undermined the promise of Dr. Triano when he said, "The chiropractic profession as a whole...is ready to step up to the plate and to let its belief systems be tested scientifically. Let the chips fall where they may."[484] Unfortunately, Triano had to fold his hand before the game ever started due to this imperfect storm.

Without a doubt, the scandal at LCC with its loss of accreditation made for a difficult defense by mainstream chiropractic educators such as Drs. Jay Triano and Alan Adams, heralded chiropractic academicians well-experienced in research and administration, who were slated to implement the chiropractic program at FSU.

The Florida Chiropractic Association and its legislative supporters knew another private college would not meet the needs of a university level research institution as the FSU proposal. However, the establishment of the Palmer Chiropractic campus in Port Orange made for an easy excuse by the Board of Governors to veto this proposal when the war became intense.

> Palmer College of Chiropractic Florida expects to graduate 188 students per year starting in 2006, which is more than sufficient numbers to cover AWI projected openings in Florida.[485]

> However, FSU does not need to implement a chiropractic degree program in order to participate in chiropractic research. Most of the extramural research funded by the

---

484 K Miller, "FSU Faculty Members Debate Chiropractic School," *Palm Beach Post* (January 14, 2005)
485 Minutes of the Florida Board of Governors, (January 27, 2005):14.

National Center for Complementary and Alternative Medicine has not been targeted at chiropractic care, and for the most part the organization's grants have been awarded to medical schools and research universities with strong biomedical programs.[486]

Apparently the Palmer tactic convinced the board that the state could avoid the $60+ million cost of establishing a new chiropractic college by having Palmer pick up the tab. To a cost-conscious governor and board with a skeptical attitude about chiropractic, they no doubt felt this was an excellent solution to this fiscal problem—have the renowned Palmer folks pay the bill, appease the medical critics at FSU, and still have a local chiropractic college to service the citizens of his state.

"Shame on those who continue to sow division within the chiropractic profession," said Representative Frank Farkas, DC, (R-St. Petersburg). "Palmer spent in excess of $100,000 hiring lobbyists to undermine our goals," claimed Farkas, himself a Palmer graduate. "Unfortunately, this is just another instance in which a few colleagues from within our profession are our own worst enemy."[487]

Understandably, the entire FCA administration and supporters were crestfallen by the governor's veto and the lobbying by Palmer to sabotage their effort. "It makes no sense for the governor to veto this funding when he approved a million dollar appropriation last year to implement planning for the school," said Ed Williams, DC, and the FCA's CEO emeritus. "Palmer's meddling clearly confused the issue," he added. Palmer's unfortunate and atrocious timing and aggressive lobbying activity gave the Governor an 'out.' This is yet another classic chiropractic scenario of shooting ourselves in the foot."[488]

"The whole purpose of this project was to provide the same in-state, low-cost educational opportunity for chiropractic students as there is for every other major profession," explained Dr. Dennis Jones, R-Treasure Island, former Florida House of Representatives Speaker Pro Tem and practicing chiropractor, who authored the original legislation. He added: "A private institution cannot increase the number of minority candidates. It cannot attract anywhere near the same level of research dollars. It will not increase the acceptance and prestige of our profession." [489]

Political Battle

This conflict of power within the state government bodies became another factor in this imperfect storm, creating a face-off between the Board of Governors and legislators. "We don't know what their authority is or isn't," said Dr. Jones.[490]

The chiropractic school became a flashpoint in the debate because traditionally, university programs are proposed and vetted by faculty members before reaching trustees

486 Ibid.p.16.
487 Editorial Staff, "FCA Fulminates over Funding Veto," *Dynamic Chiropractic* 19/16 (July 30, 2001)
488 Ibid.
489 Ibid.
490 "Board Turns Down Chiropractic School," Knight Ridder/Tribune Business News (January 2005)

for approval. Since the constitutional amendment creating the Board of Governors at the level of the State Board of Education, there had been confusion over who has oversight power in the university system: lawmakers in the legislature, the board of governors with the Board of Education or individual trustees of the University.

"This process has been turned upside down," said Larry Abele, FSU provost. The FSU's Board of Trustees eventually did not even take a position on the chiropractic school. Instead, University Trustees forwarded to the Board of Governors over the Board of Education a proposal for a chiropractic school, but said they could not support or oppose it until it had gone through the proper faculty review.[491]

Setting the stage for a showdown with the Florida Legislature, the new Board of Governors that oversees Florida's public universities, created just two years before by a constitutional amendment approved by voters, asserted that Florida State University must get its approval for a new chiropractic college, even though lawmakers had approved the college's creation and guaranteed it $9 million a year.[492]

The legislative process was "totally backward from the usual method of starting new academic programs," according to Bellamy. "This alarmed many in the state's universities as a dangerous precedent and a loss of control by those entrusted to make these decisions." [493]

Bellamy noted "because of the confusion arising out of the powers created by the new constitutional amendment, the FSU Trustees essentially punted the issue to the Board of Governors, which voted it down by a wide margin, 10 to 3. Interestingly, at the Board meeting, three chiropractors spoke out *against* the school." [494]

The whole idea of the FSU chiropractic program was to access the resources of a major university to investigate these claims. Dr. Triano pointed out: "It's not what we do, but what we *say* about what we do that matters most."[495] Triano admitted his torment with the faith-based dogma within the chiropractic profession. "How long will we let these radical few DCs drive the agenda of the majority for this profession? Who's in charge of chiropractic's destiny?"[496]

Storm Damage

The imperfect storm finally came to an end, but not before leaving destruction in its path. The Board of Governors voted down the proposal after years of hard work by the FCA and supporters in the state legislature whose hopes were capsized.

---

491 Ibid.
492 G Fineout, "Turf Battle Shapes Up For Control Of Tuition Rates At Florida Universities," The *Miami Herald* (November 2004)
493 R Bellamy via private communication with JC Smith (07-12-09)
494 R Bellamy via private communication with JC Smith (07-12-09)
495 JJ Triano, ACC-RAC Plenary Session, Las Vegas, 2005.
496 Ibid.

After the medical demagogues succeeded to kill the FSU chiropractic program, Raymond Bellamy could not hide his elation. "I'm delighted. I'm ready for the champagne," he told the media.[497]

Spoken like a conqueror touting his victory, his attitude resembled the Morris Fishbein supremacist attitude that still permeates the medical profession: *"Scientific medicine absorbs from them that which is good, if there is any good, and then they die."*[498]

Bellamy also spoke of his greatest fear–the enhanced image of chiropractors. Certainly like many MDs, he cannot tolerate any other professionals to stand aside him atop his pedestal:

> To have a 'research presence' for chiropractic on the FSU campus would be a major advance in prestige for chiropractic but would amount to chiropractic forcing themselves on the campus by political means when *all other scientific disciplines represented on campus were invited and embraced by the scientific community...*
>
> *Florida taxpayers would then be out many millions of scarce education dollars with nothing to show for it.* Or, as FSU Trustee Manny Garcia succinctly put it, "Why should we be the guinea pig?"[499] (emphasis added)

Bellamy's attitude that chiropractic should be "invited and embraced by the scientific community" is nonsense considering the political nature of medical academia. Bellamy makes FSU appear as a white country club only inviting their white friends rather than a club based on members with merit. Obviously he is more concerned about the medical "race defilement" image than advancing science.

The fact is Dr. Bellamy knows that healthcare has always been political and he politicized this program not to protect the university's image as much as to protect his own profession's dominance. Certainly, if Dr. Bellamy and the FSU faculty were so self-assured that chiropractic is placebo, why then would they not want to "let the chips fall where they may" as Triano suggested and let chiropractic hang itself?

Bellamy suggested it would be a waste of "millions of scarce education dollars" when he actually was ducking the comparative effectiveness studies that would emerge showing the superiority of manipulative therapy over medical methods. According to Bellamy:

> Especially concerned was the sciences faculty, who saw chiropractic as ignoring the scientific method and the use of the university to establish scientific credibility as inappropriate...The FSU faculty and other opponents were well aware that the proposed school was an attempt to bring scientific respectability to chiropractic.[500]

This comment is perplexing: "the proposed school was an attempt to bring scientific respectability to chiropractic." Is it a crime to bring greater respectability to any science? Considering the many international research studies that endorse spinal manipulation, the research already exists to bring respect to chiropractic care.

---

497 M Yeager, "State Board Votes Against Program," *Democrat* Staff writer, (1/28/05)
498 M Fishbein, *Medical Follies*, New York, Boni & Liveright (1925):43.
499 R Bellamy via private communication with JC Smith, 07-12-09.
500 R Bellamy via private communication with JC Smith (07-12-09)

Bellamy admitted the faculty did not vet chiropractic, nor had they studied the research like AHCPR that showed the effectiveness of chiropractic care. Nor did anyone on the faculty visit a reputable chiropractic campus to review the curriculum or meet with the faculty. Instead they assumed the worst undoubtedly from the loss of accreditation stemming from Life Chiropractic College and, of course, the AMA's belief that *"everybody knows chiropractic is an unscientific cult."* Certainly it would be difficult for members of the *most terrifying trade association on earth* to be objective about their arch rival.

Freedom of Choice

Just as Fishbein accused people who used chiropractic as suffering from "abject ignorance,"[501] Bellamy also chided the idea of freedom of choice in healthcare since he believed patients were too gullible to know what was best for themselves. In private discussion with Bellamy, he responded to my claim that he had prevented academic freedom and the right of patients to have their own treatment of choice:

> Your comments about "academic freedom" miss the mark by a wide margin. *Academic freedom does not mean that all comers get a place at the table, no matter how implausible their ideas.* If that were true the map created by the FSU professor you mentioned would become a reality. [502] (emphasis added)

If it were up to Bellamy, he might have also added, "no matter how *plausible* their ideas" since only medical methods are welcomed in his university. The FSU Science Map made that point perfectly clear. The academic dishonesty at FSU is mind-boggling.

Bellamy's brand of freedom of choice in treatment was similar to his version of academic freedom:

> You mention the "right" of the patient to choose. This "right" is illusory if the patient is without sufficient information to evaluate any particular treatment and make an informed choice. Yet chiropractors have insufficient evidence upon which to base their claims, thus requiring the help of a state university to sort things out. *Are you arguing for a "right" to choose implausible treatments?*[503] (emphasis added)

It appears Bellamy has a double standard when it comes to research: while the medical profession receives billions for research, when chiropractors want the same opportunity, he demeans this request of "requiring the help of a state university to sort things out."

Furthermore, his assertion, "Are you arguing for a 'right' to choose implausible treatments?" is unreasonable considering the volume of research supporting chiropractic care as, in fact, very plausible care. His attitude illustrates the Fishbein supremacist belief that there are *right* ways to get well (drugs and surgery) and *wrong* ways to get well (everything else).

---

501 M Fishbein, *Medical Follies*, New York, Boni & Liveright (1925):24-5
502 Ibid.
503 R Bellamy via private communication with JC Smith, 07-12-09.

Undoubtedly the most bewildering and offensive response by Bellamy concerned the lack of academic freedom at FSU: "Not opposing chiropractic presence at FSU would have been an egregious lack of academic freedom."[504]

> Do you really think that the academicians, business men and women, scientists, lawyers, journalists and others who populate these groups are such dimwits that they cannot make up their own minds? [505]

Obviously Bellamy ignored the vote of 151-1 by the Florida state legislature who made up their own minds to vote in favor of this program. In his mind, as long as he can speak out and shout down his opponents with misinformation, that alone constitutes freedom of speech.

"There are 160 of us up here with full-time professional staffs, and it passed without hardly any dissenting votes," Senator Jones said, referring to his fellow legislators. "Then you have a volunteer board of 17 with limited staff and they vote against it. What does that say to Floridians?"[506] It says mob rule supersedes the will of the legislature.

Doorway Diplomacy

Dr. Benjamin Rush warned of this repression of freedom in health care when he wrote:

> Unless we put medical freedoms into the Constitution, the time will come when medicine will organize into an undercover dictatorship.[507]

Certainly Raymond Bellamy is the embodiment of the "undercover dictatorship" at FSU. His book-burning mindset will go down in the annals of academia alongside the book-burning policy of Joseph Goebbels. Indeed, Thomas Jefferson must be turning over in his grave by this perversion of the First Amendment.

As a graduate of the University of California during the aftermath of the Free Speech Movement in the 1960s, I find Bellamy's version of academic freedom to be the antithesis of what I experienced at Berkeley—censorship is not academic freedom by any sense; denying speech to anyone due to affiliation with a political party or trade association is not the American principle of free speech.

What escapes Dr. Bellamy's sense of freedom is the fact that he does not realize we are colleagues in the battle against pain and suffering, our mutual enemy. In this light, the enemy of my enemy should make us friends. Sadly, the fact that the medical profession has yet to understand this simple truth keeps the hundred year medical war waging against chiropractors.

---

504 R Bellamy via private communication with JC Smith, July 12, 2009.
505 Ibid.
506 K Miller, "Board Snubs Legislature, Rejects Chiropractic School," *Palm Beach Post* (Jan 28, 2005)
507 ER Booth, *History of Osteopathy and Twentieth Century Medical Practice*, Cincinnati: Caxton Press, 1905 (1924):312.

The FSU project would have cleared the air on many issues and either proved chiropractic to be placebo as Bellamy contends or else it would have brought an ageless healing art to the forefront to help millions of people who suffer from both musculoskeletal disorders and those who suffer from spinovisceral reflex nerve disorders that mimic serious visceral disorders.

Bellamy contends the medical mob at FSU was acting out of academic integrity, but I believe they were actually medical bigots afraid to let the subservient class of healthcare practitioners, chiropractors, on campus.

This over-reaction to the integration of chiropractic into the medical program on the FSU campus is clearly reminiscent of the days of racial desegregation in the South. Just as former Governor George Wallace stood in the doorway at the University of Alabama in 1963 to prevent the entrance of black students after President Kennedy sent in the federal troops to desegregate the University of Alabama, Bellamy and his medical mob did the same at FSU.

While 'BAMA benefitted in the long run from integration not just on the football field, but in the classroom and in a pluralistic academic community of students of all races, so too the FSU program could have led to discoveries far beyond the present known benefits of chiropractic care into the area of neurophysiology, spinovisceral reflexes, and Type O disorders.

Gov. Wallace demonstrated his racial politics to the world and Dr. Raymond Bellamy felt justified with the same intense prejudice to keep the "nigger-chiropractors" out of FSU. Please excuse this epithet, but it seems appropriate for the dire situation at FSU to subordinate an entire profession to another on spurious grounds.

Bellamy's doorway diplomacy killed this golden opportunity to expand upon the science of chiropractic care. His demagoguery was not only hurtful to the chiropractic profession, on a larger note, considering the $100 to $200 billion dollars spent annually on spine care, the potential savings to our economy would have been enormous. [508] Indeed, the substitution of chiropractic care for medical care in this epidemic of back pain is the most overlooked potential savings in healthcare reform today.

Obviously the failure by FSU to implement the hopeful chiropractic program was a huge disappointment to members of the chiropractic profession who wanted to see an evidence-based research program that was well-funded unlike the research departments at small chiropractic colleges that, in fact, still wither on the vine for lack of funding.

The Board's veto was the final blow of a terrible storm during the FCA's five-year effort to have a chiropractic program implemented in their state's university system. Regrettably, the real damage from this imperfect storm to the FCA and the mainstream chiropractic profession was not just in the dollars spent and broken dreams, but also in academic esteem and the likelihood that chiropractic education might someday be incorporated into mainstream universities as it should be.

The hidden agenda here is not the worthiness of chiropractic science or research or treatments—the facts are clear there is validity to all three. Either way, the truth would

---

508 RD Guyer, Presidential address, "The Paradox In Medicine Today—Exciting Technology And Economic Challenges, *The Spine Journal*, 8/2 (March/April 2008):279-285.

have been found in the freedom of academia rather than killed by the hands of political medicine and academic demagogues.

Until every public university offers a pre-chiropractic program and until every state-sponsored health science program offers a graduate level chiropractic program, we must consider the medical apartheid continues and that this imperfect storm has not truly ended.

It is time to weather the storm, it is past time to stop burning books, and it is time to let there be light shined on chiropractic in our nation's universities.

Rad Science

The art, science, and philosophy of chiropractic were radical in many ways from medical science—a paradoxical philosophy with an unorthodox science that required a skillful art. The call for chiropractic care grows louder as researchers now implore for the restraint of back surgeries. The first chiropractor was not unscientific as accused by his medical opponents, but clearly a man who was ahead of his time.

Restraint & Revelations

"Low back pain has been a 20th century health care disaster.
Medical care certainly has not solved the everyday symptom of low
back pain and even may be reinforcing and exacerbating the problem."

Gordon Waddell, DSc, MD, FRCS, author of *The Back Pain Revolution* [509]

The late Robert Mendelsohn, MD, author of *Confessions of a Medical Heretic,* once quipped, "Anyone who has a back surgery without seeing a chiropractor first should also have his head examined."[510]

His concern is just as true today as it was in the 1980s before the tsunami of research began to swell in the 1990s to criticize the massive amounts of unnecessary spine surgery that began the call for restraint and reform in spinal care. Albeit long overdue, the tide is suddenly rising to new heights with increasing numbers of spine experts embracing Dr. Mendelsohn's opinion.

The AMA's war against chiropractors has been a war against all humanity for creating the pandemic of pain and the billions of dollars lost to unnecessary drugs, shots, MRIs, and back surgeries that could have been avoided by using chiropractors instead. It is unconscionable the government has not recognized the cost-effectiveness of chiropractic care, but it is a sad indictment of the power of the medical monarchy.

---

509 G Waddell and OB Allan, "A Historical Perspective On Low Back Pain And Disability, "*Acta Orthop Scand* 60 (suppl 234), (1989)
510 RS Mendelsohn, *Confessions of a Medical Heretic,* Published by Contemporary Books (1980)

"Low Back Pain Medical Industrial Complex"

Indeed, it is bitter medicine to swallow for the medical profession to realize why back surgery "has been accused of leaving more tragic human wreckage in its wake than any other operation in history."[511] The facts are clear given the research showing the dire need for a change in the treatment for back pain.

A recent distressing article, "Are We Making Progress?" by Glenn Pransky, MD, Jeffrey M. Borkan, MD, Amanda E Young, PhD, Daniel C. Cherkin, PhD, discussed the ineffective treatments, iatrogenesis, and the "Low Back Pain Medical Industrial Complex" at the Tenth International Forum for Primary Care Research on Low Back Pain in June 2010 at the Harvard School of Public Health in Boston, Massachusetts.

Concerns about ineffective treatments and iatrogenesis were discussed at greater length here than at any previous Forum since the Forums began in 1995. Research results may have led to reduction in the use of potentially harmful and unproven therapies such as bed rest and intradiscal therapy, but other harmful treatments may have taken their place, especially in the United States, such as the rise in opioids, epidural steroid injections, and spine surgery.

> Despite explosive growth in the number, range, and quality of investigations of LBP in primary care since 1990, there was a sense at recent Forums that progress in reducing the medical and economic impact or burden of suffering from LBP has been disappointing. Few treatments presented at earlier Forums withstood the test of randomized controlled trials, and the "LBP epidemic" remains a burden in Western countries. Evidence-based guidelines and systematic reviews flourished, but seem to have had little impact on actual primary care practices.[512]

This paradox highlighted the "importance of understanding what value patients find from treatments of questionable effectiveness, and what can be done to better inform patients of the benefits and risks of treatments, especially those with significant risks of adverse effects."

The authors alluded to but avoided the obvious reasons why patients select questionable treatments and what can be done to better inform them. Of course, the medical war of propaganda is the largest problem when biased PCPs refuse to refer to chiropractors and, secondly, the huge profits made from drugs, shots, and surgery also discourages the referrals to chiropractors. Indeed, professional amnesia, as Dr. Anthony Rosner mentioned, is plainly evident in this question.

---

511 G Waddell and OB Allan, "A Historical Perspective On Low Back Pain And Disability, "*Acta Orthop Scand* 60 (suppl 234),
(1989)

512 D Cherkin, FM Kovacs, P Croft, J Borkan, NE Foster, B Oberg, G Urrutia, J Zaore. "The Ninth International Forum For Primary Care Research On Low Back Pain. International Organizing Committee Of The Ninth International Forum For Primary Care Research On Low Back Pain And All The Participants," *Spine* 34 (2009):304-307

The authors were very aware that "we have an industry (a 'low back pain medical industrial complex'), not a system of health improvement, especially in the United States, seemed inescapable to many. Such a complex may have more to do with economics than with evidence-based treatment approaches."

However, the authors admitted "Given the negative impact on fragile national economies, the continued use of expensive treatments for back pain that have real risks and questionable benefits would appear to be unjustified as well as unsustainable."[513]

Despite these revelations, the call for restraint and reform in spinal care has fallen on deaf ears in America as the statistics show these spine surgeries are escalating despite the warnings, the poor outcomes, and the huge costs of these ineffective treatments. Indeed, the authors were right when they concluded this problem has "more to do with economics than with evidence-based treatment approaches."

In fact, doctors and hospitals are making huge profits off the backs of unsuspecting patients who are not told there may be a better and cheaper way to solve their back pain with chiropractic care or other non-invasive methods.

From *Dissent in Medicine: Nine Doctors Speak Out*, David Spodick, Professor of Medicine at the University of Massachusetts, stated that "Surgery is the sacred cow of our health-care system and surgeons are the sacred cowboys who milk it."[514] Indeed, spine surgery has become the cash cow in the medical world and will only grow larger unless sensibility prevails over profiteering.

The call for restraint of surgery is coming from many international spine researchers who are increasingly upset with the poor results; in fact, every major study now admits to this glaring problem. Most importantly, given the continued ineffectiveness and overuse of spine surgery, people need to understand the risks and costs before embarking on a path to potential failed back surgery. People also need to know there is a better solution—chiropractic care—that has finally gotten the recognition it has long deserved.

In his book, *The Back Pain Revolution*,[515] Gordon Waddell, DSc, MD, FRCS, and director of an orthopedic surgical clinic for over twenty years in Glasgow, Scotland, has determined that back surgery is mostly ineffective and unnecessary, and there are very disturbing reasons why this disaster has happened:

> "Low back pain has been a 20th century health care disaster. Medical care certainly has not solved the everyday symptom of low back pain and even may be reinforcing and

513 Glenn Pransky MD, Jeffrey M Borkan MD, Amanda E Young PhD, Daniel C Cherkin PhD, "Are We Making Progress?" The Tenth International Forum for Primary Care Research on Low Back Pain, Boston International Forum X, Primary Care Research on Low Back Pain, Boston, Massachusetts, United States of America, June 14–17, 2009

514 R Mendelsohn, G Crile, S Epstein, H Heinlich, A Levin, E Pickney, D Spodick, R Moskowitz, G White, *Dissent in Medicine: Nine Doctors Speak Out*, Contemporary Books, (1985)

515 G Waddell, The *Back Pain Revolution*, Philadelphia, Churchill Livingstone Inc, (1998)

exacerbating the problem...It [back surgery] has been accused of leaving more tragic human wreckage in its wake than any other operation in history."[516]

Richard Deyo, MD, MPH, a leading spine researcher and outspoken critic of spine surgery now at Kaiser Permanente Professor of Evidence-Based Family Medicine at Oregon Health and Science University in Portland, Oregon, mentioned to *The New York Times* that the spine profession is ignoring this call for restraint:

> People say, "I'm not going to put up with it," and we in the medical profession have turned to ever more aggressive medication, narcotic medication, and more invasive surgery.[517]

In his 2009 article, "Overtreating Chronic Back Pain: Time to Back Off?" Dr. Deyo speaks of the increase as well as shortcomings of the medical spine treatments in the U.S.:

> Jumps in imaging, opioid prescriptions, injections, and fusion surgery might be justified if there were substantial improvements in patient outcomes. Even in successful trials of these treatments, though, most patients continue to experience some pain and dysfunction.
>
> Prescribing yet more imaging, opioids, injections, and operations is not likely to improve outcomes for patients with chronic back pain. We must rethink chronic back pain at fundamental levels.[518]

Dr. Deyo is not alone in his call for reform in spine care. The editors of The BACK*LETTER*®, a newsletter from the Department of Orthopedic Surgery at Georgetown Medical Center in Washington, DC, agree with his frustration with the medical approach:

> *The world of spinal medicine, unfortunately, is producing patients with failed back surgery syndrome at an alarming rate...*There is growing frustration over the lack of progress in the surgical treatment of degenerative disc disease. Despite a steady stream of technological innovations over the past 15 years—from pedical screws to fusion cages to artificial discs—*there is little evidence that patient outcomes have improved...*Many would like to see an entirely new research effort in this area, to see whether degenerative disc disease and/or discogenic pain are actually diagnosable and treatable conditions.[519],[520] (emphasis added)

Dr. Deyo commented in an article in *The New York Times* when he mentioned the failings of the medical model for back pain:

> I think the truth is we have perhaps oversold what we have to offer. All the imaging we do, all the drug treatments, all the injections, all the operations have benefit for some

516 G Waddell and OB Allan, "A Historical Perspective On Low Back Pain And Disability, "*Acta Orthop Scand* 60 (suppl 234), (1989)

517 G Kolata, "With Costs Rising, Treating Back Pain Often Seems Futile" by *NY Times* (February 9, 2004)

518 RA Deyo, SK Mirza, JA Turner, BI Martin, "Overtreating Chronic Back Pain: Time to Back Off?" *J Am Board Fam Med.* 22/1 (2009):62-68. (http://www.medscape.com/viewarticle/586950)

519 *The* BACK *LETTER*, 12/7 (July 2004):79

520 *The* BACK *Page* editorial, *The* BACK *LETTER*, 20/7 (March 2005):84

patients. But in each of these situations, *we've begun using those tests and treatments more widely than science would really support.* [521] (emphasis added)

He also admitted in another interesting interview that:

> I think we need to be more careful about using our treatments in unproven circumstances. Our data, showing increasing costs without apparent benefit, may be a consequence of "promiscuous prescribing" in the broad sense. Offering poorly documented treatments may simply be counterproductive. Though some would say in the absence of proof we should do what seems reasonable, I would argue that *we may be subjecting patients to side effects and costs without knowing if there's a benefit.*" [522] (emphasis added)

Researchers Bhandari *et al.* now suggest in their article, *"Does Lumbar Surgery For Chronic Low-Back Pain Make A Difference?"* that lumbar surgery for chronic low-back pain makes no real difference in outcomes two years after surgery:

> Lumbar fusion surgery in patients with chronic low-back pain does not appear to offer any major benefit in outcomes over conservative rehabilitation programs incorporating physical activity and cognitive–behavioral therapy. Patients undergoing lumbar fusion may have a slightly lower but clinically unimportant decrease in disability scores in exchange for an increased risk of complications, higher medical costs and *no difference in quality of life at 2 years after surgery.*[523] (emphasis added)

Another study conducted by Deyo and Cherkin in 1994 compared international rates of back surgeries and found the startling fact that the rate of American surgery is unusually excessive and directly attributed to the supply of spine surgeons:

> *The rate of back surgery in the United States was at least 40% higher than any other country and was more than five-times those in England and Scotland.* Back surgery rates increased almost linearly with the per capita supply of orthopedic and neurosurgeons in that country.[524] (emphasis added)

Does this mean Americans' backs are five-times weaker than people from Great Britain or does it mean U.S. surgeons do too many unnecessary surgeries? Obviously the real difference is a profit-motivated healthcare system in the U.S. compared to the not-for-profit National Health Services in the U.K.

"While many surgeons are careful about which patients they recommend for spine operations, some are not so discriminating," says Dr. Doris K. Cope, professor and vice chair for pain medicine at the University of Pittsburgh School of Medicine. "It's a case of, if you have a hammer, everything looks like a nail."[525]

---

521 T Parker-Pope, "Americans Spend More to Treat Spine Woes," *New York Times* (February 13, 2008).
522 *The* BACK *LETTER*® 33 23/3 (2008)
523 M Bhandari, B Petrisor, JW Busse and B Drew, "Does Lumbar Surgery For Chronic Low-Back Pain Make A Difference?" *CMAJ*, 173/4 (August 16, 2005); doi:10.1503/cmaj.050884.
524 DC Cherkin, RA Deyo, *et al.* "An International Comparison Of Back Surgery Rates," *Spine*, 19/11 (June 2004):1201-1206.
525 L Carroll, "Back Surgery May Backfire on Patients in Pain," MSNBC.com, (10/14/2010)

Alf L. Nachemson, MD, regarded as the godfather of the evidence-based spine care movement, admits only one in five lumbar fusion patients are relieved of their pain:

> Fusion surgery is typically not a cure and should not be presented as such. Few patients experience complete relief of back pain following surgery. *Only one in five patients in these studies became pain-free.*[526] (emphasis added)

Dr. Deyo mentioned the sentiments of other ethical spine surgeons in his book, *Hope or Hype: The Obsession with Medical Advances and the High Cost of False Promises*:

> Some surgeons, like Dr. Edward Benzel at the Cleveland Clinic Spine Institute, believe that too much spine fusion surgery is being performed. Benzel estimated to the *New York Times* that *less than half the spinal fusions being performed were appropriate.* Dr. Zoher Ghogawala, a Yale neurosurgeon, agreed that too much fusion surgery is done, saying, *"I see too many patients who are recommended for fusion that absolutely do not need it."*[527] (emphasis added)

Other medical researchers have also concluded that spinal surgery is unnecessary in most cases. At the University of Miami Comprehensive Pain and Rehabilitation Center, Dr. HL Rosomoff concluded:

> *Low back pain in the population at large is not usually a surgical problem* and the chances of there being significant pathology requiring surgical or other forms of intervention *may be less than 1% of those affected.*...Low back pain per se is in the majority not a neurologic problem, an orthopedic problem, or a neurosurgical problem, so that consultation with these groups, unless there are strong suspicions otherwise, has limited value.[528] (emphasis added)

Dr. Rosomoff called a moratorium on back surgeries when he realized, after two weeks of rehabilitation, his back patients no longer required surgery. "Following this kind of concept, you can eliminate 99 percent of the surgical cases. In fact, the incidence of surgery if one really looks at this appropriately is one in 500."[529]

Not only can most spine surgeries be avoided, research also found that the Fortune 500 companies spend over $500 million a year on avoidable back surgeries for their workers and lose as much as $1.5 billion in indirect costs associated with these procedures in the form of missed work and lost productivity, according to a two-year study by Consumer's Medical Resource (CMR).[530]

This CMR study, "Back Surgery: A Costly Fortune 500 Burden," found one out of three workers recommended for back surgery said they avoided an unnecessary procedure

---

526 RA Deyo, A Nachemson, SK Mirza, "Spinal-Fusion Surgery—The Case for Restraint," *New England Journal of Medicine* 350/7 (February 12, 2004):643-644

527 RA Deyo and DL Patrick, *Hope or Hype: The Obsession with Medical Advances and the High Cost of False Promises* (2002):191.

528 HL Rosomoff, RS Rosomoff, "Low Back Pain. Evaluation And Management In The Primary Care Setting," *Medical Clinics of North American*, 83/3 (May 1999):643-62.

529 M Widen, "Back Specialists Are Discouraging The Use Of Surgery," American Academy of Pain Medicine, 17th annual meeting, Miami Beach, Fl. (Feb. 14-18, 2001)

530 "FORTUNE 500s Waste Over $500 Million a Year on Unnecessary Back Surgeries for Workers," Consumer's Medical Resource, (July 21, 2008)

after being given independent, high-quality medical research on their diagnosed condition and treatment options. In addition, those patients that refused surgery and opted for alternative and less invasive procedures to treat their back pain reported healthier and more personally satisfying outcomes.

According to Lynn Johnson, MD, director of the Center for Pain Medicine of North Carolina, while back surgery has a place, he admits there are too many surgeries being done, and that most doctors fail to apply conservative measures such as chiropractic, physical therapy, and minimally invasive techniques before suggesting surgery.[531] Dr. Lynn Johnson believes:

> Just about any approach is better than having surgery because all the studies have shown that, if you take a surgical population and non-surgical population, they all seem to do the same in five years.[532]

The public is rarely told by their physicians that studies now show patients are more satisfied with chiropractic care than medical care. One study confirmed that patients preferred chiropractic care than other treatments for low back pain. TW Meade, MD, of the Wolfson Institute of Preventive Medicine, London, England, surveyed patients three years after treatment and found that "significantly more of those patients who were treated by chiropractic expressed satisfaction with their outcome at three years than those treated in hospitals—84.7 percent vs. 65.5 percent."[533]

Undoubtedly, the dagger in the spine surgeon's back occurred in 1994 when the U.S. Public Health Service's Agency for Health Care Policy & Research (AHCPR) study stated the following finding printed in its Patient Guide:

> Even having a lot of back pain does not by itself mean you need surgery. *Surgery has been found to be helpful in only 1 in 100 cases of low back problems.* In some people, surgery can even cause more problems. This is especially true if your only symptom is back pain.[534] (emphasis added)

These warnings are escalating recently as more researchers investigate medical spine care and the call for restraint is growing from a whisper to a roar. Certainly when leading medical professionals from prestigious universities, journals, and the U.S. Public Health Service now openly and loudly decry the onslaught and ineffectiveness of spine surgery, this has become an epidemic of legitimate concern for patients.

Challenging Revelations

Not only is there a loud call for restraint on spine surgeries, there is growing evidence that many types of medical theories and spine treatments are now unsupported by science,

---

531 M Widen, ibid.

532 Ibid.

533 TW Meade, Letter To The Editor, *British Medical Journal* 319/57 (July 3, 1999).

534 Ibid. p. 12.

ineffective in outcomes, and very expensive. Certainly, if there is a paradox in spine care today, it rests with the medical model, not chiropractic.

Spine researcher Chien-Jen Hsu, MD, admitted in the journal *Spine*:

> By far the number one reason back surgeries are not effective and some patients experience continued pain after surgery is because the lesion that was operated on is not, in fact, the cause of the patient's pain. [535]

How can this be, considering the vast majority of spine surgeons in these cases rely almost exclusively upon the images shown by the MRI scans that clearly reveal the abnormal discs as the supposed underlying cause of back and leg pain? Patients are then routinely told disc surgery is, of course, the only solution to this problem. If the disc is the problem, and surgery is the answer, why are the results so poor?

This is the biggest paradox (and cover-up) in medicine today. Indeed, *Caveat Emptor* (Buyer Beware) is the best policy when it comes to back surgery based solely on an MRI done and performed by a surgeon who does not recommend chiropractic care first. Let the experts explain why.

Revelation #1: The Disc Theory is Dead

The Dynasty of the Disc began in 1934 when two spine surgeons, W.J. Mixter, MD, and J.S. Barr, MD, from the Massachusetts General Hospital, Boston, performed the very first spine surgery for herniated discs. William Mixter first recognized the importance of herniated intervertebral discs in causing nerve root and spinal cord compression syndromes caused by pressure from bulging or herniated discs. In collaboration with Joseph Barr, an orthopedic surgeon, this led to the first disc surgery. [536]

Most interesting in the original article by these surgical pioneers is their *recommendation to use conservative care before surgery*, a point disregarded nowadays by many surgeons. In 1941, Mixter and Barr wrote:

> "Conservative treatment should be tried in every case of suspected protrusion of the intervertebral discs unless there is obvious serious nerve-root pressure, as shown by objective sensory or motor disturbance."[537]

However, the conservative care procedures recommended by Mixter and Barr—bed rest and supports—are now deemed supportive but ineffective as standalone therapies, illustrating how conventional wisdom has changed. If Mixter and Barr had not suffered from medical bias toward chiropractic care, their patients would have certainly been

---

535 CJ Hsu, *et al.* "Clinical Follow Up After Instrumentation-Augmented Lumbar Spinal Surgery in Patients with Unsatisfactory Outcomes. In Journal of Neurosurgery," Spine 5/4 (October 2006):281-286.
536 WJ Mixter and JS Barr, "Rupture of the Intervertebral Disc With Involvement Of The *Spinal* Cord," *New England Journal of Medicine* 211 (1934):210-214.
537 WJ Mixter and JS Barr, "Posterior Protrusion Of The Lumbar Intervertebral Discs," *Journal of Bone and Joint Surgery,* 23 (1941):444-456. Orthopaedic and Neurosurgical Services of the Massachusetts General Hospital, Boston.

helped more effectively. Recall in the 1930s and 1940s that Fishbein's war against chiropractic was at its height; undoubtedly making any recommendation of manipulation by a chiropractor was a very politically-incorrect suggestion.

Today the disc theory is undoubtedly the most misleading diagnosis in American spine medicine, having been seriously questioned since 1986 and essentially disproven in 1990 by MRI research. Like Typhoid Mary, this misdiagnosis just hangs on to infect more people. It is past time to put this theory to bed because it has resulted in hundreds of thousands, if not millions, of unnecessary spine surgeries, leaving a wake of disability and suffering.

The fundamental flaw of the spine surgeons rests with their emphasis on MRIs to detect *pathoanatomical* disorders (disc abnormalities, arthritis, bone spurs) rather than the emphasis on *pathophysiologic* disorders (malfunctioning due to a combination of joint dysfunction, malalignment, loss of flexibility, muscle weakness, and compression). What matters most, as studies now confirm, is how the spine bears weight and functions, not just the amount of disc degeneration.

This renaissance in spine diagnosis began in 1990 when research by Scott Boden *et al.*[538] followed in 1994 by a supportive study by Maureen Jensen *et al.*[539] found no clear correlation between disc abnormalities and back pain.

Dr. Boden's study performed MRI scans of sixty-seven asymptomatic patients who had *never* had low-back pain, sciatica, or neurogenic claudication. These scans were interpreted by three neuro-radiologists who had no knowledge about the subjects. About one-third of the subjects had a substantial abnormality. In the sixty years or older group, the findings were abnormal on about 57 percent of the scans: 36 per cent had a herniated nucleus pulposus and 21 per cent had spinal stenosis. 35 per cent had degenerative or bulging discs.[540] *Yet none of these patients had any symptoms.*

The authors concluded:

> In view of these findings in asymptomatic subjects, we concluded that abnormalities on magnetic resonance images must be strictly correlated with age and any clinical signs and symptoms before operative treatment is contemplated.

In a follow-up study in 2003, Boden reaffirmed his previous findings:

> It should be emphasized that back pain is not necessarily correlated or associated with morphologic or biomechanical changes in the disc. The vast majority of people with back pain aren't candidates for disc surgery.[541]

---

538 SD Boden, DO Davis, TS Dina, NJ Patronas, SW Wiesel, "Abnormal Magnetic-Resonance Scans of the Lumbar Spine in Asymptomatic Subjects: A Prospective Investigation," *J Bone Joint Surg Am.* 72 (1990):403–408.
539 MC Jensen, MN Brant-Zawadzki, N Obuchowski, MT Modic, D Malkasian, JS Ross, "Magnetic Resonance Imaging Of The Lumbar Spine In People Without Back Pain," *N Engl J Med.* 331 (1994):69–73.
540 SD Boden, *et al.* ibid.
541 SD Boden, *et al.* "Emerging Techniques For Treatment Of Degenerative Lumbar Disc Disease," *Spine* 28(2003):524-525.

Dr. Jensen's study confirmed early suspicions that herniated discs were "coincidental" and not the holy grail of back pain causation:

> The relation between abnormalities in the lumbar spine and low back pain is controversial. We examined the prevalence of abnormal findings on magnetic resonance imaging (MRI) scans of the lumbar spine in people without back pain.
>
> On MRI examination of the lumbar spine, many people without back pain have disk bulges or protrusions but not extrusions. Given the high prevalence of these findings and of back pain, *the discovery by MRI of bulges or protrusions in people with low back pain may frequently be coincidental.*[542] (emphasis added)

The Boden and Jensen studies showed that disc abnormalities were not the sole cause of back pain since many asymptomatic patients have the very same disc abnormalities. In fact, it is part of the normal aging process, like graying hair. Per Kjaer, PT, PhD, also found more than half the people 40-years and older have abnormalities on MRI scans.[543]

The low incidence of actual disc herniations coincides with the mechanism that Nikolai Bogduk, MD, PhD, proposes in his text, *Clinical Anatomy of the Lumbar Spine and Sacrum*.[544] In his text he mentions the difficulty of producing a herniated disc on fresh cadaver spines simulating normal positions and ranges of motion that would occur during typical activities of daily living.

He argues that an inflammatory reaction must change the consistency of the nucleus (disc degradation), then the annulus begins to tear due to the increased/faulty load it must endure (internal disc disruption), and only then can the nucleus actually herniate outside the boundary of the annulus.

The low incidence of cervical herniation is even easier to support. Reviewers Jull *et al.*[545] have found that by the third decade the cervical disc nucleus is almost completely fibrotic. This is logical because the cervical disc, unlike the lumbar, is not designed primarily for load bearing and the need for compression force dissipation is less necessary. Yet most spine surgeons will use the evidence of cervical disc degeneration to warrant fusion when, in fact, it is a natural part of the aging process.

Very few of these studies followed subjects for more than a year or two. However, it is known that the consequences of surgical fusion in the cervical spine are accelerated degenerative changes and recurrence of radiculopathy or myelopathy at adjacent levels in

---

542 MC Jensen, MN Brant-Zawadzki, N Obuchowski, MT Modic, D Malkasian, and JS Ross, "Magnetic Resonance Imaging of the Lumbar Spine in People without Back Pain," *NEJM*, 331/2 (July 14, 1994):69-73

543 P Kjaer *et al.*, "Magnetic Resonance Imaging And Low Back Pain In Adults: A Diagnostic Imaging Study Of 40-Year-Old Men And Women," *Spine* 30 (2005):1173-80.

544 N Bogduk, *Clinical Anatomy of the Lumbar Spine and Sacrum*, Churchill Livingstone (2005)

545 G Jull, E Kristjansson, P Dall'Alba, "Impairment in the Cervical Flexors: A Comparison Of Whiplash And Insidious Onset Neck Pain Patients," *Manual Therapy* 9 (2004):89-94

the ensuing years—consequences not accounted for in studies with follow-up periods of under 10 years. [546,547]

Many studies now admit the fallacy of using MRIs to detect abnormal discs to justify spine surgery:

> You may have a bulging disc that shows up on an MRI scan, but that may not be the cause of your leg pain. You can have disc degeneration or other anatomical lesions that show up on the scan, but are not causing pain. *Studies have shown that many people with no pain or other symptoms often have some sort of disc problem show up on an MRI scan.*[548] (emphasis added)

Raj Rao, M.D., director of spine surgery in the Department of Orthopaedic Surgery at the Medical College of Wisconsin, also spoke of this paradox in spine imaging:

> You can look at the MRIs of two people, both showing degenerative discs, but in one case there is little to no pain, while in the other, extreme pain. On the other hand, you can see a healthy spine but the patient has severe pain.[549]

Not only is the bulging disc theory unreliable, many other long held beliefs about discs are wrong. It is widely thought that once herniated or bulging, disc material cannot naturally move back; therefore, surgery is the only definitive treatment if the severity of symptoms warrants it.

Researchers now recognize a lesser known fact that disc bulges and herniations often undergo some degree of regression without surgery. In the past decade, research has shown that discs do, in fact, move back, and do so to a significant degree (70 percent or more).[550,551,552]

Another surprising discovery has shown that clinical improvement does not generally correlate with regression, indicating that the "ruptured disc pinching nerves" concept may also be wrong. Just as Boden and Jensen found, patients with obvious bulging discs often had no back or leg pain.

Indeed, the Dynasty of the Disc has been investigated and disproven for the most part as the singular cause of back pain, but this theory has remained alive because it is

546 A Katsuura, S Hukuda, MK Saruhashi, "Kyphotic Malalignment After Anterior Cervical Fusion Is One Of The Factors Promoting The Degenerative Process In Adjacent Intervertebral Levels," *Eur Spine J* 10 (2001):320-324.

547 AS Hilibrand, GD Carlson, MA Palumbo, PK Jones, HH Bohlman, "Radiculopathy and Myelopathy At Segments Adjacent To The Cite Of A Previous Anterior Cervical Arthrodesis," *J Bone Joint Surgery* 81-A 4 (1999):519-528

548 www.spine-health.com...pain.../s1-sciatica-numbness-how-long-does-it-last

549 P Garfinkel, "The Back Story," *AARP: the magazine*, (July & August 2009)

550 E Ilkko, S Lahde, ER Heikkinen, "Late CT Findings In Nonsurgically Treated Lumbar Disc Herniations," *Eur J Radiol*. 16/3 (1993):186-189.

551 MR Ellenberg, ML Ross, JC Honet, *et al*. "Prospective Evaluation Of The Course Of Disc Herniations In Patients With Proven Radiculopathy," *Arch Phys Med Rehab* 74/1 (1993):3-10,

552 K Bush, N Cowan, DE Katz, *et al*. "The Natural History Of Sciatica Associated With Disc Pathology," *Spine* 17/10 (1992):1205-1212.

has been drummed into the public narrative as a valid reason to warrant surgery. Sadly, modern surgeons know better, but ignore this revelation because they make too much money to be totally honest with patients.

Revelation #2: MRI Scan for Disc Abnormalities

After the MRI was invented in 1977, spine researchers began examining its ability to detect spine abnormalities, and MRI imaging has become a burgeoning industry onto itself. Unfortunately, the MRI has been the main weapon in the medical war that has perpetuated this disc fallacy despite the emerging evidence to the contrary. In essence, MRI scans make it much easier to lie to patients.

Indisputably, MRI scans have been used as effective selling points and have greatly increased the number of unnecessary surgery. "In fact," according to Dr. Richard Deyo, *"back surgery rates are highest where MRIs are the highest*. In a randomized trial, we found that doing an MRI instead of a plain x-ray led to more back surgery, but didn't improve the overall results of treatment."[553]

Dr. Deyo again debunked the disc theory that often leads to a "false positive" misdiagnosis when he concluded that "many of these abnormalities are trivial, harmless, and irrelevant, so they have been recently dubbed "incidentalomas," because it may be *incidental* to your pain:

> And *we know that bulging, degenerated, and even herniated discs in the spine are common among healthy people with no symptoms.* When doctors find such discs in people with back pain, *the discs may be irrelevant,* but they are likely to lead to more tests, patient anxiety, and perhaps even unnecessary surgery.[554] (emphasis added)

Evidence-based medicine (EBM) also questions whether or not scans are necessary in light of the ubiquitous nature of disc abnormalities, but most MDs still prescribe an MRI as a standard initial test rather than waiting at least a month as recommended while conservative care is used. Unfortunately, the outdated disc theory remains very much alive in the medical profession in America due to MRI scans, the best sales pitch tool ever made for surgeons. Until the "herniated or degenerated disc causes back pain and requires surgery" mindset is publicly denounced, this epidemic of failed back surgery will continue to plague the public.

To the surprise of spine surgeons, even a 2009 Stanford University study found the abundance of MRI scans lead to excessive back surgeries. According to Stanford University Medical Center,[555] patients who live in areas with more MRI scanners are more likely to undergo spine surgery. "The worry is that many people will not benefit from the surgery, so heading in this direction is concerning," said senior author Laurence Baker, PhD.[556]

---

553 Richard A. Deyo, MD, MPH and Donald L. Patrick, PhD, MSPH, *Hope or Hype: The Obsession with Medical Advances and the High Cost of False Promises,* AMACOM books, (2005): 36-37
554 Ibid.
555 M Brandt, Stanford University Medical Center, "MRI Abundance May Lead To Excess In Back Surgery," (Oct. 14, 2009)
556 JD Baras and LC Baker, "Magnetic Resonance Imaging And Low Back Pain Care For Medicare Patients," *Health Aff* (Millwood) 28/6 (2009):1133–40.

Between 2000 and 2005, the MRI availability in the United States more than tripled from 7.6 machines per one million persons to 26.6 machines. Each machine costs more than $2 million, and each low back scan costs $1,500. A General Accounting Office report concluded that it costs efficient MRI centers only $262 to $399 to do the test.[557] Obviously there is a huge markup on this imaging.

According John Birkmeyer, MD, professor of surgery and a health policy researcher at the University of Michigan, the Stanford study *confirms fears that greater access to MRI technology leads to more back surgeries.* "The net result is increased risks of unnecessary surgery for patients and increased costs for everybody else."[558]

Not only are patients scanned more often, they are inappropriately scanned within the first month of the onset of pain when guidelines suggest this should not be done since many cases resolve spontaneously or by conservative care practitioners. Even having a lot of pain does not mean you need to jump into surgery.

Dr. Deyo in his 2009 article, "Overtreating Chronic Back Pain: Time to Back Off?: Imaging for Low Back Pain," cites the huge *307 percent* increase of CT and MRI scans and concluded "one-third to two-thirds of spinal computed tomography (CT) imaging and MRI may be inappropriate."[559] This is a huge increase for an unnecessary test that leads to many unnecessary and ineffective spine surgeries.

Regrettably, the images seen on scans are convincing selling points to the naïve public by surgeons who know better, but profit greatly, by pointing to these misleading images: "I can show you your problem right here (a herniated or degenerated disc), and the only solution is surgery. And whatever you do, don't go to a chiropractor who might rupture it." This is another Big Lie told too often to unsuspecting patients who take this bait, succumb to surgery, and suffer for the rest of their lives in many cases.

This debunked disc theory leaves the question: if an abnormal disc is not the issue, then what is the underlying problem causing most back and leg pain?

Revelation #3: Paradigm Shift from Discs to Joints

While the medical model of back pain focuses on *pathoanatomical* disc problems, the chiropractic model and justification for manipulation focuses on joint function and *pathophysiological* issues like structure, alignment, movement, gait, and muscle imbalances. Even foot abnormalities like excessive pronation or fallen arches may lead to spinal problems. Obviously there is more to the diagnosis of back pain than merely disc abnormalities or spinal arthritis as the root causes, and this is the untold story of back pain whose sufferers need to know.

It requires a lot of unfounded faith to believe in the medical model for back pain. Most physicians preach and lay-people still believe in "pulled muscles" and "slipped

---

557 E Rosenthal, "MRI Scanner Industry Faces a Shakeout," *NY Times*, (December 10, 1993)

558 Brandt, ibid.

559 RA Deyo, SK Mirza, JA Turner, BI Martin, "Overtreating Chronic Back Pain: Time to Back Off?" *J Am Board Fam Med.* 22/1 (2009):62-68

discs" when it comes to back pain, ignoring the role of spinal joints and altered spinal mechanics in this pain process. This simplistic misunderstanding is the underlying cause of mistreatment for back pain that has perpetuated far too long.

Most people fail to understand the importance of joint dysfunction, a disorder not even detectable on imaging as the New Zealand Report mentioned. Although spinal misalignments, curvatures, and scoliosis are seen on imaging, these obvious malalignments alone may not be problematic.

The key rests with how well the joints move and how well the spine bears weight—in other words, how well the spine functions. Although the areas of misalignments may point to possible areas of joint problems, as long as the joints are functioning with proper movement or *joint play*, it may not necessarily be painful.

Joint dysfunction is not detectable on an MRI or x-ray image, just as any locked, buckled, twisted, or wrenched joint cannot be seen on imaging. The New Zealand Inquiry remarked about this phenomenon:

> *The problem is a functional not a structural one... the medical profession simply fails to see the direction and subtlety of the chiropractic approach towards spinal dysfunction.* Because the chiropractor uses x-ray extensively the medical practitioner thinks he is looking for a gross bony change, and when the medical practitioner cannot see this on the x-ray the chiropractor is using he immediately becomes skeptical. *He might as well expect to see a limp, or a headache or any other functional problem on x-ray.*[560] (emphasis added)

The role of joint play in this back pain process is a primary concern as John Mennell, MD, suggested in his testimony at the *Wilk* trial:

> Eight out of ten patients that come out of any doctor's office complain of a musculoskeletal system problem, regardless of what system the pain is coming from...*I will say 100 percent of those complaints...are due to joint dysfunction in the musculoskeletal {system}.*
>
> The science of mechanics demands that joint play movement is prerequisite to normal pain-free functioning of movement...in the spine there are about 137 synovial joints [this has been revised] between the lamina facets, the occipital condyles, the bottom of the skull as it rests on the atlas, the sacroiliac joints, the sacrococcygeal joints, the z-joints, even the joints of the fundusca in the neck. [561] (emphasis added)

Even those researchers who criticize the disc theory often fail to mention the role of joint dysfunction as the underlying causation due to their limited understanding of spinal mechanics and, of course, their ingrained bias against chiropractors and manipulative therapy as evident during the *Wilk* trial.

Foremost, spinal problems are *dynamic* type of injuries according to Drs. David R. Seaman and James F. Winterstein who explained that joint complex dysfunction (JCD) is associated with spinal misalignment and aberrant joint motion that may subsequently

---

560 Ibid. p. 55.
561 Transcript of testimony of John McMillan Mennell, MD, *Wilk v AMA* transcript, pp. 2090-2093.

cause a cascade of events such as reflex muscle spasms, disc inflammation, nerve compression, neurological dysafferentiation, vascular vaso-constriction, muscle spasm, localized pain, and joint stiffness.[562,563] Evidently JCD is not as simple to understand as the slipped disc theory, but essential to comprehend why manipulative therapy is so effective.

This JCD is not a *static* problem like a thorn in the paw, a broken bone, or a slipped disc. Rather than looking at back pain as a static problem caused primarily by disc degeneration or pathologies, another approach is to view the spine as a dynamic, mechanical, weight-bearing column susceptible to overloads, injuries, repetitive stress, prolonged compression, and leverage issues.

The possibility of JCD is enormous considering the anatomy of the spinal column. For the last few decades, researchers believed the number of spinal joints to be 137, such as we heard in Dr. Mennell's testimony at the *Wilk* trial, but that count has changed. Counting all the vertebral joints, sacroiliac joints, rib heads, and the pubic symphysis, new research now suggest the total is 313, a fact that is lost to most physicians. This total includes all synovial, symphysis, and syndesmosis joints according to Gregory D. Cramer, DC, PhD, Dean of Research at National University of Health Sciences.[564]

The number of spinal joints includes: [565]

Joints by Region

	Synovial	Symphysis	Syndesmosis	Total
Cervical Spine	17	6	39	62
Thoracic Spine	68	12	116	196
Lumbar Spine	10	5	29	44
Sacrum/Pelvis	2	3	6	11
Total	97	26	190	313

When any of the 313 joints in the spine become dysfunctional, misaligned, and develop abnormal motion, this may lead to pain, stiffness, inflammation, and the surge of irregular neurological events. Although spinal misalignments are obvious clues where this spinal dysfunction may occur, not all spinal misalignments are problematic considering many people with scoliosis are pain free.

---

562 DR Seaman, JF Winterstein. "Dysafferentiation, a Novel Term To Describe The Neuropathophysiological Effects of Joint Complex Dysfunction: A Look at Likely Mechanisms of Symptom Generation," *J. Manipulative Physiol Ther* 21 (1998):267-80.

563 DR Seaman, "Joint Complex Dysfunction, A Novel Term To Replace Subluxation/Subluxation Complex. Etiological And Treatment Considerations," *J. Manip Physiol Ther* 20 (1997):634-44.

564 G Cramer, Dean of Research, National University of Health Sciences, via personal communication with JC Smith (April 29, 2009)

565 G Cramer via private communication with JC Smith (May, 2009)

Imagine these interconnecting 24 vertebrae sitting atop the three pelvic bones, with these gliding joints all balancing a ten-pound head, withstanding gravity compression, and resisting bad leverage, and you can see why this unstable, weight-bearing spinal column is susceptible to many types of forces, such as falls, twisting, prolonged sitting, lifting with bad leverage, or impacts from outside forces like football, which alone may the single largest source of spinal injuries for most players.

Recent research has shown the accumulative effect from traumatic injuries during childhood may compound and be aggravated as adults. Prolonged sitting/standing, improper lifting, and accidents can develop a functional spinal problem may cause a "segmental buckling effect," according to research by Jay Triano, DC, PhD, *et al.* while at the Texas Back Institute, an interdisciplinary clinic offering comprehensive spinal care.

The buckling effect is a function of overloading rather than a static misalignment of vertebrae:

> Several characteristics of buckling behavior are known. *An obvious causative factor is a single overload event that exceeds critical load for the conditions.* For less severe tasks, the process is more complex. *Normal creep deformity occurs with prolonged static posture.* Creep alters the constitutive properties of the tissue and the relative critical load. *Under the right conditions, even a small additional load will cause the joint to buckle.* Rapidly applied loads also are associated with buckling and vibration reduces the threshold necessary to achieve it. *Finally tissues that are damaged, as in discopathy, may buckle sooner and reach maximum displacement (deformation) under lower peak loads than do healthy tissues.*[566] (emphasis added)

Anyone versed in spinal mechanics realizes that the disc is a shock absorber and is a secondary player in the back/leg pain syndrome. A disc is not muscle that moves, but it is cartilage that can swell, bulge, degenerate, dehydrate, and even crack when the mechanical forces and leverage cause it to react. In essence, a disc does nothing until it is forced to do so by the mechanics of the spinal column itself.

A revealing study by orthopedist JL Shaw, MD, suggests most low back pain and disc abnormalities began after the sacroiliac joint (SIJ) becomes dysfunctional. This joint is a butting type of joint and has no disc or interlocking joints—just synovial lining between the flat joint surfaces. Once the SIJ slips, it causes intense pain in the buttock area that may also go into the upper thigh or groin area, but will not go below the knee:

> "The conventional wisdom is that herniated discs are responsible for low back pain, and that sacroiliac joints do not move significantly and do not cause low back pain or dysfunction. *The ironic reality may well be that sacroiliac joint dysfunctions are the major cause*

---

566 JJ Triano, *et al.* "Biomechanics of Spinal Manipulation," *Spine* 1 (2001):121-30

of low back pain, as well as the primary factor causing disc space degeneration, and ultimate herniation of disc material."[567] (emphasis added)

In fact, SIJ dysfunction has been implicated as a common cause of back pain in more than 30 percent of American children.[568] Additionally, a study involving the correction of SIJ dysfunction in patients at a chiropractic center in one day found an incidence of 57 percent for SIJ dysfunction.[569]

Another study[570] done in Germany investigated the role of SIJ dysfunction in back and leg pain. Since there are no intervertebral discs in the SIJ, spine surgeons ignore this as the cause of back or leg pain, but the research now shows a SIJ dysfunction is a prominent source of pain in many patients. The aim of this study was to evaluate the frequency and significance of SIJ dysfunction in patients with low back pain and sciatica and imaging-proven disc herniation.

Researchers examined the SIJs of 150 patients with low back pain and sciatica; all of these patients had herniated lumbar disks, but none of them had sensory or motor losses. Forty-six patients were diagnosed with dysfunction of the SIJ. The remaining 104 patients had no SIJ dysfunction. Dysfunctions were resolved with mobilizing and spinal manipulative techniques. Regardless of SIJ findings, all patients received intensive physiotherapy throughout a 3-week hospitalization.

At the 3 weeks follow-up, 34 patients of group with SIJ dysfunction (73.9%) reported an improvement of lumbar and ischiadic pain; 5 patients were pain free. Improvement was recorded in 57 of the patients with no SIJ problems (54.8%); however, nobody in this group that only received intensive physiotherapy was free of symptoms.

Clearly this study confirmed what Dr. Shaw found—the importance of the SIJ dysfunction in low back and leg pain syndromes. The German study also showed that spinal manipulative therapy proved superior to physiotherapy alone in these cases; again demonstrating the need to adjust spinal joints first and foremost.

Just imagine the millions of patients with SIJ pain who underwent spine surgery that was ineffective and left them disabled when, in all possibility, if they had seen a chiropractor first to have their SIJ joints adjusted, this tragedy could have been avoided as many chiropractors well know.

---

567 JL Shaw, "The Role Of The Sacroiliac Joints As A Cause Of Low Back Pain And Dysfunction," proceedings of the First Interdisciplinary World Congress on Low Back Pain and its Relation to the Sacroiliac Joint, University of California, San Diego, (Nov.5-6, 1992)

568 DR Mierau *et al.* "Sacroiliac Joint Dysfunction and Low Back Pain in School Aged Children," *JMPT* 7/2 (1984):81-84.

569 HA Gemmell, BJ Heng, "Low Force Method of Spinal Correction and Fixation of the Sacroiliac Joint," The Amer Chiro (Nov 1987):28-32.

570 R Galm, M Fröhling, M Rittmeister, E Schmitt Sacroiliac, "Joint Dysfunction in Patients with Imaging-Proven Lumbar Disc Herniation," *Eur Spine J.* 7/6 (1998):450-3. Spine Clinic, Bad Homburg, Germany.

Remember: you don't slip discs as much as you slip joints. To overlook joint play and spinal function (pathophysiology) and to focus on the secondary effect of disc pathology (pathoanatomical) is putting the proverbial cart before the horse.

Revelation #4: Knowledge of Ignorance

"Many of our ideas about low back pain have been wrong," said Aage Indahl, MD. "The slow pace of change in giving up old ideas is probably a result of the lack of new ideas."[571]

Is it really a "lack of new ideas" or is it actually the result of intense bias by the medical industrial complex against alternative treatments like chiropractic care? Dr. Indahl's admission is honest, albeit it naïve considering the lengthy medical war to suppress chiropractic care.

Paul H. Goodley, MD, author of *Release from Pain*, founder of the American Association of Orthopaedic Medicine, leading orthopedic physician and champion of manual medicine/spinal manipulation, has also experienced the bias that has deterred the integration of manual medicine into the mainstream. He admits that most MDs do not even understand the source of their skepticism: "while the schism's origin was lost like dark legend," an attitude developed that he has coined as the *Fundamental Flaw*—the bias of medicine toward manipulative therapy and, specifically, against "its most despised competitor—chiropractic":

> Eventually, the prejudice against manipulation self-perpetuated, and evidence was always available to justify this attitude. There have always been charlatans. So, *instead of the manipulative fundamental dynamically developing as a cohesive, trustworthy guide within traditional medicine, it was discredited as the synonymous derelict symbol of its most despised competitor-chiropractic.* And future generations born into a hardening tradition of pervasive belligerence against anything manipulative unquestioningly accepted this verdict.[572] (emphasis added)

Admittedly, Dr. Goodley is right in that there has always been a small percentage of chiropractors who can be viewed as charlatans—those DCs who make outrageous claims of cure and those who are unprofessional in their practices. This is the fundamental flaw in chiropractic's reputation that has been self-inflicted.

The chiropractic profession has had its share of out of the ordinary characters, but they are dwindling in numbers as the state licensing boards become stronger, accreditation agencies improve the curriculum, and the chiropractic colleges matriculate better students.

Indeed, sometimes the chiropractors have added fuel to the fire of skepticism by their own desperate actions. Considering the segregation, demonization, and boycott chiropractors have experienced in the medical war, their desperation may have been understandable as a reaction to oppression.

---

571 *The BACKLETTER*, 23/5 (2008):55.
572 PH Goodley, *Release from Pain*, www.DrGoodley.com (2005): xiv.

George McAndrews addressed this very point during the *Wilk* trial:

> There are a lot of faults attributed to people that have been ghettoized. But you don't look to the person that has been placed in that position for the blame. You look to the medical societies with all of their resources and all of their so-called education for the blame. When you put someone in that condition you can't argue then that the outgrowth of that condition is something that they can use to destroy them. [573]

Nonetheless, considering the medical bias that has thwarted the use of chiropractic care and the adherence to the disproven pathoanatomical disc model, it is easy to understand why progress has been so slow in spinal care.

Daniel Cherkin, PhD, mentioned the dilemma facing spine researchers:

> Over the past 13 years, the back pain research movement has made important discoveries about the nature and course of low back pain. However, if anything, low back pain appears to be a more complex, variable, and mysterious condition than it did 13 years ago. *"If nothing else, we have increased our knowledge of our ignorance."*[574] (emphasis added)

Certainly this ignorance stems not only from the ingrained medical bias fostered by political medicine, but also from the lack of education in medical schools on problems of the musculoskeletal system. This becomes a huge challenge considering most MDs are not schooled in musculoskeletal disorders (MSDs) according to many experts.

Recall Dr. John C. Wilson, chairman of the American Medical Association's Section on Orthopedic Surgery, testified at the *Wilk* trial about the poor training of medical students, "MDs often displayed a disturbing ignorance of the cause and treatment of low back and sciatic pain, one of mankind's most common affliction."[575]

Although most low back pain patients initially seek help from their primary care physicians, research has shown the *primary care physicians are the least educated to diagnose musculoskeletal problems.* This is a huge admission considering conditions affecting the musculoskeletal system are the primary reason patients seek medical care from physicians, accounting for nearly 100 million office visits per year in America.[576],[577]

New studies have confirmed that most primary care physicians are inept in their training on musculoskeletal disorders,[578] more likely to ignore recent guidelines[579],

---

573 G McAndrews closing arguments, *Wilk v. AMA*, (June 26, 1987):3093-97.

574 Ibid. pp. 49.

575 JC Wilson, "Low Back Pain and Sciatica: A Plea for Better Care of the Patient, Chairman's Address," *JAMA*, 200/8, (May 22, 1967):705-712.

576 A Praemer, S Furner, DP Rice, *et al.* "Musculoskeletal conditions in the United States," Rosemont, IL, American Academy of Orthopaedic Surgeons (1999)

577 AD Woolf, B Pfleger, "Burden of Major Musculoskeletal Conditions," *Bull World Health Organ* 81/09 (2003):646-656.

578 EA Joy, S Van Hala, "Musculoskeletal Curricula in Medical Education-- Filling In the Missing Pieces, The Physician And Sports Medicine," 32/11 (November 2004).

579 PB Bishop *et al.*, "The C.H.I.R.O. (Chiropractic Hospital-Based Interventions Research Outcomes) part I: A Randomized Controlled Trial On The Effectiveness Of Clinical Practice Guidelines In The Medical And Chiropractic Management Of Patients With Acute Mechanical Low Back Pain," presented

and more likely to suggest spine surgery than surgeons themselves.[580] As well, biased physicians suffer from "professional amnesia" when they inexcusably forget to inform patients that chiropractic care is a recommended option to the often ineffective medical methods.

Scott Boden, MD, currently director of the Emory Orthopaedic and Spine Center in Atlanta, admits that "Many, if not most, primary care providers have little training in how to manage musculoskeletal disorders."[581] His belief is supported by the consensus that the poor medical outcomes stem from an antiquated disc theory, too many MRIs detecting incidentalomas, ineffectual medical treatments, and primary care physicians who are ill-trained to diagnosis. Indeed, the major obstacle to overcome in this epidemic of back pain originates with medical doctors themselves.

This "doctor problem" begins with "medical students who are not trained to think critically," according to Michael Wilkes, vice dean of education at U.C. Davis. Apparently the only thing they are taught to be critical of is chiropractic care. He contends medical students are required to memorize a huge number of facts—such as anatomy, physiology, structure of the body to tests, diagnoses, and treatments—that "they do not have time to critique the information they must cram into their heads."[582] Certainly reliable information about spinal care is one issue not crammed into their minds.

In 1998, Kevin B. Freedman, MD, and Joseph Bernstein, MD, published a landmark study in *Journal of Bone and Joint Surgery* wherein they administered a validated musculoskeletal competency examination to recent medical graduates who had begun their hospital residency; *82 percent of these medical doctors failed to demonstrate basic competency on the examination,* leading the authors to conclude, "We therefore believe that medical school preparation in musculoskeletal medicine is inadequate." [583]

In their 2004 review published in *Physician and Sports Medicine*, Elizabeth A. Joy, MD, and Sonja Van Hala, MD, MPH, described the formal training of a sample of medical graduates. "The average time spent in rotations for courses devoted to orthopedics during medical school was only 2.1 weeks. One third of these examinees graduated without any formal training in orthopedics. As would be expected, these *data suggest that limited educational experience contributes to poor performance."* [584]

at the annual meeting of the International Society for the Study of the Lumbar Spine Hong Kong, 2007; presented at the annual meeting of the North American Spine Society, Austin, Texas, 2007; *Spine*, in press.
580 SS Bederman, NN Mahomed, HJ Kreder, *et al.* In the Eye of the Beholder: Preferences Of Patients, Family Physicians, And Surgeons For Lumbar Spinal Surgery," *Spine* 135/1 (2010):108-115.
581 S Boden, *et al.* "Emerging Techniques For Treatment Of Degenerative Lumbar Disc Disease," *Spine* 28 (2003):524-525.
582 J Lenzer and S Brownlee, "Reckless Medicine," *Discover* (Nov. 2010):68-69
583 KB Freedman, J Bernstein, "The Adequacy Of Medical School Education In Musculoskeletal Medicine," *J Bone Joint Surg Am.* 80/10 (1998):1421-7
584 Joy ibid.

Many physical therapists hold themselves out to be spine therapists, but a study by JD Childs *et al.*[585] on the physical therapists' knowledge in managing musculoskeletal disorder (MSD) conditions found that only 21 percent of students working on their Master's degree in physical therapy and 25 percent of students working on their doctorate degree in physical therapy achieved a passing mark on the Basic Competency Exam.

Even those physicians with a special interest in low back pain were more likely to believe in outdated concepts such as narcotics, complete bed rest, and avoidance of work are appropriate for acute low back pain—concepts now regarded as inappropriate. Oddly, there were no important differences in back pain beliefs between those with and without a special interest in musculoskeletal medicine.[586] It appears that any MD with an interest in back pain can hang out a "pain clinic" shingle even when poorly trained in this area.

The Bishop study published in *Spine* scored the content of the family physician-directed care and found it to be "highly guideline-discordant." The three studies by Bishop *et al.* provide an excellent illustration of the slow pace of implementation of evidence-based spinal care into primary care settings.

"Typically, the family physician-based care involved excessive use of passive therapies such as massage and passive physical therapy, excessive bed rest, and excessive use of narcotic analgesics," said Paul B. Bishop, DC, MD, PhD, Clinical Associate Professor in the Department of Orthopaedics at University of British Columbia.[587]

Despite this lack of education, the average MD still poses as an expert to patients. As attorney McAndrews mentioned during the *Wilk* trial, this typifies a quack:

> They use the definition of quackery: somebody who pretends to knowledge they do not have. Chiropractors that pretend to medical knowledge are quacks. And medical physicians who pretend to universal knowledge of human anatomy and biomechanics on this record should be called quacks if the definition is: somebody who pretends to knowledge they don't not have. That's quackery. We all agree on that.[588]

Unfortunately, medical quacks are still prescribing ineffectual medications, ordering expensive MRIs looking for "incidentalomas," only then to refer to a spine surgeon. If and when patients ask for an opinion on chiropractic care, many are discouraged or even ridiculed for asking. Typically, the usual MD-patient encounter is one of a misdiagnosis, mistreatment, and misinformation about options to the best care available—specifically, chiropractic care.

Millions of patients are mistaken when they are led to believe their primary care physician actually knows something about the best management of back disorders. In

585 JD Childs, JM Whitman, PS Sizer, ML Pugia, TW Flynn, A Delitto, "A Description Of Physical Therapists' Knowledge In Managing Musculoskeletal Conditions," BMC *Musculoskelet Disord* 6 (2005):32.
586 R Buchbinder, M Staples, D Jolley, "Doctors With a Special Interest in Back Pain Have Poorer Knowledge About How to Treat Back Pain," *Spine*, 34/11 (May 2009)
587 Bishop, ibid.
588 Ibid. p. 3051-52.

fact, a truly ethical primary care practitioner should admit his inadequacies and refer these cases to chiropractors who are the foremost spine specialists, just as he would refer you to a dentist for tooth pain.

When it comes to musculoskeletal conditions, chiropractors are by far the experts and receive the most formal education in this subject that includes an average of 4,800 hours of in-classroom instruction, laboratory, diagnosis, and clinical experience compared to the miniscule classroom time spent by medical students in musculoskeletal issues. They also have the most practical, hands-on, in-office experience—delivering more than 90 percent of the manipulations reimbursed by health insurance.[589]

Don Nixdorf, DC, co-author of *Squandering Billions*, challenged health ministers in Canada as to why they continued to use MDs instead of chiropractors for musculoskeletal disorders knowing their incompetence in this area:

> Since 30 percent of all visits to medical doctors and health professionals are for spine-related illnesses and injuries, why does the system not insist that primary diagnoses and care is delivered by those most thoroughly trained to recognize and treat these problems?[590]

Dr. Deyo also blamed the medical profession for creating false hope among some patients looking for a miracle cure to end their suffering:

> I think many people have unrealistic expectations of medical care. We live in a culture that wants quick, easy fixes. Many people seem to think that they should never have pain if they're getting good medical care.

These expectations didn't rise in a vacuum. The marketing of new products to patients and physicians may help create those expectations. *We in the medical profession are also probably guilty of creating unrealistic expectations.*[591]

The 200+ various treatments available for low back pain only compound their misery.[592] To make matters worse for patients, surgeons often have a conflict of interest. Many doctors ignore evidence-based guidelines, some physicians practice outdated methods, and many still hold a bias against what is proven to be effective—spinal manipulative therapy.

The bias against chiropractors by orthopedists was noted in a survey of North American orthopedic surgeons' attitudes toward chiropractic that found "44.5% endorsing a negative impression, 29.4% holding favorable views, and 26.1% being neutral."[593] Considering the

589 W Meeker, S Haldeman, ibid.

590 G Bannerman and D Nixdorf, Squandering Billions; Health Care in Canada, Hancock House, (2005):15.

591 *The BACKLETTER®* 33 23/3 (2008)

592 S Haldeman, S Dagenais, "Evidence-Informed Management of Chronic Low Back Pain Without Surgery," The *Spine Journal* 8/1 (January/February 2008):258-65.

593 J Busse, C Jacobs, T Ngo, R Rodine, D Torrance, J Janey, A Kulkarni, B Petrisor, B Drew, M Bhandari, "Attitudes Toward Chiropractic: A Survey of North American Orthopedic Surgeons," *Spine*, 1 34/25 (Dec 2009):2818-25.

medical industrial complex bias toward any competition, especially toward chiropractors, the results were not surprising.

Despite this admitted bias, "approximately half of respondents referred patients for chiropractic care each year, mainly due to patient request." This demand by patients for referral to a chiropractor is troublesome when the orthopedist has to be urged by his patients for a referral. Indeed, it is somewhat surprising intimidated patients found the nerve to confront their surgeon for a referral to a chiropractor considering the intimidation most surgeons use to sway patients to surgery.

Even more surprising was the fact that "the majority of surgeons believed that chiropractors provide effective therapy for some musculoskeletal complaints (81.8%)." If that is true, why do they not refer to chiropractors before surgery is considered? Furthermore, what does this suggest about the remaining 18.2 percent who refuse to refer to chiropractors? Is their bias so profound that they withhold this non-surgical solution in order to profit?

However, the survey also showed that orthopedists "disagreed that chiropractors could provide effective relief for non-musculoskeletal conditions (89.5%)."[594] Certainly their lack of understanding of neurophysiology, spinal visceral reflexes, or the effects of spinal stress upon the chemistry and circuitry of the brain may contribute to this misunderstanding how spinal manipulation may help some Type O disorders.

The survey also touched on controversial issues that have plagued the medical warfare for nearly a century. "The majority endorsed that chiropractors provide unnecessary treatment (72.7%), engage in overly-aggressive marketing (63.1%) and breed dependency in patients on short-term symptomatic relief (52.3%)."[595]

This survey might have questioned what percent of the same orthopedists felt their spine surgeries were unnecessary or if their opioids created a dependency in patients as well. Certainly a survey of chiropractors concerning similar issues might have been revealing to the shortcomings of the medical industrial complex.

Consequently, the dilemma for spine patients remains daunting with medical bias, conflicting diagnosis, divergent treatments, huge surgical costs, insurance limits or non-coverage for alternative treatments, serious surgical and drug side-effects, lack of informed options, and common medical treatments unsupported by current research. Compounding this dilemma are surgeons and hospitals motivated by the profit motive to do what is most expensive rather than recommending cheaper and more effective non-surgical solutions.

The potential for realistically lowering costs with chiropractic care may be a large reason why hospitals controlled by a biased medical society may not want to include lower cost providers such as doctors of chiropractic. When hospitals can charge $50,000 or *more* for radical back surgeries, the incentive to utilize lower cost services is compromised. Realistically, why would a hospital want a chiropractor on staff who will earn a mere $800

594 J Busse, ibid.
595 Ibid.

per case on the average?[596] While the patient might enjoy this inexpensive resolution, the hospital administration surely would not.

Unfortunately, instead of the truth, we see a continuation of misleading research by some who stand to profit by spine surgery. The deceptive nature of spine research was evident in the 2008 study by WC Peul, MD, *et al.*,[597] "Prolonged Conservative Care Versus Early Surgery In Patients With Sciatica Caused By Lumbar Disc Herniation: Two-Year Results Of A Randomized Controlled Trial," that compared prolonged conservative *medical* care versus early microdiscectomy surgery in patients with sciatica caused by lumbar disc herniation.

There are many concerns about this Peul study, most prominently, the definition of "conservative care" and his belief that "There are no proven nonoperative treatments for sciatica":

> Treatment methods were straightforward. Those allocated to disc surgery underwent microdiscectomy and removal of loose degenerated disc material from the disc space. *General practitioners supervised conservative care. There are no proven nonoperative treatments for sciatica*, so the treatment approach was empirical. It included information, reassurance, pain control, and encouragement to return to normal activity. Those who were fearful of movement were referred for physical therapy. Both groups had access to research nurses for advice and encouragement.[598] (emphasis added)

Dr. Peul's statement "There are no proven nonoperative treatments for sciatica" and his omission of chiropractic care is clearly an example of dishonesty considering one quick scan of Medline[599] for sciatica/herniated discs/manual medicine revealed a plethora of studies showing the effectiveness of spinal manipulative therapy, flexion-distraction, and non-surgical spinal decompression for leg pain/herniated discs.

Here is a short sampling of research supporting manual therapy (SMT, Flexion/distraction, non-surgical spinal decompression) for LBP/leg pain:

- Henderson RS The treatment of lumbar intervertebral disk protrusion: an assessment of conservative measures, *Br. Med J* 2 (1952):597-598.

---

596 M Mushinski, "Average Hospital Charges For Medical And Surgical Treatment Of Back Problems: United States, 1993," Statistical Bulletin. Metropolitan Life Insurance Co., Health and Safety Division, Medical Dept. (April-June 1995)

597 WC Peul, HC van Houwelingen, WB van den Hout, R Brand, JAH Eekhof, JT Tans, RTWM Thomeer, BW Koes, for the Leiden–The Hague Spine Intervention Prognostic Study Group, "Prolonged Conservative Care Versus Early Surgery In Patients With Sciatica Caused By Lumbar Disc Herniation: Two-Year Results Of A Randomized Controlled Trial," *BMJ*, 23/6 (2008)

598 "Balancing Costs and Benefits: Is Disc Surgery Cost-Effective?" *The* BACK *LETTER*, 23/6 (June 2008):61

599 MedlinePlus - Health Information from the National Library of Medicine, Health information from the National Library of Medicine. Easy access to Medline and Health topics, medical dictionaries, directories and publications. http://www.nlm.nih.gov/medlineplus/

- Mensor MD, "Non-operative Treatment, Including Manipulation, For Lumbar Intervertebral Disc Syndrome," *J Bone Joint Surg* 37A (1955):926-935.
- Kuo PP, Loh Z, "Treatment of Lumbar Intervertebral Disc Protrusions by Manipulation," *Clin Orthop* 215 (1987):47-55.
- Cassidy JD, Thiel HW, Kirkaldy-Willis WH, "Side Posture Manipulation For Lumbar Intervertebral Disk Herniation," *J Manipulative Physiol Ther.* 16/2 (Feb 1993):96-103.
- Troyanovich SJ, Harrison DD, Harrison DE, "Low Back Pain and The Lumbar Intervertebral Disk: Clinical Considerations for The Doctor Of Chiropractic," *J Manipulative Physiol Ther.* 22/2 (Feb 1999):96-104.
- Quon JA, Cassidy JD, O'Connor SM, Kirkaldy-Willis WH, "Lumbar Intervertebral Disc Herniation: Treatment By Rotational Manipulation," *J Manipulative Physiol Ther.* 12/3 (Jun 1989):220-7.
- Cox JM, Hazen LJ, Mungovan M, "Distraction Manipulation Reduction Of An L5-S1 Disk Herniation," *J Manipulative Physiol Ther.* 16/5 (Jun 1993):342-6.
- Schneider MJ, "Distraction Manipulation Reduction Of An L5-S1 Disk Herniation," *J Manipulative Physiol Ther.* 16/9 (Nov-Dec 1993):618-20
- Slosberg M, "Side Posture Manipulation For Lumbar Intervertebral Disk Herniation Reconsidered," *J Manipulative Physiol Ther.* 17/4 (May 1994):258-62.
- Bergmann TF, Jongeward BV, "Manipulative Therapy In Lower Back Pain With Leg Pain And Neurological Deficit," *J Manipulative Physiol Ther.* 21/4 (May 1998):288-94.
- Shealy, CN, MD, PhD, and Borgmeyer, V, RN, MA, "Emerging Technologies: Preliminary Findings, Decompression, Reduction, And Stabilization Of The Lumbar Spine: A Cost-Effective Treatment For Lumbosacral Pain," *AJPM* 7/2 (April 1997).
- Gose EE, Naguszewski WK, Naguszewski RK, "Vertebral Axial Decompression Therapy For Pain Associated With Herniated Or Degenerated Discs Or Facet Syndrome: An Outcome Study," Department of Bioengineering, University of Illinois at Chicago, USA. *Neurol Res.* 20/3 (April 1998):186-90.

This list is just a quick scan, so obviously Peul failed to do his homework when he stated "there are no proven nonoperative treatments for sciatica."

A recent 2010 study in Calgary, Alberta, Canada, by Gordon McMorland *et al.* compared spinal manipulation against microdiscectomy in patients with sciatica secondary to lumbar disc herniation.[600] The authors found sixty percent of patients with sciatica benefitted from spinal manipulation.

---

600 G McMorland, E Suter, S Casha, SJ du Plessis, and RJ Hurlbert, "Manipulation or Microdiskectomy for Sciatica? A Prospective Randomized Clinical Study," *JMPT* 33/8 (Oct 2010):576-584.

Dr. Peul is Director of the Spine Intervention Prognostic Study Group at Leiden University Medical Center. Since 2004, he has been a full time spinal neurosurgeon in The Hague and Chairman of the Spine Center in The Netherlands. Certainly his vested interest in discectomies should be a clue as to his inclination.

Despite the call for restraint among American and European spine experts, Peul inexplicably concluded:

> From a societal perspective, disc surgery is cost-effective. It earns money for society. Based on the cost-effectiveness data only, a health economist might say "You should do as much disc surgery as possible."[601]

Considering the call for restraint, Peul's conclusion was more than shocking, but not surprising considering the fact that he is a neurosurgeon. He ought to have just said, "It earns money for me!"

Peul's conclusion is even more perplexing when he suggested discectomies for sciatica were preferable and cost-effective over conservative care in the short term (six weeks), but he also admitted discectomies were not more effective in the long term (six months). [602] Peul offered no explanation for this obvious problem.

Peul's use of conservative *medical* care also prevented a true comparison in that it failed to offer the most effective *chiropractic* conservative treatments such as a combination spinal manipulative therapy, flexion-distraction, non-surgical spinal decompression, along with active rehab therapies.

Obviously this was a sham comparison of spine surgery to "conservative care" since not all conservative care is alike. In effect, the medical conservative care offered— reassuring advice and pain pills—is certainly misleading. To suggest this represents the *best* of conservative care is another Big Lie.

Yet, even the use of those weak conservative medical treatments still proved comparable in the long run with spine surgery!

Peul admitted there were no significant differences between treatment groups beyond six months, and his follow-up results for surgery were even worse. Results of the two groups were identical at one-year follow-up in terms of pain, disability, and global outcome. Over the course of the first year, 95 percent of both groups reported complete recovery, but *this worsened in the surgical group over the next few years.*

In a subsequent interview, Peul also admitted the downside of microdiscectomy:

> "However, some patients had recurrent complaints. And at one year 13% had bad outcomes. And at two years, the proportion of patients with unsuccessful outcomes rose to 20%. This is a huge issue. We are not doing something right."[603]

---

601 Ibid.

602 Ibid.

603 "Balancing Costs and Benefits: Is Disc Surgery Cost-Effective?" The BACK LETTER 23/6 (June 2008):61

Peul finally speaks the truth—what these surgeons are "not doing something right" is treating a secondary disc issue and ignoring the mechanical dynamics of the spine as a functioning unit that caused the disc to herniate in the first place. Peul attempts to view back pain as primarily a pathoanatomical disc problem with surgery as the logical solution when, in reality, most spine pain is now believed to be a pathophysiologic problem, primarily as a joint complex dysfunction.

Bearing in mind the enormous number of spinal vertebrae and spinal joints, the likelihood is great that joint dysfunction may be a commonplace source of back pain that must be treated before expensive imaging, shots, drugs, and invasive surgery are considered.

No doubt in many cases, both pathoanatomical (pathological anatomical changes such as disc abnormalities, arthritis, bone spurs) and pathophysiological (altered biomechanics) problems exist—long standing joint dysfunction as well as disc abnormalities. To address only the disc issue with surgery still leaves the joint dysfunction uncorrected, which may explain why surgical patients have recurrent back pain. As Dr. Mennell testified, until the joint play is restored, back pain will not cease.

The differential diagnosis and management of musculoskeletal disorders are assuming this new direction, according to Gwen Jull, PhD:

> The focus on pathoanatomical diagnoses is generally shifting towards a more pathophysiological approach in the recognition that in the majority of neck disorders *a definitive pathoanatomical cause may not be able to be readily identified in up to 80% of neck pain patients.*[604] (emphasis added)

Her remarks echo Dr. Deyo when he opined that 85 percent of low back pain cannot be attributed to pathoanatomical findings either:

> Up to 85% of patients cannot be given a definitive diagnosis because of weak associations among symptoms, pathological changes, and imaging results.[605]

Dr. Goodley answered Dr. Deyo's admission with his belief that the fundamental bias against manipulative therapy is the main reason for this pandemic of pain. "I accuse that a big slice of the 85 percent of undetermined diagnosis of back pain is ignorance and is accountable for the rejection of the thinking involved in manipulative approaches."[606]

This argument exemplifies the pathoanatomical view that Deyo and Peul have taken rather than the emphasis on pathophysiologic perspective such as joint dysfunction as Goodley and Mennell have done. The New Zealand Inquiry recognized this difference when it mentioned, "The problem is a functional not a structural one...He might as well expect to see a limp, or a headache or any other functional problem on x-ray."[607]

---

604 G Jull, *et al. Whiplash, Headache, and Neck Pain,* (Churchill Livingstone, 2008).
605 RA Deyo, "Conservative Therapy for Low Back Pain: Distinguishing Useful From Useless Therapy," *Journal of American Medical Association* 250 (1983):1057-62.
606 Ibid. p. 517.
607 Ibid. p. 55.

Considering 85 percent of spine problems are admittedly misdiagnosed and, consequently, mistreated, it should not come as a surprise that research now shows spine surgeries offer no long term benefits over conservative care. Spine surgery is also now hugely expensive and increasing at an astronomical rate despite the call for restraint.

Dr. Deyo and his colleagues tracked the U.S. national trends in lumbar fusion surgery for degenerative conditions from 1990–2000 and found shocking increases of 220 percent between 1990 and 2001:

> In 2001, approximately 122,000 lumbar fusions were performed in the U.S. On a population basis, this represented a *220% increase from 1990 in fusions* per 100,000. The slope of the rising rate increased in 1996, when fusion cages were approved. From 1996 to 2001, the number of lumbar fusions increased over 113%, compared with 13-15% for hip replacement and knee arthroplasty. Rates of lumbar fusion rose most rapidly among patients aged 60 and above. In this group, rates increased 230% over the decade, compared with 180% among adults aged 40-59, and 120% among adults under age 40. The proportion of all lumbar operations involving a fusion increased for all diagnoses.[608] (emphasis added)

A study by James N. Weinstein *et al.*, "Trends and Regional Variations in Lumbar Spine Surgery in the United States," indicated the shocking cost increases of 500 percent between 1992 and 2002. Recall this period followed the attack on the 1994 AHCPR guideline #14 on acute low back pain in adults that urged a restraint on spine surgery.[609] Once this US Public Health Service guideline was dismantled, instead of moderating their surgeries, they escalated tremendously:

> *Spending for lumbar fusion increased more than 500%,* from $75 million to $482 million. In 1992, lumbar fusion represented 14% of total spending for back surgery; by 2003, lumbar fusion accounted for 47% of spending.[610]

Ironically, despite the high costs and poor outcomes of spine surgery, they continue to be permitted by Medicare and many insurance programs. "If we stopped paying for everything that had no evidence of benefit, we would be a very unpopular organization," said Dr. Steve Phurrough, director of Medicare's coverage and analysis group. "Back pain is an increasing problem in our country and people want something done."[611]

---

608 RA Deyo, *et al.*, "Epidemiology of Spinal Surgery: Rates and Trends, Comparative Costs, Effectiveness, and Outcomes," Research Center, University of Washington, http://depts.washington.edu/ccor/studies/SpineSurgEpi.shtml: Accessed (February 23, 2010).

609 SJ Bigos, O Bowyer, G Braea, K Brown, R Deyo, S Haldeman, *et al.* "Acute Low Back Pain Problems in Adults: Clinical Practice Guideline no. 14." Rockville, MD: U.S. Department of Health and Human Services, Public Health Service, Agency for Health Care Policy and Research; (1992) AHCPR publication no. 95-0642.

610 JN Weinstein, JD Lurie, PR Olson, KK Bronner, ES Fisher, "United States' Trends and Regional Variations in Lumbar Spine Surgery: 1992-2003," *Spine* 31/23 (1 November 2006):2707-2714

611 A Dembner, "Spine tuning, Innovative Surgeries Raise Hope, Concern," *Boston Globe* Staff, (September 3, 2007)

While something is being done, it often is the wrong thing to do. As Dr. Waddell, warned, "Medical care certainly has not solved the everyday symptom of low back pain and even may be reinforcing and exacerbating the problem."[612]

Drugs, shots, and spine surgery have not stopped the rising tide in the tsunami of back pain, and reliance upon these treatments may actually be worsening the problem; indeed, medical spine care today is a shot in the dark with suspect treatments and unreliable outcomes. Not only have spine surgeries skyrocketed, so has another, newer treatment that has not proven effective, although it has become very profitable.

The recent growth in "pain management" clinics featuring epidural steroid injections (ESI) have gotten troubling criticism from medical experts like Robert J. Barth, a neuropsychologist, who believes these ESI treatments "reliably fail, the treatments seems to lead to a progressive worsening of the claimant's presentation, the ineffective treatment never ends, and the original treating doctors refer the claimants into pain management simple as a means of escaping from or 'dumping' a problematic patient."[613]

Barth believes "pain management does not accomplish anything but getting the patient addicted." He concludes that "pain management situation in the U.S. is, indeed, horrific."[614] Nonetheless, it is among the fastest growing segments in medicine today.

A similar review of pain management via ESI was regarded as "goofy" by R. Norman Harden, MD, in the *American Pain Society Bulletin*:

> We practice at a time when unproven experimental, invasive, and expensive procedures are often compensated without question. Many of the surgical and interventional techniques have never been subjected to evidence based inquiry. Oddly, the FDA approves devices and procedures relatively easily...in this context, there has been a proliferation of extremely goofy therapies, which are expensive at best, and downright dangerous at worst.[615]

Another criticism of ESI appeared in the *American Pain Society Bulletin* by Steven H. Sanders, PhD, who revealed nerve blocks for back pain are not supported by scientific research: "From the current review, we must conclude injections and nerve blocks produce a large amount of money with very little science to support their application."[616]

Not only have epidural injections come under criticism, so has the widespread use of opioids in the long-term treatment of back pain. "There is increasing recognition

---

612 G Waddell and OB Allan, "A Historical Perspective On Low Back Pain And Disability, "*Acta Orthop Scand* 60 (suppl 234), (1989)

613 RJ Barth, "Saying No!—Unjustified Surgeries, Pain Management and Tests," *For the Defense* 48/3 (March 2006):33-39. Washington & Lee Law School Current Law Journal Content

614 Barth, ibid. p. 33

615 RN Harden, "Chronic Opioid Therapy: Another Reappraisal," *APS Bulletin* 12/1 (January/February 2002) Pain and Public Policy, Corey D. Fox, PhD, Department Editor

616 SH Sanders and P Vicente, "Medicare and Medicaid Financing For Pain Management: The Wrong Message At The Right Time," *The Journal of Pain*, 1/3 (September 2000):197-198.

that this massive treatment movement may have been a mistake," opined the editors of ᵀᴴᴱBACK*LETTER.* "The proven benefits of opioids do not extend to the long-term treatment of chronic pain...Editorials and commentaries in medical journals are starting to pose the question 'How could this have happened?'" [617]

A new study on opioid use from Denmark reveals more disturbing news. Although proponents of opioid drugs speculate they provide significant pain relief, improve function, and enhance quality of life over the long term, a new study by Per Sjøgren, MD, and colleagues refute this claim. They found the use of opioids was associated with inadequate pain relief, poor quality of life, long-term unemployment, and high levels of medical care-seeking.[618]

"Furthermore, the results indicated that individuals with chronic pain using strong opioids had a higher risk of death than individuals without chronic pain," according to Sjøgren."[619]

Paul Goodley, MD, commented on the change in spine care and the sudden rise of pain management clinics:

> Much has recently changed since I began writing this book in 1992. Among the more notable: Leaders in chiropractic have remarkably advanced the merits of its professionalism, in some states, in extraordinary ways. In traditional medicine, some, at long last, are beginning to, at least, listen.
>
> At the same time, unhappily, "pain management," a new discipline, is increasingly equated with specialized injection techniques absent understanding (yet) that biomechanical fundamentals related to the beginnings of many pain syndromes must be appreciated by any professional who professes to treat pain. Regardless, the beginnings of the shift in restoring balance are now noticeable.[620]

Other spine specialists are noticing the change in treatments, but Dr. Richard Deyo openly admits that too many people are still getting risky and expensive back surgery when more minimal approaches would work.[621] Overuse of spine surgery is a huge reason why the nation's health bill was so high. He concluded that "More people are interested in getting on the gravy train than on stopping the gravy train."[622]

---

617 "How Could This Have Happened?" *The* BACK*LETTER* 26/1 (2011):7

618 Per Sjøgren *et al.,* "A Population-Based Cohort Study On *Chronic Pain*: The Role Of Opioids," Clinical Journal of Pain, 26/9 (2010):332-9

619 "Long-Term Opioid Therapy for Chronic Pain: Dismal Results in Real-World Settings?" *The* BACK*LETTER* 26/1 (2011):1

620 PH Goodley, *Release from Pain,* www.DrGoodley.com (2005):2

621 J Silberner, "Surgery May Not Be The Answer To An Aching Back," *All Things Considered*, National Public Radio, Melissa Block, host. (April 6, 2010)

622 R Abelson, "Financial Ties Are Cited as Issue in Spine Study," *NY Times* (January 30, 2008)

Few people realize the enormous costs for medical spine procedures (not including hospital cost): [623]

- lumbar fusion with hardware can cost as high as $169,000,
- lumbar laminectomy: $82,614,
- lumbar discectomy: $39, 836,
- cervical laminectomy: $60,304,
- cervical fusion with hardware: $112,480.
- lumbar MRI: $2,000
- discogram: $4,500
- epidural steroid injections: $2-3,000
- intradiscal electrothermal therapy (IDET): $6,500

RD Guyer, MD, former North American Spine Society president, in his 2008 presidential address, "The Paradox In Medicine Today—Exciting Technology And Economic Challenges," admitted the huge money involved in the spine business. "The stakes are great as there is big money in spine…in 2005 dollars, between $100 and $200 billion per year are spent on spine care…U.S. spinal device manufacturers was estimated at $2.5 billion." [624]

Be certain the medical industrial complex has no interest in slowing down this gravy train. After Weinstein *et al.* showed the shocking increase in spine costs and usage from 1992 to 2002, Deyo *et al.* reiterated the large increase in the rate of spine surgery in their recent study of the subsequent five years. "The most complex type of back surgery has increased dramatically between 2002 and 2007 with a *15-fold increase.*"[625]

Deyo discovered that the more-complex type of spine surgery was associated with substantially higher risk of life-threatening complications. He and his colleagues found the mean hospital costs for surgical decompression and complex fusions ranged from $23,724 for the former and $80,888 for the latter.

Deyo also noted, "It seems implausible that the number of patients with the most complex spinal pathology increased 15-fold in just six years." Among the various reasons for such a large increase, he mentioned one strong motivation included *"financial incentives involving both surgeons and hospitals."*[626]

For the ninety minutes or so it takes to do a simple decompression surgery to clean out the boney growth that can compress nerves, the surgeon is typically reimbursed around $600 to $1,000. The fee for a five or six-hour fusion of multiple vertebrae is

623 A Schlapia, J Eland, "Multiple Back Surgeries And People Still Hurt." Available at http://pedspain. nursing.uiowa.edu/CEU/Backpain.html Accessed April 22, 2003.

624 RD Guyer, Presidential address, "The Paradox In Medicine Today—Exciting Technology And Economic Challenges, *The Spine Journal*, 8/2 (March/April 2008):279-285.

625 J Silberner, "Surgery May Not Be The Answer To An Aching Back," *All Things Considered*, NPR (April 6, 2010)

626 "New Study Demonstrates A Three-Fold Increase N Life-Threatening Complications With Complex Surgery," *The BACKLETTER*, 25/6 (June 2010):66

ten times as high, $6,000 to $8,000 for the complex fusion, which explains the sudden increase in these surgeries.[627,628]

Eugene J. Carragee, MD, from Stanford University, admitted the "fundamental failing" with unnecessary spine surgery:

> The proliferation of risky and expensive practice beyond reasonable supporting evidence is commonly mentioned as a *fundamental failing of medical practice* in the United States.[629]

> New and more complex technologies are being used for patients with little specific indication for the approaches and for whom there is *good evidence that simpler methods are highly effective.*[630] (emphasis added)

Despite the much higher cost for complex fusion, there was no evidence of superior outcomes, but there was greater morbidity associated with the complex fusion. They found that those who underwent complex spinal fusion had roughly *three times the risk of developing a life-threatening complication* compared with those who had decompression alone.[631]

Indeed, there are "simpler methods" that are highly effective for back pain, namely chiropractic care as many studies have indicated. If it were not for the medical war to eliminate and defame chiropractic care, the utilization of this effective, time-proven method would certainly help to decrease the costs and usage of back surgery. Unfortunately, the medical profession is not interested in cooperation as much as it is focused on domination and profits. Nor is it, apparently, interested in its Hippocratic Oath to "do no harm" to patients.

In fact, spine surgeries are doing much harm, more than any other surgery in history as Dr. Waddell has warned.[632] Experts estimate that nearly 600,000 Americans opt for back operations each year. But for many, surgery is just an empty promise that can backfire, leaving patients in more pain, according to an article by Linda Carroll, "Back Surgery May Backfire on Patients in Pain."

In 2010, researchers reviewed records from 1,450 patients in the Ohio Bureau of Workers' Compensation database who had diagnoses of disc degeneration, disc herniation

---

627 RA Deyo, SK Mirza, BI Martin, W Kreuter, DC Goodman, JG Jarvik, "Trends, major medical complications, and charges associated with surgery for lumbar spinal stenosis in older adults," *JAMA.* 303/13 (Apr 7, 2010):1259-65.

628 J Silberner, "Surgery May Not Be The Answer To An Aching Back," *All Things Considered*, National Public Radio, Melissa Block, host. April 6, 2010

629 "Spike in Complex Spinal Surgery Sets Off a Wave of Serious Complications and Exorbitant Costs," *The* BACK*LETTER*, 25/6 (June 2010):61,67

630 EJ Carragee, "The Increasing Morbidity of Elective Spinal Stenosis Surgery: Is It Necessary?" *JAMA* 303 (2010):1309-10

631 EJ Carragee, ibid.

632 G Waddell and OB Allan, "A Historical Perspective On Low Back Pain And Disability, "*Acta Orthop Scand* 60 (suppl 234), (1989)

or radiculopathy, a nerve condition that causes tingling and weakness of the limbs. Half of the patients had surgery to fuse two or more vertebrae in hopes of curing low back pain. The other half had no surgery, even though they had comparable diagnoses. [633]

After two years, only 26 percent of those who had surgery returned to work compared to 67 percent of patients who did not have surgery. Of the lumbar fusion subjects, 36 percent had complications, and the reoperation rate was 27 percent for surgical patients. Permanent disability rates were 11 percent for cases and 2 percent for nonoperative controls. In what might be the most troubling finding, researchers determined that there was a 41 percent increase in the use of painkillers, with 76 percent of cases continuing opioid use after surgery. Seventeen surgical patients died by the end of the study. [634]

The study provides clear evidence that for many patients, fusion surgeries designed to alleviate pain from abnormal discs do not work according to the study's lead author Dr. Trang Nguyen, MD, PhD, researcher at the University of Cincinnati College of Medicine. His study concluded: "Lumbar fusion for the diagnoses of disc degeneration, disc herniation, and/or radiculopathy in a Workers Compensation setting is associated with *significant increase in disability, opiate use, prolonged work loss, and poor return to work status.*" [635]

"The outcomes of this procedure for degenerative disc disease and disc herniation make it an unfortunate treatment choice," according to Nguyen.[636]

According to the editors of ᵀᴴᴱBACK*LETTER*, "This form of surgery in workers' compensation subjects appears to be a gamble at best." In another workers' compensation study from Kentucky by Leah Carreon, MD, *et al.,* only 19 percent of patients had a clinically significant improvement in disability after fusion surgery. "Surgeons should be cautious in discussing the effectiveness of lumbar fusion for patients on workers' compensation," said Carreon.[637]

Dr. Steven Atlas, MD, shared his thoughts with the editors of ᵀᴴᴱBACK*LETTER*:

> In my experience, patients don't want spinal fusion when they're given good information—that is why I favor a shared decision-making approach. Others would argue that we should stop doing this expensive procedure until we show that it provides a benefit. But that is not how we do things at present in the United States. But if we don't see rates of spinal fusion dropping—then maybe it would be time to simply say no.[638]

---

633 L Carroll, "Back Surgery May Backfire on Patients in Pain," MSNBC.com, (10/14/2010)

634 TH Nguyen, DC Randolph, J Talmage, P Succop, R Travis," Long-term Outcomes of Lumbar Fusion Among Workers' Compensation Subjects: An Historical Cohort Study," *Spine*, (Aug 23, 2010)

635 Nguyen, ibid.

636 "Dismal Results for Spinal Fusion Among Patients with Workers' Compensation Claims," *The* BACK*LETTER* 25/11 (November 2010):121

637 Ibid. p. 127.

638 "Fusion Surgery for Injured Workers: An Opportunity for Shared Decision-Making?" *The* BACK*LETTER* 25/11 (November 2010):129.

Not only are most spine surgeries unnecessary, costly, and life-threatening, they are also disabling for many. Another study in *Surgical Neurology* by E. Berger showed that 71 percent of patients with a single surgery and 95 percent of lumbar fusion patients who had multiple surgeries never returned to work.[639]

Another extensive 2006 study, "The Spine Patient Outcomes Research Trial (SPORT)," led by James N. Weinstein, Director of the Dartmouth Institute for Health Policy and Clinical Practice, shows that patients with low back and leg pain who underwent spinal discectomy surgery fared no better two years later than those who used non-invasive therapies.[640]

The SPORT study is the latest to suggest that America is losing its battle against back pain and that many medical treatments may be ineffective or overused. Dr. Weinstein said the rapid growth in surgical procedures, coupled with the lack of hard evidence, points to the need to spell out all the risks and benefits for patients and let them choose—in other words, to end the medical stranglehold on the back pain treatments of drugs, shots, and surgery.

"As in most of medicine, there isn't as much evidence as we would like," said Dr. Weinstein. "We need to be clear that there is a choice of treatments," he said, and "that one isn't necessarily better than the other."[641]

Quite an admission from an orthopedist undoubtedly tormented that the profitable spinal surgeries cannot be well substantiated in this era of evidence-based medicine. Dr. Weinstein admits that medicine does not always follow the best evidence and noted that better information would benefit patients:

I think if patients were well-informed, they would choose the right thing. We've done lots of studies with shared decision-making. Where patients are given good information, *they generally choose the least invasive, less risky procedure.*[642] (emphasis added)

Of course, the "least invasive, less risky procedure" certainly alludes to chiropractic care. As with many medical researchers, Dr. Weinstein has trouble admitting this truth publicly, undoubtedly fearing a backlash from his surgeon colleagues just as Richard Deyo experienced a similar wrath after the AHCPR episode.

Despite these admonitions from experts, their message is slow getting to the public in the popular press, and many gullible patients are still being fooled by their spine surgeon. Additionally, some surgeons stoop to scare tactics to persuade unsuspecting patients. Many surgeons often frighten patients that if they delay surgery they may risk permanent nerve damage, perhaps a weakened leg, or even losing bowel or bladder control, yet nothing like that occurred in the two-year study with nearly 2,000 patients comparing surgery with waiting.

---

639 E Berger, "Later Postoperative Results in 1000 Work Related Lumbar Spine Conditions," *Surgical Neurology* 54/2 (August 2000):101-106.

640 JN Weinstein *et al.,* "Surgical vs. Nonoperative Treatment For Lumbar Disc Herniation: The Spine Patient Outcomes Research Trial (SPORT) Observational Cohort," *Journal of the American Medical Association* 296 (2006):2451–9.

641 A Dembner, "Spine Tuning, Innovative Surgeries Raise Hope, Concern," *Boston Globe* Staff (September 3, 2007).

642 JN Weinstein transcript from National Public Radio, (April 6, 21010)

Fear that delaying an operation could be dangerous "was the 800-pound gorilla in the room," according to Eugene Carragee, professor of orthopedic surgery at Stanford, in an interview in *The New York Times*.

> The worry was not knowing. If someone had a big herniated disk, can you just say, "Well, if it's not bothering you that much, you can wait." It's kind of like walking on eggshells. What if something terrible did happen?[643]

Dr. Carragee said that he had never believed it himself, but that the concern was widespread among patients and doctors. However, in most cases, nothing did happen although the fright forced many patients into unnecessary surgery.

Not only are many spine surgeries often unnecessary, the research shows the majority rarely require immediate action, many are ineffective in the long term, and new research now suggests they may only have a placebo effect. Ironically, the placebo effect was an aspersion—"it's all in your head"—used by MDs in regards concerning patients who improved with chiropractic care. During the *Wilk* trial, Dr. Ernest K. Howard, the AMA president at that time, testified that chiropractic care was only "psychosomatic,"[644] the prevailing medical slander touted by most MDs.

Now, it appears the table has turned. Not only do their scare tactics cause many unnecessary back surgeries, a 2005 study from Switzerland suggests that a surgeon's optimistic attitude may be unrealistic compared to actual patient outcomes and illustrates the "curabo effect" of surgery.[645]

According to a University of Lausanne study done of 197 patients who had surgery for low back pain or sciatica, surgeons forecasted "excellent or at least moderate improvement" for nearly all (99 percent) of patients. Rather than the optimistic 99 percent prediction by surgeons, in fact, the majority (56 percent) of the patients showed no significant improvements in their general health a year after their back surgery.

The Swiss team concluded that "surgeons tended to give overly optimistic predictions that were not correlated with patient outcome." The researchers believed the "more optimistic physician expectation was associated with better improvement of psychological dimensions," what they referred to as the "curabo effect." The power of the surgeon's suggestion, not unlike the "placebo effect" makes patients think they improved without any real corrective intervention.

Despite these studies and warnings, the rates of spine surgery in the U.S. have only increased as the costs have soared, which shows that evidence-based spine care is ignored when it conflicts with the economic-based profit motive of spine surgeons. Many surgeons continue to ignore the guidelines or ridicule the researchers, just as they did when the North American Spine Society attacked the AHCPR guideline on acute low back pain.

---

643 G Kolata, "Surgery Need Is Questioned In Disk Injury," *New York Times* (November 12, 2008)

644 Deposition of Ernest K. Howard by George McAndrews, (Dec. 15, 1980):1052.

645 B Graz, V Wietlisbach, F Porchet, JP Vader, "Prognosis or "Curabo Effect"?: Physician Prediction and Patient Outcome of Surgery for Low Back Pain and Sciatica," *Spine* 30/12 (June 15, 2005):1448-1452

Considering the plethora of evidence today showing the questionable diagnostics, poor outcomes, and high costs of spine surgery, it is hard to imagine spine surgeons are unaware of these issues and warnings. Any "overly optimistic predictions" may have more to do with salesmanship rather than clinical reality.

On the other hand, there are ethical orthopedists who are well aware of the misfortune of back surgery. Jens Ivar Brox, MD, lead investigator of the Norway Spine Study, reported that he and his colleagues "no longer perform spinal fusion specifically for 'degenerative disc disease' because they do not regard it as a clearly diagnosable entity."[646]

Dr. Brox admitted some of the orthopaedic surgeons in his department have recurrent back pain and disc degeneration, but these surgeons refuse to have fusion surgery or recommend fusion surgery for their family members.

"So the question is: Why should we recommend these procedures for our patients?" Finally, an honest surgeon speaks.

Every American spine surgeon should ask himself the same question: will he be so quick to do surgery on his own family members (or have it done on oneself) as he does on his patients?

Addendum: A very important event has occurred as this book goes to press; BlueCross/BlueShield of North Carolina announced that as of January 1, 2011, it would no longer provide reimbursement for lumbar spinal fusion with the sole indication of degenerative disc disease as well as three other conditions. The official North Carolina BC/BS website[647] states:

Lumbar spinal fusion is also considered not medically necessary if the sole indication is any one or more of the following conditions:

- Disk Herniation
- Degenerative Disk Disease
- Initial diskectomy/laminectomy for neural structure decompression
- Facet Syndrome

If and when this policy goes nationwide, it will save billions of dollars and help millions of patients from failed back surgery syndrome. Indeed, this policy change could become the tipping point chiropractors have long awaited—the day when clinical and cost-effectiveness overcome the profit motive in medicine. Hopefully this evidence-based trend continues to restore sanity to spine care.

---

646 JI Brox, R Sørensen, A Friis, *et al*. "Randomized Clinical Trial Of Lumbar Instrumented Fusion And Cognitive Intervention And Exercises In Patients With Chronic Low Back Pain And Disc Degeneration," *Spine* 28 (2003):1913–1921.

647 http://www.bcbsnc.com/assets/services/public/pdfs/medicalpolicy/lumbar_spine_fusion_surgery.pdf

Call for Reform

"There is an overwhelming body of evidence
indicating that chiropractic management of low back pain
is more cost-effective than medical management."

Pran Manga, PhD, health economist[648]

The back pain business is huge in both the number of patients and treatments; moreover, it is tainted by the lure of high surgical fees. Medical experts now admit that it is also rampant with a smorgasbord of treatments most of which most are unproven and ineffective according to a study on chronic low back pain headed by Dr. Scott Haldeman.[649]

This smorgasbord of treatments for low back pain includes:[650]

- 60+ pharmaceutical products
- 32 different manual therapies
- 20 different exercise programs
- 26 different passive physical modalities
- 9 educational and psychological therapies
- 20+ different injections therapies

648   P Manga, D Angus, C Papadopoulos, W Swan, "The Effectiveness and Cost-Effectiveness of Chiropractic Management of Low Back Pain," (funded by the Ontario Ministry of Health) (August, 1993):104

649   S Haldeman, S Dagenais, "Evidence-Informed Management of Chronic Low Back Pain Without Surgery," The Spine Journal 8/1 (January/February 2008):258-65.

650   S Haldeman and S Dagenais, "What Have We Learned About The Evidence-Informed Management Of Chronic Low Back Pain?" The Spine Journal 8/1 (January-February 2008):266-277.

- 11 more traditional and newer surgical approaches
- Extensive lifestyle products sold for chronic low back pain, including braces, beds, chairs, and ergonomic aides
- Complementary and alternative medical approaches to chronic low back pain

Dr. Haldeman believes that "navigating this selection without an informed guide is analogous to shopping in a foreign supermarket without understanding the product labels."[651] Dr. Haldeman also admitted not much has changed since the AHCPR report in 1994:

> This interpretation of the best available evidence is not materially different than the recommendations from the Practice Guidelines on Acute Low Back Pain in Adults that were published by the Agency for Health Care Policy and Research in 1994...*it is somewhat disappointing to note that 14 years {since AHCPR} after dozens of highly promoted* new interventions, thousands of studies, millions of lost work days, and billions of dollars spent on its care, *so little has changed in the evidence available to guide stakeholders and support treatments for chronic low back pain.*[652] (emphasis added)

When one of the most astute spine authorities in the world admits the confusion about back pain treatments and the intransigence to change, undoubtedly there is a big problem for consumers trying to understand the myriad treatments as well as doctors trying to keep track of this assortment.

Dr. Haldeman did state his confidence in chiropractic care for this epidemic of chronic low back pain. "It also shows the positive effects of preventive chiropractic treatment in maintaining functional capacities and reducing the number and intensity of pain episodes after an acute phase of treatment."[653]

Despite the smorgasbord of treatments, there is no confusion about one thing: *In the American healthcare system, everyone agrees there is too much spine surgery.* The call for restraint has led to a loud call for reform in the treatment of musculoskeletal disorders, and leading the way is the chiropractic profession.

Chiropractors to the Rescue

Today, the proof is positive that manual therapy is helping to relieve this epidemic. In an article, "Are There Any Effective Nonsurgical Treatments for Painful Disc Herniations?", Jo Jordan, PhD, wrote that spinal manipulation may be the "lone ray of light" for back pain treatment:

> *The lone ray of light among nonsurgical treatments in this review concerned spinal manipulation.* With regard to non-drug treatments, spinal manipulation seems to be

---

651 S Haldeman and S Dagenais, "A Supermarket Approach To The Evidence-Informed Management Of Chronic Low Back Pain," *The Spine Journal* 8/1 (January-February 2008):1-7.
652 Ibid. pp. 266-277.
653 Ibid.

more effective at relieving local or radiating pain in people with acute back pain and sciatica with disc protrusion compared with sham manipulation, although concerns exist regarding possible further herniation from spinal manipulation in people who are surgical candidates.[654] (emphasis added)

By the end of the 1990s, evidence-based research from Europe and America recommended major changes to the management of patients with low back pain, including those diagnosed with disc herniation. Studies in the U.S.[655], U.K.[656], Canada[657], and Denmark[658] all concluded: back surgeries were excessive, and conservative care such as spinal manipulative therapy and active rehab were the best initial approaches to the vast majority of low back pain (LBP) problems.

"No clear evidence emerged that primary spinal fusion surgery was any more beneficial than intensive rehabilitation," according to Jeremy Fairbank, MD, lead investigator, British Spine Study (UK BEAM). "And *spine care providers should offer intensive rehabilitation enthusiastically*, as it finds clear support in the scientific literature, and will prevent unnecessary surgery in a substantial proportion of patients."[659]

The BACK*LETTER* editorial staff also noticed the stubbornness of physicians to implement the new guidelines for low back pain, which includes the use of spinal manipulation as a first route of treatment before surgery:

> Numerous international guidelines have endorsed the use spinal manipulation as a treatment for acute back pain—as part of an evidence-based treatment algorithm. But researchers have been slow to examine the impact of guidelines-based care in rigorous clinical trials—"to see if an evidence-based approach actually works in real-world clinical settings."[660]

Perhaps American surgeons are reluctant "to see if an evidence-based approach actually works in real-world clinical settings" because spinal manipulation and other hands-on therapies done by chiropractors would certainly take a lot of money out of the surgeons' pockets and the hospitals' coffers.

---

654 J Jordan, *et al.*, "Herniated Lumbar Disc," *BMJ* Clinical Evidence, quote in The BACK*LETTER*® 25/7 (July 2010):76-77

655 S Bigos et al.

656 Her Majesty's Stationery Office in London in its Report of a Clinical Standards Advisory Group Committee on Back Pain (1994)

657 P Manga and D Angus, "Enhanced Chiropractic Coverage Under OHIP As A Means Of Reducing Health Care Costs, Attaining Better Health Outcomes And Achieving Equitable Access To Select Health Services." Working paper, University of Ottawa, 98-02.

658 C Manniche *et al.* "Low-Back Pain: Frequency, Management And Prevention From An HDA Perspective," Danish Health Technology Assessment 1/1 (1999)

659 J Fairbank, *et al.*, "Randomized Controlled Trial To Compare Surgical Stabilisation Of The Lumbar Spine With An Intensive Rehabilitation Programme For Patients With Chronic Low Back Pain: The MRC Spine Stabilisation Trial," Spine Stabilisation Trial Group, *BMJ* (2005):330:1233 (28 May), doi:10.1136/bmj.38441.620417.8F (May 23, 2005)

660 "Evidence-Based Care That Includes Chiropractic Manipulation More Effective Than Usual Medical Care," *The* BACK*LETTER* editorial, 23/1 (2008):3.

Pran Manga, PhD, health economist from Ontario, Canada, conducted two studies in the 1990s and noted, "There is an overwhelming body of evidence indicating that chiropractic management of low back pain is more cost-effective than medical management."[661] There is now broad agreement internationally that surgery should not generally be considered until there has been a trial of conservative non-surgical care.[662,663,664]

According to the 1993 Manga Report, "The Effectiveness and Cost-Effectiveness of Chiropractic Management of Low-Back Pain,"[665] this evidence-based study concluded spinal manipulation was the "therapy of choice for most low back pain":

In our view, the constellation of the evidence shows:

- The effectiveness and cost-effectiveness of chiropractic management of low-back pain.
- The untested, questionable or harmful nature of many current medical therapies.
- The economic efficiency of chiropractic care for low-back pain compared with medical care.
- The safety of chiropractic care.
- The higher satisfaction levels expressed by patients of chiropractors.

Dr. Manga was very realistic about the turf warfare in the healthcare business:

There should be a shift in policy now to encourage the utilization of chiropractic services for the management of LBP, given the impressive body of evidence on the effectiveness and comparative cost-effectiveness of these services, and on the high levels of patient satisfaction.

The shift in utilization from physician to chiropractic care should lead to significant savings in healthcare expenditures judging from evidence in Canada, the U.S., the U.K. and Australia, and even larger savings if a more comprehensive view of the economic costs of low back pain is taken.

Unnecessary or failed surgery is not only wasteful and costly but, *ipso factor*, low quality medical care. The opportunity for consultations, second opinions and wider treatment options are significant advantages we foresee from this initiative which has been employed with success in a clinical research setting at the University Hospital, Saskatoon.

A prominent medical organization, the North American Spine Society, has recently concluded that spinal manipulation, and specifically chiropractic adjustment, is an

661 P Manga, ibid.

662 H Weber, "The Natural History Of Disc Herniation And The Influence Of Intervention," *Spine* 19 (1994):2234-2238.

663 J Saal, "Natural History And Nonoperative Treatment Of Lumbar Disc Herniation," *Spine* 21(1996):2S-9S.

664 F Postacchini, "Results of Surgery Compared With Conservative Management For Lumbar Disc Herniations," *Spine* 21(1996):1383-1387.

665 P Manga, ibid.

acceptable and effective treatment for most patients with lumbosacral disorders. *This review, when coupled with more thorough analysis by prestigious institutions such as RAND Corporation, adds measurably to the growing credence in spinal manipulation as a therapy of choice for most low back pain.*[666] (emphasis added)

A study commissioned by The Foundation for Chiropractic Progress[667] enabled Niteesh Choudhry, MD, PhD, from Harvard Medical School and Arnold Milstein, MD, from Mercer Health and Benefits consulting firm, to investigate an important issue: "Do Chiropractic Physician Services for Treatment of Low-Back and Neck Pain Improve the Value of Health Benefit Plans?" They found in terms of clinical effectiveness and cost together, "chiropractic physician care for low back and neck pain is *highly cost-effective*, represents a good value in comparison to medical physician care and to widely accepted cost-effectiveness thresholds."[668]

Not only is manual therapy more clinically effective, another study shows it is less costly than medical care. A study published in 2010 revealed data over a two-year span from 85,000 Blue Cross Blue Shield beneficiaries with low back pain in Tennessee. The patients had open access to MDs and DCs through self-referral, and there were no limits applied to the number of visits allowed and no differences in co-pays. Results show that paid costs for episodes of care initiated by a chiropractor were almost 40 percent less than care initiated through an MD. They estimated that allowing DC-initiated episodes of care would have led to an annual cost savings of $2.3 million for BCBS of Tennessee.[669]

The truth about the effectiveness of spinal manipulation is emerging in the aftermath of the medical war, but the public remains mostly unaware due to the lack of media attention. Certainly, the medical profession is also ignoring this call for reform despite the growing evidence from around the world.

The following is a review of the numerous international and American guidelines that recommend spinal manipulation for both acute and chronic low back pain:

- 1978: New Zealand Royal Commission on Chiropractic
- 1990: RAND study on appropriateness of spinal manipulation
- 1990: Meade Study (UK) comparing manipulation vs. hospital care
- 1993: Manga Report Ontario (Canada) Ministry of Health

---

666 P Manga, *et al.* "The Effectiveness and Cost-Effectiveness of chiropractic Management of Lob-Back Pain, "Ontario Ministry of Health (1993)

667 www.f4cp.com

668 Arnold Milstein and Niteesh Choudhry, "Do Chiropractic Physician Services for Treatment of Low-Back and Neck Pain Improve the Value of Health Benefit Plans? An Evidence Based Assessment of Incremental Impact on Population Health and Total Healthcare Spending." Funded by the Foundation for Chiropractic Progress, http://www.f4cp.com/pr/2009/1.pdf

669 R L Liliedahl, David V. Axene, Christine M. Goertz, "Cost of Care for Common Back Pain Conditions Initiated With Chiropractic Doctor vs. Medical Doctor/Doctor of Osteopathy as First Physician: Experience of One Tennessee-Based General Health Insurer," *Journal of Manipulative and Physiological Therapeutics* (October, 2010)

- 1994: AHCPR Acute Low Back Pain Guideline
- 1994: Clinical Standards Advisory Group (UK)
- 1995: Council on Chiropractic Guidelines and Practice Parameters
- 2003: Ontario Workers' Safety and Insurance Board
- 2003: Norway Spine Study
- 2004: European Back Pain Guidelines.
- 2004: The UK Back Pain Exercise And Manipulation (UK BEAM) Trial
- 2004: Swedish Lumbar Spine Study
- 2007: Guideline on Back Pain: American College of Physicians
- 2008: Decade of Bone & Joint Disorders: CLBP
- 2008: The Bone and Joint Decade Task Force on Neck Pain and Its Associated Disorders
- 2009: The National Institute for Clinical Excellence (UK-NICE)

As well, an editorial in the *Annals of Internal Medicine* published jointly by the American College of Physicians and the American Society of Internal Medicine (1998) noted that "spinal manipulation is the treatment of choice":

> The Agency for Health Care Policy and Research (AHCPR) recently made history when it concluded that spinal manipulative therapy is the most effective and cost-effective treatment for acute low back pain[670]. The 1994 guidelines for acute low back pain developed by AHCPR concluded that spinal manipulation hastens recovery from acute low back pain and recommended that this therapy be used in combination with or as an alternative to non-steroidal anti-inflammatory drugs. At the same time, AHCPR concluded that various traditional methods, such as bed rest, traction, and other physical and pharmaceutical therapies were less effective than spinal manipulation and cautioned against lumbar surgery except in the most severe cases.
>
> *Perhaps most significantly, the guidelines state that unlike nonsurgical interventions, spinal manipulation offers both pain relief and functional improvement.* One might conclude that for acute low back pain not caused by fracture, tumor, infection, or the cauda equina syndrome, *spinal manipulation is the treatment of choice.* [671] (emphasis added)

The American College of Physicians and the American Pain Society published in 2007 a *Joint Clinical Practice Guideline for the Diagnosis and Treatment of Low Back Pain* that also concluded:

> Recommendation 7: For patients who do not improve with self-care options, clinicians should consider the addition of nonpharmacologic therapy with proven

---

670 SJ Bigos, O Bowyer, G Braea, K Brown, R Deyo, S Haldeman, *et al.* "Acute Low Back Pain Problems in Adults: Clinical Practice Guideline no. 14." Rockville, MD: U.S. Department of Health and Human Services, Public Health Service, Agency for Health Care Policy and Research; 1992. AHCPR publication no. 95-0642.

671 MS Micozz, "Complementary Care: When Is It Appropriate? Who Will Provide It?" *Annals of Internal Medicine* 129/1 (July 1998):65-66

benefits—for acute low back pain, *spinal manipulation*; for chronic or subacute low back pain, intensive interdisciplinary rehabilitation, exercise therapy, acupuncture, massage therapy, *spinal manipulation*, yoga, cognitive-behavioral therapy, or progressive relaxation (weak recommendation, moderate-quality evidence). [672] (emphasis added)

More spine experts are emerging from the medical closet to express their support for chiropractors, although most remain cautious with the fear of reprisal from their surgical peers who profit greatly from spine surgery.

William Lauerman, MD, chief of spine surgery, professor of orthopedic surgery at Georgetown University Hospital states: "I'm an orthopedic spine surgeon, so I treat all sorts of back problems, and I'm a big believer in chiropractic."[673]

Richard Deyo, MD, MPH, mentioned chiropractic as a solution: "Chiropractic is the most common choice, and evidence accumulates that spinal manipulation may indeed be an effective short-term pain remedy for patients with recent back problems."[674]

Gordon Waddell, MD, also suggested chiropractic care as a solution: "There is now considerable evidence that manipulation can be an effective method of providing symptomatic relief for some patients with acute low back pain."[675]

Surprisingly, although most MDs and many in the public remain convinced that a disc problem requires surgery, most guidelines now recommend non-surgical care before surgery. The North American Spine Society (NASS), the same organization that attacked the AHCPR findings in 1994, has now published online a Public Education Series that includes "Spinal Fusion." Remarkably, this explanation proved to be very accurate, including the opinion that "Fusion under these conditions is usually viewed as a last resort and should be considered only after other conservative (nonsurgical) measures have failed."

The NASS stated:

> A major obstacle to the successful treatment of spine pain by fusion is the difficulty in accurately identifying the source of a patient's pain. The theory is that pain can originate from painful spinal motion, and fusing the vertebrae together to eliminate the motion will get rid of the pain.
>
> Unfortunately, current techniques to precisely identify which of the many structures in the spine could be the source of a patient's back or neck pain are not perfect. Because it can be so hard to locate the source of pain, treatment of back or neck pain alone by spinal fusion is somewhat controversial. *Fusion under these conditions is usually viewed as*

---

672 R Chou, *et al.*, "Diagnosis and Treatment of Low Back Pain: A Joint Clinical Practice Guideline from the American College of Physicians and the American Pain Society," Low Back Pain Guidelines Panel, *Annals of Internal Medicine* 2 147/7 (October 2007):478-491

673 B McClain, "Mainstream Makes Adjustment," *The Washington Post*, (July 17, 2007).

674 RA Deyo, "Low -Back Pain," *Scientific American*, (August 1998):49-53

675 G Waddell and OB Allan, "A Historical Perspective On Low Back Pain And disability, "*Acta Orthop Scand* 60 (suppl 234), (1989)

> *a last resort and should be considered only after other conservative (nonsurgical) measures have failed.* [676] (emphasis added)

The admission by NASS that fusion should be a *last resort* is a huge warning that has been unheard by the public. More surprisingly, the NASS again admitted that spinal manipulation should be considered before surgery in the October, 2010, edition of *The Spine Journal*:

> Several RCTs (random controlled trials) have been conducted to assess the efficacy of SMT (spinal manipulative therapy) for acute LBP (low back pain) using various methods. *Results from most studies suggest that 5 to 10 sessions of SMT administered over 2 to 4 weeks achieve equivalent or superior improvement in pain and function* when compared with other commonly used interventions, such as physical modalities, medication, education, or exercise, for short, intermediate, and long-term follow-up. *Spine care clinicians should discuss the role of SMT as a treatment option for patients with acute LBP who do not find adequate symptomatic relief with self-care and education alone.*[677] (emphasis added)

Indeed, it is past time for every physician to follow this advice and stop with the pain pills, muscle relaxers, epidural steroid injections, and MRI scans that lead to unnecessary spine surgeries. It is time for all primary care MDs to refer patients to chiropractors for their hands-on care before any drugs, shots, or surgery are suggested.

Pain in the Neck

Not only is low back pain an epidemic, so too is neck pain. Whether caused by whiplash in car accidents, and sports injuries, aggravated by sleeping incorrectly or sitting for prolonged periods at a computer, neck disorders are huge.

A recent seven-year, international study, *The Bone and Joint Decade 2000-2010 Task Force on Neck Pain and Its Associated Disorders,* found that some alternative therapies such as acupuncture, neck manipulation, and massage are better choices for managing most common neck pain than many current practices.[678]

The study also found that corticosteroid injections and surgery should only be considered if there is associated pain, weakness or numbness in the arm, fracture or serious disease according to Task Force president Dr. Scott Haldeman:

> Neck pain is not a trivial condition for many people. It can be associated with headaches, arm and upper back pain, and depression. Whether it arises from sports injuries, car collisions, workplace issues or stress, it can be incapacitating. Understanding

---

676 "Spinal Fusion," North American Spine Society Public Education Series, www.spine.org/documents/fusion

677 MD Freeman and JM Mayer "NASS Contemporary Concepts in Spine Care: Spinal Manipulation Therapy For Acute Low Back Pain," *The Spine Journal* 10/10 (October 2010):918-940

678 S Haldeman, L Carroll, JD Cassidy, J Schubert, Å Nygren, "The Bone and Joint Decade 2000-2010 Task Force on Neck Pain and Its Associated Disorders: Executive Summary," 33/ 4S (February 15, 2008): Neck Pain Task Force Supplement.

the best way to diagnose and manage this problem is of high importance for those who are suffering and for those who manage and pay for its care.

> *One thing that became very clear to us is that the classic model we use in clinical practice doesn't work.* We tend as clinicians to see a person with neck pain, try to diagnose the cause of the problem, prescribe treatment, and hope the patient has no more pain. What we found is that this model just doesn't fit the evidence. *Given the existing evidence, management models based on the effective diagnosis and treatment of neck pain are simply "doomed to failure."* [679] (emphasis added)

The Task Force admitted that surgery has a role to play in the treatment of neck problems, but there are huge gaps in the evidence on surgery's role:

> There is some evidence that surgery can lead to substantial relief of pain and disability over the *short-term* in the treatment of cervical radiculopathy. *But there is no compelling evidence from high-quality clinical trials that surgery is superior to nonsurgical care or that any form of surgery is clearly superior to others in the treatment of radiculopathy.* And there is currently very little compelling evidence that surgery is an effective treatment for axial neck pain in the absence of radicular (arm) symptoms. [680] (emphasis added)

In addition, another review study found the lack of support for surgery for neck pain caused by an injured nerve:

> When neck pain happens because of pressure on a nerve, doctors sometimes suggest surgery to relieve the pressure. *However, there's no evidence that surgery can help people with neck pain caused by nerve problems.* More research is needed into this treatment.
>
> One study (a randomized controlled trial) found that people who had surgery were in just as much pain one year later as those who had a steroid injection or rested their neck in a soft collar.[681] (emphasis added)

The *British Medical Journal* group has published recommendations for neck pain and found manipulation plus exercise works best. "Combining an exercise programme to strengthen your neck with manipulation by a chiropractor or osteopath can help long-term pain. The combination may work better than either treatment on its own."[682]

The case is clear that chiropractic care for Type M (musculoskeletal disorders) is the best treatment for the vast majority of these spinal pain problems, notwithstanding the small percentage of cases involving cancer, fractures, infections, or true disc protrusions that do not respond to manual therapy.

---

679 The Bone and Joint Decade Task Force Questions Common Assumptions About Neck Pain; *The BACKLETTER*; Published by Lippincott Williams & Wilkins 23/2 (February 2008):1

680 EJ Carragee *et al.*, Treatment of Neck Pain: Injections And Surgical Interventions, *Spine* 33/S4 (2008): S153–S169.

681 LC Persson, CA Carlsson, JY Carlsson. "Long-lasting Cervical Radicular Pain Managed with Surgery, Physiotherapy, or a Cervical Collar: A Prospective Randomised Study," *Spine*, 22 (1997):751-758

682 Neck Pain: What Treatments Work? *BMJ* Publishing Group Limited ("BMJ Group") (2010) http://www.guardian.co.uk/lifeandstyle/besttreatments/neck-pain-treatments

Modern Revelations

Although most doctors understand that chiropractic care may help Type M disorders, there remains much confusion how Type O disorders may be helped. Today modern research has increased our knowledge of the relationship between manipulative therapy, the nervous system, organic disorders, and the circuitry and chemistry of the brain.

According to Dr. Keating, "Whether or not Palmer's theories would stand up in light of present day knowledge of neuroanatomy and physiology remains to be seen."[683] Fortunately, that day has finally arrived in regards to Type M disorders and there is a promising future for Type O and Type B problems as researchers reveal more of the fascinating aspects of the complex spine and nervous system.

New research now shows that manipulative therapy may also have an effect on Type O (organic disorders). This contention has always certainly been a leap into controversy for many people who are unschooled in neurophysiology, and it may have taken a century for science to explain DD Palmer's quaint claims, but modern neurophysiologists now give a clearer understanding of the impact of the spine upon the physiology and homeostasis of the body.

The treatment by manipulation of Type O disorders has been supported by clinical experience and case reports according to an article in the *Annals of Internal Medicine* by William Meeker, DC, MPH, and Scott Haldeman, DC, MD, PhD, FRCP(C).[684] These include randomized clinical trials for primary dysmenorrhea[685,686], hypertension[687,688], chronic asthma[689,690], enuresis[691], infantile colic[692], and premenstrual

683 JC Keating, "Toward a Philosophy of the Science of Chiropractic," ibid, pp. 30.

684 WC Meeker and S Haldeman, "Chiropractic: A Profession At The Crossroads Of Mainstream And Alternative Medicine," American College of Physicians-American Society of Internal Medicine, *Ann Intern Med.* 136 (2002):216-227

685 MA Hondras, CR Long, PC Brennan, "Spinal Manipulative Therapy Versus A Low Force Mimic Maneuver For Women With Primary Dysmenorrhea: A Randomized, Observer-Blinded, Clinical Trial," *Pain* 81 (1999):105-14. [PMID: 10353498]

686 K Kokjohn, DM Schmid, JJ Triano, PC Brennan, "The Effect Of Spinal Manipulation On Pain And Prostaglandin Levels In Women With Primary Dysmenorrhea," *J Manipulative Physiol Ther.* 15 (1992):279-85. [PMID: 1535359]

687 JP Morgan, JL Dickey, HH Hunt, PM Hudgins., "A Controlled Trial Of Spinal Manipulation In The Management Of Hypertension," *J Am Osteopath Assoc.* 85 (1985):308-13. [PMID: 3900016]

688 RG Yates, DL Lamping, NL Abram, C Wright, "Effects of Chiropractic Treatment On Blood Pressure And Anxiety: A Randomized, Controlled Trial," J Manipulative *Physiol Ther.* 11 (1988):484-8. [PMID: 3075649]

689 J Balon, PD Aker, ER Crowther, C Danielson, PG Cox, D O'Shaughnessy, *et al.* "A Comparison Of Active And Simulated Chiropractic Manipulation As Adjunctive Treatment For Childhood Asthma," *N Engl J Med.* 339 (1998):1013-20. [PMID: 9761802]

690 NH Nielsen, G Bronfort, T Bendix, F Madsen, B Weekes, "Chronic Asthma And Chiropractic Spinal Manipulation: A Randomized Clinical Trial," *Clin Exp Allergy.* 25 (1995):80-8. [PMID: 7728627]

691 WR Reed, S Beavers, SK Reddy, G Kern, "Chiropractic Management Of Primary Nocturnal enuresis," *J Manipulative Physiol Ther.* 17 (1994):596-600. [PMID: 7884329]

692 JM Wiberg, J Nordsteen, N Nilsson, "The Short-Term Effect of Spinal Manipulation in the Treatment of Infantile Colic: A Randomized Controlled Clinical Trial with a Blinded Observer," *J Manipulative Physiol Ther.* 22 (1999):517-22. [PMID:10543581]

syndrome.[693] "The outcomes of these completed studies have provided varied but promising results," according to the authors.

One mechanism mentioned by Dr. Haldeman involved the possible ability of manual therapy to influence reflex activity in the central nervous system. This somatovisceral reflex, in his view, holds possibly the greatest interest for those trying to establish a role for manual therapy like chiropractic care for Type O complaints.[694] The suggestion is that sensory input to one part of the nervous system can influence physiologic function in other parts of the body.

The original and rather archaic "pinched nerve" theory has been abandoned and replaced by the "reflex-based" theory. While this was investigated by the New Zealand Commission in 1978-79, it too has been modified by recent investigators.[695]

The "somatovisceral reflex" or, in regards to the spine, the "spinovisceral reflex," is at the core of this explanation. Spinovisceral reflexes refer to a specific type of somatovisceral reflex that stems from the spinal components. Reflex effects have been demonstrated throughout the cardiovascular system, in the digestive system, urinary system, endocrine system, and immune system, which explains why many patients—seven percent in the New Zealand Inquiry—admitted they felt improvement after chiropractic care.[696]

Recent research by Brian S. Budgell, DC, supports an explanation for the neurophysiologic concept that abnormal stimulation of spinal or paraspinal (brain) structures may lead to reflex responses of the autonomic nerve system, which in turn may alter organ function.[697] In other words, a back injury can cause the nerves in that region of the spinal column to have a reflex reaction in the organs that are innervated by them.

This is where chiropractic care can help patients with misdiagnosed problems who are not responding to medical care. For many, examination of the somatic system of the spinal column (muscles, joints, nerves, and ligaments) can hold the answer to visceral conditions that are unresponsive to medical care.

Consider, for example, a neurogenic cause of a heart attack. Most understand that one sign of a heart attack is referral of pain into the chest wall and down the left arm. Many patients think they are having a heart attack when this type of pain strikes them. They have the electrocardiogram (ECG) and cardiac catheterization (heart cath) only to be told

693   MJ Walsh, BI Polus, "A Randomized, Placebo-Controlled Clinical Trial On The Efficacy Of Chiropractic Therapy On Premenstrual Syndrome," *J Manipulative Physiol Ther.* 22 (1999):582-5. [PMID: 10626701]

694   BD Inglis, B Fraser, BR Penfold, Commissioners, *Chiropractic in New Zealand Report 1979*, PD Hasselberg, Government Printer, Wellington, New Zealand, (1979):101-2

695   D Nansel and M Szlazak, "Somatic Dysfunction And The Phenomenon Of Visceral Disease Simulation: A Probably Explanation For The Apparent Effectiveness Of Somatic Therapy In Patients Presumed To Be Suffering From True Visceral Disease," *JMPT* 18/6 (July 1995):379-397.

696 A Sato, Y Sato, RF Schmidt, "The Impact of Somatosensory Input on Autonomic Functions," *Reviews of Physiology Biochemistry and Pharmacology* 130 (Berlin, 1997):1–328.

697 BS Budgell, "Reflex Effects Of Subluxation: The Autonomic Nerve System," *J Manipulative Physiol Ther* 23/2 (Feb. 2000):104–6.

everything is okay, but they remain in pain. Once again it may be condition known as spinovisceral reflex stemming from the spine.

Drs. Dale Nansel and Mark Szlazak from Palmer College of Chiropractic-West in San Jose, California, did an in-depth study of somatovisceral theories of over 350 articles spanning the last 75 years and found that it has been firmly established that somatic dysfunction is notorious in its ability to create obvious signs and symptoms that can mimic or simulate rather than cause internal organ disease. In fact, they believe as much as 10 percent of supposed heart attacks may be caused by this syndrome.[698] This is a huge revelation that may affect thousands of people who think they are having a heart attack, but are having a spinovisceral reflex that spinal adjustments may help.

During the *Wilk v. AMA* trial, witness John Mennell, MD, used the term "cardiac invalid" to describe patients suffering from referred chest pains due to spinovisceral reflex. "They are being given drugs for something they do not have because the cardiologist thinks it is angina and what it is, in fact, is referred pain."[699]

In his closing argument at the *Wilk* trial attorney George McAndrews summarized this problem of referred pain being misdiagnosed by MDs and the frustration by patients:

> You remember Dr. Mennell and Dr. Haldeman on referred pain. They referred to a person who goes to a medical physician and he has a Type O disorder and the medical physician not having been trained in school to look for joint dysfunction or neurological components to a disease process will take care of the patient chemically and in a great number of cases that's totally adequate.
>
> But when the medical physician runs into what they call "crocks"—hypochondriacs or malingers—the patient who doesn't get well under that chemical care. Dr. Mennell says that's because they have been misdiagnosed. They have been told they have kidney problems, angina, liver disease, and they do not.
>
> What they have is an aberrant neurological signal coming from another portion of the body that gives all of the indicia that a diagnostician would define as an organic problem. They go to the medical physician and in desperation finally say, "You cannot help me." They go to the chiropractor who manipulates the spinal vertebrae and removes the referred pain syndrome.
>
> The patient walks out saying, "The medical physician told me I had liver disease, kidney disease, bladder disease. I went to the chiropractor and in two adjustments he cured me of my disease."
>
> Now where is the problem? *The problem is that because the medical profession has failed to even look for this referred pain syndrome and has no knowledge of spinal manipulative therapy, so* they have told that the patient they have a disease and when they cannot help them, the

---

698 D Nansel and M Szlazak, "Somatic Dysfunction And The Phenomenon Of Visceral Disease Simulation: A Probably Explanation For The Apparent Effectiveness Of Somatic Therapy In Patients Presumed To Be Suffering From True Visceral Disease," *JMPT* 18/6 (July, 1995):379-397.
699 G McAndrews closing argument, *Wilk v. AMA*, p.6809.

patient still has the problem, but the medical profession labels them crocks, malingerer, or hypochondriac.

This is a problem. It is referred pain, and this is another reason why you have to have cooperation. Somewhere along the line those people, as Mennell says, become cardiac invalids.[700] (emphasis added)

Other researchers speak of the misdiagnoses stemming from the referred pain caused by spinovisceral reflexes that mimic organic problems. In their research, Drs. David Seaman and James Winterstein suggest that spinovisceral reflex caused by spinal joint complex dysfunction should be included in the differential diagnosis of pain and visceral symptoms because "joint complex dysfunction can often generate symptoms which are similar to those produced by true visceral disease."[701]

Research in the 1960-70s by Irvin M. Korr, PhD, from Princeton University introduced on a new concept in neurophysiology concerning the *trophic* function of nerves. He and his associates produced exciting work revealing that nerves not only conduct bio-electrical impulses to tissues, but also supply chemical nourishment to organs through continuous transfer of proteins and other substances along the nerve fibers by altering the neurochemicals that flow along the nerves themselves.

This research demonstrated that nerve compression may interrupt or reduce the *axoplasmic flow* of material from nerve to muscle, influencing muscle structure, excitability, contractile properties, and metabolism. Korr postulated that one mechanism by which spinal manipulation achieves its effects may be by removing this obstruction to trophic function in compromised nerves:[702]

Deformations of nerves and roots, such as compression, stretching, angulation, and torsion that are known to occur all too commonly in the human being...are subject to manipulative amelioration and correction.[703]

Aside from disruption of axoplasmic flow along the nerves, Korr also mentioned the disturbance primarily at the spine would cause "cross-talk" of meaningless commands by joining the real nerve commands with "gibberish" causing uncoordinated motor and autonomic responses. In turn, this might cause disruption in the function of organs and muscles; therefore, therapy like spinal adjustments to correct vertebral subluxations directed at reducing the gibberish in the affected sympathetic pathways is often helpful.[704]

---

700 Ibid. p. 6807-09.

701 DR Seaman and JF Winterstein, "Dysafferentiation: A Novel Term To Describe The Neuropathophysiological Effects Of Joint Complex Dysfunction. A Look At Likely Mechanisms Of Symptom Generation," *JMPT* 21/4 (May 1998):267-80.

702 IM Korr, "The Collected Papers of Irvin M. Korr," American Academy of Osteopathy, Newark Ohio (1979)

703 IM Korr, GSL Appeltauer. "Trophic Functions of Nerves," In: Beal MC, ed. *1994 Yearbook: Louisa Burns Memorial.* Indianapolis, Ind: American Academy of Osteopathy; (1994):52 -60.

704 V Strang, ibid. p. 57.

In this light, DD Palmer's quaint concept was not too distant from Korr's concept of gibberish: "In disease, mental impulses are not impeded, hindered, stopped or cut off–they are *modified*. An impingement does not obstruct; it is either an excitor or a depressor."[705] While this explanation of neurophysiology may be simplistic by today's standards, it certainly was not conceptually much different to Korr's concept.

The founder of osteopathy, Andrew Still, also alluded to axoplasmic flow and attributed the cause of dysfunction to "partial or complete failure of the nerves to properly conduct the fluids of life." [706]

Chiropractic for Heart Health

Research by HT Vernon, DC, PhD, and MS Dhami, PhD, perhaps best summarizes the impact of the effects of spinal adjustments upon the whole body:

> There is now good evidence that spinal adjustment decreases pain, increases range of movement, increases pain tolerance in the skin and deeper muscle structures, raises beta-endorphin levels in the blood plasma and... has potent impact on a variety of nerve pathways between the soma and viscera that regulate good health.[707]

Not surprisingly today, most Americans have fallen into the allopathic trap about their health analysis, depending solely upon blood analysis as the guiding factor in their diagnosis. Not only do organs require proper blood flow to function, but proper nerve energy also is required to sustain the organs. Few people understand that the essential blood flow is also controlled by the nerve system and, thus, any interference in these regulating nerves can cause blood circulation problems.

Once again, let Dr. Vernon explain this physiological fact:

> Every function in the human body, be it conscious or otherwise, depends upon nerve energy. *This energy has its source in the cells of the brain and spinal cord. Even the caliber of the blood vessels throughout the entire body is under the control of the nervous system.* The blood aspect of disease permits the use of an interesting illustration which applies to many other disease processes.
>
> For example, *if the nerves supplying the blood vessels are disturbed, then normal generation, transmission, distribution, or expression of the nerve energy is interfered with,* and the vessels become either contracted or dilated as the case may be. This contraction or dilation prevents normal blood circulation, and this insufficient or excessive blood supply, technically known as ischemia or hyperemia, may cause the organ which it supplies to become diseased.

---

705 DD Palmer, ibid. p. 57.

706 AT Still. *Autobiography of Andrew T. Still*. Kirksville, Mo: AT Still; 1897.

707 HT Vernon, MS Dhami *et al.*, "Spinal Manipulation and Beta-Endorphin: A Controlled Study on the Effect of a Spinal Manipulation on Plasma Beta-Endorphin Levels in Normal Males," *J. Manipulative Physio Ther* 9/2 (1986): 115-123.

It should be understood that this is merely one of the many possibilities of nerve disturbance: What applies to this, likewise applies to all the nerves that regulate the ductless glands, the digestive and respiratory systems, and every other tissue, gland, organ, and system in the body. *Interference with the nerve supply may cause disease in any of these tissues, glands, organs, and systems.*[708] (emphasis added)

As proof in point, in December, 1989, a provocative article by Mark E. Jarmel, DC, "Possible Role of Spinal Joint Dysfunction in the Genesis of Sudden Cardiac Death" broached the relationship between heart attack and the spine.[709] He noted that sudden cardiac death causes about 15 percent of all natural fatalities in the industrially developed countries. In the United States alone, it claims over 400,000 lives each year. Anecdotal reports from the chiropractic and osteopathic professions have indicated the beneficial effects of manipulation in the management of arrhythmias, coronary arterial spasm, and premature ventricular contractions. Dr. Jarmel's study suggests that nerve irritation from the spine will cause heart problems:

> "Numerous researchers have concluded that strategies for prevention of sudden death should be focused on controlling neurophysiologic factors which may enhance ventricular vulnerability. By removing a source of destabilizing neural input to the heart, correction of vertebral dysfunction may prove of value in reducing susceptibility to sudden cardiac arrest."

Explaining organ function, dysfunction or failure as a result of vertebral subluxation is conceptually alien to the allopathic mindset and often is too high-tech for most lay people to understand. Few people ever think of heart disease in terms of dysfunction of their nerve system. Instead, they focus on other important contributors such as smoking, lack of exercise, junk foods and the "bad blood" concepts like cholesterol and triglyceride levels.

Even being physically fit and eating correctly may not be assurance enough to avoid a sudden heart attack. Dr. Jarmel noted in his study of 79 cases of sudden cardiac death in people 18-35 years of age, three of them were competitive athletes. "This may suggest," according to Jarmel, "that so-called 'physical fitness' may provide little cardiovascular protection when asymptomatic coronary artery disease is combined with neurally induced vasomotor disturbance." In other words, it is equivalent to a race car with a big engine that fails because of faulty electrical wiring although nothing is mechanically wrong with the engine itself.

Dr. Jarmel's main premise that nerve irritation may lead to a sudden heart attack and that spinal adjustments may help alleviate or prevent such problems should come as no surprise to any chiropractor or researcher with an understanding of neurophysiology and spinal mechanics.

---

708 Vernon, ibid.

709 ME Jarmel, a paper, "Possible Role of Spinal Joint Dysfunction in the Genesis of Sudden Cardiac Death," *Journal of Manipulative and Physiological Therapeutics*, 12/6 (Dec. 1989).

Along the same concept by Korr concerning ectopic gibberish, another article by Jarmel along with Judith Zatkin, Ph.D., of Cleveland College of Chiropractic in Los Angeles titled "Improvement of Cardiac Autonomic Regulation Following Spinal Manipulative Therapy" suggests the magnitude of this problem.

Their paper mentioned a trial about heart conditions and chiropractic care, which may substantiate the claim of vertebral subluxations as a plausible explanation of sudden heart attacks:

> Unbalanced activation of cardiac sympathetic nerves plays a crucial role in the pathogenesis of sudden cardiac death. It has been proposed that *mechanical irritation of upper thoracic vertebral joints may create an ectopic source of unbalanced cardiac sympathetic nerve activation.* Spinal manipulative therapy is hypothesized to modulate mechanically induced sympathetic activity by restoring proper mobility to dysfunctional vertebral joints. This study evaluated the possibility that spinal manipulative therapy may have value in treating a previously unrecognized source of unbalanced cardiac autonomic regulation.

> Eleven patients without a prior history of myocardial infarction who were found to have signs of dysrhythmic abnormalities on Holter monitoring, received a one month course of chiropractic manipulative treatment. After one month of spinal manipulative therapy, follow-up 24 hour ECG recordings were performed. A positive trend was noted in the number of ventricular beats, number of ischemic events, maximum time of ST segment depression, elimination of after-depolarizations, and enhanced heart rate variability. *These preliminary results suggest that spinal manipulative therapy may significantly enhance cardiac autonomic balance.*

> *The results of this study suggest that upper thoracic spinal joint dysfunction may be a previously unrecognized source of cardiac sympathetic activation.* The results of this study may have implications for developing a novel nonpharmacological treatment which may have value in reducing risk of sudden cardiac death.[710] (emphasis added)

Again it appears the more research is done, the more it leads to DD Palmer's early but quaint ideas of "functionating" and "tone" that are affected by nerve interference from the spine.

Rebooting the Brain

The research is clear that chiropractic care is effective for most Type M back pain disorders, and the emerging research on spinovisceral reflexes and Type O disorders is promising. There is another benefit from chiropractic care that I have taken the liberty to label *Type B*—disorders of the brain stemming from spinal issues. Although much

---

710 M Jarmel, J Zatkin, *et al.,* "Improvement of Cardiac Autonomic Regulation Following Spinal Manipulative Therapy," Cleveland College of Chiropractic, LA, a paper presented at the Conference Proceedings of the Chiropractic Centennial Foundation, July 6-8, 1995.

research must be done, the emerging neuroscience reveals more about the value of chiropractic's type of spinal care than even DD Palmer might have expected.

There are many emerging models in neurophysiology that indicate how the central nervous system is affected by the altered mechanics of the spine. The more neuroscientists discover, the clearer it becomes that many health problems can be triggered by spinal stresses. Even the memory of a spinal injury can lead to non-specific low back pain from altered nervous system processing.

Not only can spinal dysfunction affect organ physiology by way of spinovisceral reflexes or axoplasmic flow, research in a new trial study has now shown that back problems may also affect the cortical circuitry functioning and the actual size and health of the brain itself.

Scientists have long understood prolonged mental stress can cause cortical problems and immune cells to age prematurely. In a study of mothers of chronically ill children that required constant care, the cells of the most stressed-out women showed signs of about ten years' worth of accelerated aging.[711]

Now other researchers have discovered back pain stress also causes the brain circuitry to malfunction and actually degenerate. These are the Type B disorders that have never been understood until recently with the use of EEG and MRI scans, and these findings open up an entirely new array of possible help for many "mental" patients by chiropractic care.

Often patients will tell their chiropractors after receiving a cervical adjustment, "I can think more clearly now." Although this is a common reaction many chiropractors have heard before, the explanation of this phenomenon was unknown until it caught the interest of two chiropractors-turned-researchers in New Zealand who found a novel explanation.

Heidi Haavik-Taylor, PhD, and Bernadette Murphy, DC, PhD, from the New Zealand College of Chiropractic in Auckland, conducted a study consisting of 24 patients with a history of neck stiffness and sometimes neck pain (but sometimes no neck pain) that measured the central nervous system activity in the brainstem and spinal cord of the participants before and after cervical adjustments.[712]

Since the nerve system is often equated to the body's own computer, sometimes our brain malfunctions just like a computer and we need to reboot the hard drive to clean up and clear out the accumulation of unnecessary nerve "gibberish" caused by vertebral subluxation and spinal lesions.

This remarkable study found that the sensitive measurements in the brain (called sensory evoked potentials) indicated that neck adjustments may "reboot the nervous system" to help it to function better. This is the first time that anyone has used

711 ES Epel, E H Blackburn, J Lin, FS Dhabhar, NE Adler, JD Morrow and R Cawthon, "Accelerated Telomere Shortening In Response To Life Stress," *PNAS* 101/49 (December 7, 2004)
712 HH Taylor, B Murphy, "Altered Sensorimotor Integration with Cervical Spine Manipulation," *J Manipulative Physiol Ther.* 31/2 (Feb 2008):115-26.

electroencephalograph (EEG) [incidentally, a diagnostic machine invented by BJ Palmer[713]] to prove that there are definite changes to the way the brain processes information after chiropractic care.

Dr Haavik-Taylor has spent years researching the effects of chiropractic adjustments on the nervous system. In her latest research, she and Dr. Murphy were able to measure how brain waves are altered before and after spinal adjustments.

"The process of a spinal adjustment is like rebooting a computer. The signals that these adjustments send to the brain, via the nervous system, reset muscle behaviour patterns," said Dr. Haavik-Taylor. "By stimulating the nervous system we can improve the function of the whole body. This is something that chiropractors and their patients have known for years; and now we have some scientific evidence to prove it."[714]

In computerese, the technical language of those involved in computer technology, this resembles "GIGO" which stands for "garbage in, garbage out." In other words, when there is nerve interference or gibberish due to vertebral subluxations, this causes the brain to change its feedback to the viscera and muscles.

According to Dr. Haavik-Taylor,

> It is a bit like trying to do homework with the radio blasting in the background, plus the TV going at full volume as well. Harder to concentrate and get it right. Because the dysafferentiation is coming from the spine, which changes the way the CNS interprets and controls the rest of the body, even though the rest of the body may well be sending perfectly accurate afferent info.[715]

In this Haavik-Taylor and Murphy study, after chiropractic adjustments of the cervical spine the nervous system firing patterns became more normal, suggesting that the brain can relearn normal firing patterns, thereby improving the person's overall functioning. Obviously the loss of the central nervous system's ability to adapt and recover with an impaired homeostasis regulation has now become a critical lynch pin in maintaining good health.

It may have taken over 100 years to come to this milestone, but this work by Haavik-Taylor and Murphy may confirm what DD Palmer said about "functionating," a concept he intuitively understood but had no means to prove it without the high-tech tools that now available.

The Shrinking Brain

Aside from re-booting the brain with spinal adjustments, other research shows another Type B disorder stemming from the spine has an impact upon the chemistry of the brain and nerve system.

---

713 JC Keating, *B.J. of Davenport: The Early Years of Chiropractic*, (1997):279.

714 Press Release: "New Science Behind Chiropractic Care," *NZ Chiropractors Association*, (January 27, 2008)

715 H Taylor via private communication with JC Smith on 5-18-2010.

Unlike the dry electrical system in your home, the human electrical system is wet with neurochemicals that influence the action of the nerve system which, in turn, affects the function of organs and your homeostasis. The brain is more than a source of electrical conduction like a battery; it is an organ that secretes chemicals to change the action of your organs and body.

Researchers now better understand how the alterations of neurochemicals and hormones influence the physiology of your overall health. Nerves secrete chemical substances called neurotransmitters that are endogenous chemicals that relay, amplify, and modulate signals between a neuron and another cell. Neurotransmitters are stored in nerve endings or terminals located in the brain. They are also found at the axon endings of motor neurons, where they stimulate the muscle fibers to contract. They and their close relatives are produced by glands such as the pituitary and the adrenal glands.

The brain controls the regulation of your body functions via these neurotransmitters that have different actions. The problem of some disorders begin when these hormones are out of control or balance due to diet, lack of exercise, depletion of vitamins, stress, or spine injury, which is a relatively new concept.

Unlike other parts of the neuromusculoskeletal system, the spine is complex with hundreds of joints supported by soft tissues, and when the central nervous system, spinal cord, and peripheral nerves are included, the spine is the most complicated entity in the human body. Any study of this cortical-spinal system is a multifaceted task that stretches the furthest reaches of science today.

Exciting new research by A. Vania Apkarian, PhD, from Northwestern University has shown the impact of pain upon brain tissue in ways never known before, including creating "noise" similar to the "gibberish" mentioned by Haavik-Taylor and Murphy:

> Moreover, psychological research and recent investigation of neurophysiological processes in chronic pain highlight the fact that the pain of many patients with NSLBP(nonspecific low back pain) depends not only on the "signal" of a structural lesion in the spine, but also on the "noise" introduced by altered nervous system processing.[716]

Another factor that influences neurochemistry has been found, but this one starts in your back and ends up affecting your brain. In an article published in *The Journal of Neuroscience,* Dr. Apkarian, *et al.* has shown that long standing back pain may lead to altered neurotransmitters and serious brain degeneration. He found in MRI studies that chronic back pain can shrink the brain by as much as 11 percent, equivalent to the amount of gray matter lost in 10 to 20 years of aging.[717]

---

716   JP Robins and AV Apkarian, "Low Back Pain," *Functional Pain Syndromes: Presentation and Pathophysiology*, EA Mayer and MC Bushnell, editors, IASP Press, Seattle, © (2009):23.

717   AV Apkarian *et al.* "Chronic Back Pain Is Associated with Decreased Prefrontal and Thalamic Gray Matter Density," *The Journal of Neuroscience* 24/46 (November 17, 2004):10410-10415.

Using magnetic resonance imaging brain scan data and automated analysis techniques, chronic back pain patients were divided into neuropathic, exhibiting pain because of sciatic nerve damage, and non-neuropathic groups.

In an interview, Dr. Apkarian said:

> We basically studied 26 chronic back pain patients…and compared them to 26 normal subjects who had similar age and sex distribution. And we looked at the overall volume of the gray matter of the cortex. And *essentially we find significant decrease in the overall volume of the brain gray matter in the back pain patients.*
>
> Patients with chronic back pain showed 5-11% less neocortical gray matter volume than control subjects. The magnitude of this decrease is equivalent to the gray matter volume lost in 10-20 years of normal aging. The decreased volume was related to pain duration, indicating a 1.3 cm^3 loss of gray matter for every year of chronic pain…Our results imply that chronic back pain is accompanied by brain atrophy and suggest that the pathophysiology of chronic pain includes thalamocortical processes. [718] (emphasis added)

Apkarian says one of the areas of the brain impacted by chronic back pain is the prefrontal cortex:

> The prefrontal cortex is important because it's a region that has to do with cognition. *It's the highest area of the brain and has to do with a lot of decision making, rational thinking, and decisions along those lines.* Obviously that's an important area of the brain to become dysfunctional. (emphasis added)

His discovery adds support to the research by Haavik-Taylor and Murphy's concept of rebooting the brain to think more clearly. Apparently for those who live with chronic back pain, the consequence is not only the "noise" sensory nerve conduction, but damage to the brain itself. "The results imply that chronic pain is accompanied by cerebral atrophy."[719]

When asked if the brain can regenerate itself, Apkarian answered:

> We don't really know the answer. There are some new studies suggesting that at least some of this loss of tissue might be reversible. There are a couple of studies showing that when the pain is dramatically decreased, some regional gray matter density is recovered. So some of it is clearly reversible.[720]

In another study published in 2008, Apkarian *et al.* concluded "these findings demonstrate that chronic pain has a widespread impact on overall brain function."[721] In

---

718 B Cosgrove, Northwestern University Newsfeed, Dr. Vania Apkarian on "Chronic Back Pain and the Brain," (November 29, 2004)

719 AV Apkarian, J Scholz, "Shared Mechanisms Between Chronic Pain And Neurodegenerative Disease," *Drug Discovery Today: Disease Mechanisms* 3/3 (2006):319-326

720 Is It Possible to Regain Brain Tissue Lost to Chronic Back Pain? 26/2, THEBACK*LETTER* (Jan 2011)

721 MN Baliki, PY Geha, AV Apkarian, and DR Chialvo, "Beyond Feeling: Chronic Pain Hurts the Brain, Disrupting the Default-Mode Network Dynamics," *The Journal of Neuroscience* 28/6 (February 6,

other words, that there is more to a patient's suffering with back pain than merely a hurting sensation called pain—it may become a chemical degeneration of the cerebral cortex:

> In conclusion, these findings suggest that the brain of a chronic pain patient is not simply a healthy brain processing pain information, but rather is altered by the persistent pain in a manner reminiscent of other neurological conditions associated with cognitive impairments.[722]

Dr. Apkarian says he hopes his study causes those who suffer from chronic back pain to seek out solutions. He explained how chronic pain may be the result of an injury/ dysfunction of the spine, or the result of more complex processes involving nervous system processing of sensory information where old "memory traces" get stuck in the brain's prefrontal cortex, which controls emotion and learning. This process is called neuroplasticity, and may explain how an acute problem becomes a chronic, painful problem despite being completely healed.[723]

"In some way, you can think of chronic pain as the inability to turn off the memory of the pain," said Dr. Apkarian.[724] As a result, the brain seems to remember the injury as if it were fresh, even long after it is healed, so some people continue to suffer chronic pain that cannot be totally relieved through traditional analgesic drugs, such as aspirin and morphine derivatives:

> You should try to seek ways to reduce the pain, and that one should not live with the pain. *The longer you live with the pain, the worse the impact on the brain.* So one needs to actively find methods or therapies that would diminish the suffering as much as possible.[725]

Of course, we chiropractors believe "therapies that would diminish the suffering" speaks of spinal manipulative therapy.

Perhaps this study affirms that a sequential pattern exists in the brain and nerve system: spinal injuries causing stress creates neurochemical changes and nerve "noise," and together these chemical and neurological stresses slowly lead to cerebral malfunction that manifests itself first as neurologic and neurochemical disorders and, secondly, as degeneration.

In this light, chiropractic spinal adjustments that reduce joint dysfunction and eliminate back pain would possibly reduce altered neurotransmitter changes that may cause damage to the brain and, thus, improve the brain circuitry of pain and dysfunction that leads to gibberish and noise.

2008):1398-1403

722 MN Baliki, ibid.

723 M Millecamps, MV Centeno, HH Berra, CN Rudick, S Lavarello, T Tkatch, AV Apkarian, "D-Cycloserine Reduces Neuropathic Pain Behavior Through Limbic NMDA-Mediated Circuitry Q," *Pain* 132 (2007):108–123

724 M Hawryluk, "Managing Pain," The *Bulletin*, (September 03. 2009) BendBulletin.com

725 Cosgrove, ibid.

Chiropractic Care for Fibromyalgia

Not only can chronic back pain shrink the brain, other scientists now believe degenerative disorders of the central nerve system may be responsible for fibromyalgia (FMS).

Researchers found similar degeneration of the brains in women with fibromyalgia, which has traditionally been classified as either a musculoskeletal disease or a psychological disorder. But accumulating evidence now suggests that fibromyalgia may be associated with central nervous system (CNS) dysfunction via altered neurotransmitters stimulated by spinal column lesions or vertebral subluxations.

In a study published in *The Journal of Neuroscience* in 2007 by Anil Kuchinad *et al.*, MRI scans of the brains of ten female fibromyalgia patients and ten healthy controls found that fibromyalgia patients had significantly less total gray matter volume and showed a 3.3 times greater age-associated decrease in gray matter than healthy controls:

> The longer the individuals had had fibromyalgia, the greater the gray matter loss, with each year of fibromyalgia being equivalent to 9.5 times the loss in normal aging. In addition, fibromyalgia patients demonstrated significantly less gray matter density than healthy controls in several brain regions...The neuro-anatomical changes that we see in fibromyalgia patients contribute additional evidence of CNS involvement in fibromyalgia.
>
> In particular, *fibromyalgia appears to be associated with an acceleration of age-related changes in the very substance of the brain.* Moreover, the regions in which we demonstrate objective changes may be functionally linked to core features of the disorder including affective disturbances and chronic widespread pain. [726]

Fibromyalgia's defining features (chronic widespread pain and tenderness to palpation) may be explained by the mechanism known as "sympathetically maintained pain." After a triggering event (physical or emotional trauma, infections), relentless sympathetic hyperactivity may develop in susceptible individuals. This hyperactivity induces excessive norepinephrine (also known as noradrenalin) secretion that could in turn sensitize central and peripheral pain receptors and thus induce widespread pain and tenderness.

Altered tone is now associated with FMS. Patients with fibromyalgia have relentless hyperactivity of the sympathetic nerve system. Irwin Korr, PhD, referred to this as *sympathicotonia*, stating that this long-term hyperactivity may have general clinical significance as well as specific manifestations, depending on which organs or tissues receive innervation from the involved sympathetic pathways.[727]

At the same time, such individuals have sympathetic hypo-reactivity to stress, which could explain the profound fatigue, morning stiffness, and other complaints associated

---

726 A Kuchinad, *et al.* "Accelerated Brain Gray Matter Loss in Fibromyalgia Patients: Premature Aging of the Brain?" The *Journal of Neuroscience*, 27/15 (April 11, 2007):4004-4007

727 IM Korr, "Sustained Sympathicotonia as a Factor in Disease." In: IM Korr, ed. The Neurobiologic Mechanisms in Manipulative Therapy. New York: Plenum, (1978):229-268.

to low blood pressure. This autonomic nerve system dysfunction could induce other symptoms of fibromyalgia such as irritable bowel, urinary discomfort, limb numbness, anxiety, and dryness of the eyes and mouth.[728]

According to Robert A. Leach, DC, FICC, author of *The Chiropractic Theories*:

> Amazingly, Palmer's concept of altered "tone" of the nervous system being the cause of disease then has some support in the current neurophysiologic literature regarding facilitation and sympathicotonia. While ischemia may or may not be the link, it is apparent that through various mechanisms abnormal sympathetic tone leads to aberrant functioning of sympathetic nerves that innervate visceral smooth muscle.

FMS in the Medical Trap

Drs. Michael Schneider, David Brady, and Stephen Perle wrote a compelling paper suggesting that patients with fibromyalgia may often be misdiagnosed. To the average MD, the authors suggest, this presents a "diagnostic conundrum because of generally poor knowledge about musculoskeletal disorders within primary care medicine."[729]

Unfortunately, some misinformed MDs like NM Hadler still believe FMS is "a learned illness, taught over time by a number of actors, including physicians:"

> Despite a concerted effort for some time, no abnormality in any organ system has been identified as associated with fibromyalgia, nor does one become manifest during its prolonged course. Absence of proof of a pathobiological cause, of course, is not proof of its absence. Some clinical investigators continue to pursue this will-o'-wisp with enthusiasm that far outstrips the yield. Perhaps there is no biological abnormality. Fibromyalgia is a learned illness, taught over time by a number of actors, including physicians. [730]

Obviously Hadler is caught in the allopathic trap. What he fails to realize is that it may have to do with neurophysiologic disorders as Apkarian, Baliki, Haavik, or Schneider suggest. Instead of looking for a pathoanatomical "abnormality in any organ system," he ought to look for the pathophysiology component. Sadly, Hadler's myopia is not uncommon for many medical physicians unschooled in neurophysiology or spinovisceral reflexes.

Unfortunately, the diagnosis of facet and sacroiliac joint dysfunction is not a simple matter for those clinicians who rely solely upon imaging studies because there is not necessarily any pathoanatomical changes in these joints associated with the referred pain

---

728 M Martinez-Lavin, AG Hermosillo, C Mendoza, et al. "Orthostatic Sympathetic Derangement In Individuals With Fibromyalgia," *J Rheumatol* 24 (1997):714.

729 MJ Schneider, DM Brady, and SM Perle, "Commentary: Differential Diagnosis Of Fibromyalgia Syndrome: Proposal Of A Model And Algorithm For Patients Presenting With The Primary Symptom Of Chronic Widespread Pain," *J Manipulative Physiol Ther* 29 (2006):493- 501.

730 NM Hadler, *Stabbed in the Back, Confronting Back Pain In An Overtreated Society*, The University of North Carolina Press, Chapel Hill, NC, (2009):25.

patterns. Actually, for decades the medical profession believed the sacroiliac joints could not move, which proved to be wrong, and, secondly, because there are no discs in these joints, many ignored the sacroiliac as a source of pain, which is another big trap.[731],[732]

Consequently, these unusual patterns of back or neck pain coupled with negative diagnostic imaging studies might lead the unwary medical clinician to declare FMS as the diagnosis when, in reality, the pain is emanating from the spinal facet or sacroiliac joints, conditions helped greatly by spinal manipulation. Some physicians believe as Hadler that "Fibromyalgia is a learned illness," only to compound the patient's suffering with unnecessary worry and depression.

Schneider and his colleagues concluded:

> Lastly, many common musculoskeletal conditions can mimic FMS. It is imperative that the clinician understand the many musculoskeletal sources of unusual referred pain patterns that could be misdiagnosed as FMS. A careful physical examination by a clinician with experience in musculoskeletal differential diagnosis would help to sort out more of these cases, which could potentially reduce the error rate of FMS misdiagnosis...collaborative patient management between clinicians, chiropractors, osteopaths, and physical therapists would seem to be the best way to ensure that patients with these musculoskeletal causes of widespread pain would receive the appropriate diagnosis and therapy, without resorting to a default diagnosis of FMS in all cases of widespread pain. [733]

To the surprise of many, important guidelines that rely on evidence-based criteria now recommend chiropractic care for the treatment of fibromyalgia.

The American College of Occupational and Environmental Medicine (ACOEM) recommends chiropractic care in its *Occupational Medicine Practice Guidelines* treatments for several chronic pain conditions including complex regional pain syndrome (CRPS), neuropathic pain, trigger points/myofascial pain, chronic persistent pain, fibromyalgia, and chronic low back pain. The recommendations are based on more than 1,500 references, including 546 randomized, controlled trials.[734]

ACOEM's latest chronic pain guidelines represent a step in the right direction in terms of recognizing the value of chiropractic care. The guidelines also recommend manipulation for chronic, persistent low back or neck pain, and cervicogenic headache.

---

731   JL Shaw, "The Role Of The Sacroiliac Joints As A Cause Of Low Back Pain And Dysfunction," proceedings of the First Interdisciplinary World Congress on Low Back Pain and its Relation to the Sacroiliac Joint, University of California, Sand Diego, (Nov.5-6, 1992)

732   R Galm, M Fröhling, M Rittmeister, E Schmitt," Sacroiliac Joint Dysfunction In Patients With Imaging-Proven Lumbar Disc Herniation," *Eur Spine J.* 7/6 (1998):450-3. Spine Clinic, Bad Homburg, Germany.

733   D M Brady, MJ Schneider, "A New Paradigm For Differential Diagnosis And Treatment," *JMPT*, 24/8 (October 2001):529-541

734   Occupational Medicine Practice Guidelines: Evaluation and Management of Common Health Problems and Functional Recovery in Workers, 2nd Edition, 2008 revision.

The American Academy of Family Physicians (AAFP) published "Treating Fibromyalgia" and admitted this elusive disorder is not psychosomatic as Hadler believes, but is directly associated with "musculoskeletal pain unrelated to a clearly defined anatomic lesion" and that chiropractic treatment has proven effective. [735] The AAFP Guideline now recommends chiropractic treatment for fibromyalgia, citing a pilot study by KL Blunt *et al.* in which following four weeks of treatment, twenty-one patients with fibromyalgia improved compared with control subjects receiving medication only.[736]

Again, the mechanism of this improvement—the how and the why—may lie deep within the cranium initiated by neurotransmitters and spinal stress years before; it may be an imbalance of the autonomic nerve system or a spinovisceral reflex, but the evidence suggests that reducing back pain may decrease the degeneration at the core of this malady as Apkarian and Kuchinad suggest. Indeed, these FMS patients may need to reboot their brains via spinal manipulative therapy as Haavik-Taylor and Murphy recommend removing the gibberish as Korr also mentioned.

The research suggesting chronic back pain may lead to altered circuitry and/or degeneration of the brain is a good example of finally seeing the neurological forest through the anatomical trees. What may have begun as a common childhood fall off a bicycle that injures the spine may later lead to a life of chronic back pain, which in turn may develop into fibromyalgia or degeneration as the researchers now suggest.

Today's explanations of chiropractic are not the quaint concepts of "pinched nerves" from yesteryear. Neurophysiologists now suggest the effects of a bad back may lead to a myriad of problems such as somatovisceral reflexes, neuroplasticity, and cerebral degeneration via altered neurotransmitters. In fact, the research vindicates what DD Palmer tried to explain as "functionating" although much more has yet to be discovered.

Now you can better understand the complex madness behind chiropractic's methods. This research now emerging validates the importance of a healthy spine and the role chiropractic care may have upon pain syndromes and organic disorders.

Chiropractic Conclusions

Considering the plethora of new research of the spine, imagine the possibility of problems stemming from a neck or back pain injury:

- Spinal joints become dysfunctional causing pain and stiffness as well as muscle reflex spasms and nerve root compression.
- This may lead to the altered spinal-cortical circuitry issues.
- Nerve compression may lead to nerve and tissue degeneration by the disruption of axoplasmic flow of protein.
- Disturbed neurological conduct results in pathophysiology, disintegration of homeostasis, and eventually the intrusion of disease.

---

735 P Millea and R Holloway, "Treating Fibromyalgia," *Amer Family Physician* 62/7 (Oct 2000)
736 KL Blunt, MH Rajwani, RC Guerriero. "The Effectiveness Of Chiropractic Management Of Fibromyalgia Patients: A Pilot Study," *J Manipulative Physiol Ther* 20 (1997):389-99.

- Prolonged back pain may lead to cortical degeneration and premature aging.
- Nerve interference in the spine may cause somatovisceral or spinovisceral reflex disorders.

Few people understand the enormity of problems that can be generated from back pain. This research has opened up an entirely new dimension to health and disease, not unlike that of the new science of the human genome. Hopefully, as science discards its institutional bias, it will continue to discover other new aspects of the spine and nervous system's impact upon our health and lives. Indeed, this exciting new research may simply be the tip of the iceberg.

In conclusion, DD Palmer was right when he asked, "Is it possible that the science of Chiropractic has arrived before its time?"[737]

Imagine the amount of pain and disease that could have been alleviated by chiropractors if the medical boycott had not forced people into the allopathic trap and prevented people from receiving chiropractic spinal care. Indeed, the boycott of chiropractic care caused more than the pandemic of back pain; it has led to possible organic/visceral problems and brain damage beyond imagination.

Now you can understand when the Juice Man came knocking, the pioneer chiropractors stood their ground despite the skepticism stemming from medical harassment. These stalwart chiropractors had seen the remarkable results of their art and fought to maintain its practice despite the arrests, beatings, humiliation, and imprisonment. Thankfully, many did survive the medical war to keep alive an ageless healing art for people today to benefit.

---

737 DD Palmer, *The Chiropractor's Adjuster: The Text-Book of the Science, Art and Philosophy of Chiropractic* (Portland, Oregon: Portland Printing House) (1910):847

Epilogue

Let this plea be heard by all
in the court of public opinion:
Chiropractors v. the Medical Profession.

In the Court of Public Opinion

"The ultimate objective of the AMA, theoretically,
is the complete elimination of the chiropractic profession."

Robert Youngerman, attorney for the AMA's Department of Investigation[738]

Ladies and Gentlemen of the Jury:

As the author of this book, I have told you an incredible story of chiropractic from persecution to vindication. Very few Americans have heard this story nor have Americans realized the medical war against chiropractors entailed such deplorable actions by the American Medical Association.

I now want to summarize the evidence presented so you can act as jurors to come to a fair decision to exonerate chiropractors from the slander and defamation heaped upon them by an unmerciful medical opponent.

First of all, let me ask each of you to forget everything you were ever told about chiropractors before this trial began. Let's start with a clean slate because up to this point, there is a great possibility what most people have heard are the boldface medical lies as the evidence in this case has shown. From now on, I want each of you to listen to the truth that we have learned at trial and then come to a fair decision.

To the Committee on Quackery, chiropractors were not colleagues in the fight against pain and suffering, but they were enemies to be eliminated by any means. Just as any MD might prescribe an antibiotic to kill a germ without giving it a second

---

738 Memo from Robert Youngerman to Robert Throckmorton, 24 September 1963, PX 173, *Wilk v. AMA.*

thought, this Committee tried to wipe out chiropractors with the same indifference. In order to do that, the AMA's Committee on Quackery created the most extensive defamation campaign ever used in America to slander and to destroy the chiropractic profession.

Even if everything the AMA had said about chiropractors were true, is this not a case of the pot calling the kettle black? They said chiropractic was dangerous, but could not find one person to testify to that fact during the *Wilk* trial. On the other hand, let me ask: how many deadly medical treatments have American endured, such as mastectomies, back surgeries, super germs, and innumerable medications that have been withdrawn because their side effects were too dangerous? Too many to count.

Dr. Barbara Starfield told us that as many as 225,000 Americans die from medical mistakes annually, but has the AMA Committee on Quackery ever pointed their accusatory fingers at themselves? Never once did the same alarmists tell the public about these deadly medical methods although they knew medicine was inherently more dangerous than anything chiropractors did.

Attorney J. Minos Simon from Louisiana mentioned this duplicity when he described the attitude of the medical monarchists there: "While chiropractic is good for some things, it is not good for all things, and, therefore, Chiropractors should not be permitted to attend the sick for anything. Such chameleonic versatility is destined to doom…" and now that doomsday has arrived for you to be the judge.

You have heard a lengthy discourse how the chiropractic profession suffered by the hands of the American Medical Association. It has been a lengthy story covering many topics involving several players for nearly a century. If you had not seen the evidence with your own eyes and heard the testimonies of witnesses with your own ears, you would not have believed this stranger-than-fiction medical war against the chiropractic profession. But this unbelievable story is all too true.

Please bear with me now as I summarize the evidence so you can come to a reasonable conclusion that the AMA is guilty of its attempted assassination of the chiropractic profession, guilty of fomenting unwarranted public skepticism, and guilty of impugning the reputations of thousands of decent, hard-working chiropractors.

More importantly are the incriminating testimonies the medical experts have given: how the medical profession has perpetuated a "pandemic of pain" as Paul Goodley mentioned and "left a wake of disability" as Gordon Waddell wrote. You also heard Bruce Charlton speak of "zombie scientific theories" in medicine based purely on greed. All of these men are renowned medical doctors who were honest about the rampage of unnecessary back surgeries.

You also heard the admissions of guilt by the medical culprits themselves, such as the mastermind behind this war, Morris Fishbein, who was known as the Medical Mussolini by his contemporaries. He was not coy when he wrote of his evil intention: "Scientific medicine absorbs from them that which is good, if there is any good, and then they die."[739] Many alternative practitioners have died in the medical wars, and many more were left gravely wounded or emotionally scarred for life.

Morris Fishbein terrorized chiropractors for no reason other than to create a medical monarchy. He was the voice and face of political medicine for a quarter of a century, and his propaganda and tactics have lived on long past his death to impugn the good men and women who sought to help patients without drugs or surgery. Indeed, whenever you may hear someone say, *"I don't believe in chiropractic,"* be assured that is Fishbein speaking from the grave.

You also heard Joseph A. Sabatier say, "Rabid dogs and chiropractors fit into about the same category...they killed people."[740] You recall Robert Youngerman admitted, "The ultimate objective of the AMA, theoretically, is the complete elimination of the chiropractic profession."[741]

If these admissions are not frightening, David Stevens, member of the Committee on Quackery, put it more bluntly, "We weren't out to be fair. We were advocates. Our job was to destroy chiropractic."[742]

Despite the lack of evidence to prove their accusations, the medical monarchy had the audacity to write "The Right and Duty of Hospitals to Exclude Chiropractors," all based on falsehoods to keep chiropractors out of public hospitals.

Now you can understand why writer Milton Mayor dubbed the AMA "...the most terrifying trade association on earth."[743] Little did he know the true intention of the AMA was to inflict a mortal wound on the entire chiropractic profession as these association leaders have so clearly stated. As many astute Americans understood, the AMA was up to no good with the chiropractors. Like the cancer of racism, medical bigotry was plainly obvious from the bad treatment of chiropractors by the medical professionals.

Thankfully, the truth is finally emerging after years of this medical war, not only about the attempted murder of the chiropractic profession, but of the value of chiropractic spinal care. Without a doubt, the art of manual manipulation has helped millions of people around the world throughout the centuries. Despite this outstanding history, the American medical profession has virtually ignored chiropractic except to irrationally condemn it.

The most unforgiving violation of the Hippocratic Oath to *"do no harm"* is the fact the AMA has fought tooth and nail to prevent each of you from reaping the benefits of this healing art. Considering 90 percent of American adults will suffer from acute low back pain, to deny you the benefit of safe and natural chiropractic care is, indeed, causing you harm.

---

739 Morris Fishbein, Medical *Follies*, New York, Boni & Liveright (1925):43.

740 JA Sabatier, Minutes from the "Chiropractic Workshop," Michigan State Medical Society, held in Lansing on 10 May 1973, exhibit 1283, *Wilk*.

741 Memo from Robert Youngerman to Robert Throckmorton, 24 September 1963, plaintiff's exhibit 173, *Wilk v.AMA*.

742 Ibid. p. 3055

743 MS Mayer, "The Rise and Fall of Dr. Fishbein," *Harper's Magazine* (Nov. 1949):76-85.

Few people have ever appreciated the heroism and perseverance required to be a chiropractor. Just as black Americans were forced to sit in the back of the bus, chiropractors were thrown under the medical bus. Historian Russell Gibbons told us that "chiropractors felt the brunt as one of the first grass roots movements in America."[744] And for this effort to attain social justice in healthcare, they paid a heavy price.

In the first half of the twentieth century, over 12,000 chiropractors were prosecuted 15,000 times and 3,300 were sent to prison for helping sick people get well using only their hands. As the testimonies showed, you never heard any public outcry against chiropractors to warrant these arrests; instead, many courageous supporters picketed the jails where their favorite chiropractor was imprisoned.

You learned how Fishbein's successors, Robert Throckmorton, H. Doyl Taylor, Robert Youngerman, and Joseph A. Sabatier, were the spin doctors who headed the Committee on Quackery and used propaganda as a weapon to destroy chiropractic, including such schemes as distributing Quack Packs to educators and editors, tampering with committeemen during the Medicare legislation debate, and sponsoring many public figures like columnist Ann Landers to misinform the public about chiropractic.

Certainly the turning point in this dark episode of American history occurred when a few brave chiropractors sued the AMA and thirteen co-conspirators in federal court. You have seen the compelling evidence during the *Wilk et al. v. AMA et al.* trial presented by attorney George McAndrews that convinced a federal judge to find the AMA guilty of the boycott of chiropractors.

This trial revealed the war was not simply an antitrust case where one competitor tried to corner the market by spreading incriminating truths or ugly rumors; it was a blitzkrieg of cultural, economic, and political might by the AMA to completely *"eliminate"* the chiropractic profession as Youngerman said. The federal court described this conspiracy as "systematic, long-term wrongdoing, and the long-term intent to destroy a licensed profession."[745]

You also learned of the extensive research done by workers' compensation studies that showed a 2:1 superiority rate for chiropractors getting injured patients back to work. The New Zealand Inquiry into Chiropractic also concluded that chiropractic care was safe, effective, and should be embraced by the mainstream health care system. In fact, the New Zealand study found chiropractors were better educated and clinically trained to handle back pain cases than the average general practitioner. At trial, many medical doctors including a member of the AMA's board, Dr. Irwin Hendryson, testified in behalf of the chiropractor-plaintiffs.

Despite this legal victory and these landmark studies, you learned how the AMA misinformers continued to ignore these facts and later worked to thwart progress in the back pain treatments. Most notably, you saw how the medical monarchy killed

---

744 Gibbons, ibid. p. 67.

745 *Associated Press*, "U.S. Judge Finds Medical Group Conspired Against Chiropractors," *New York Times* (1987)

the AHCPR guideline #14 on acute low back pain in adults that recommended spinal manipulation over back surgery. It is a prime example how the AMA remains the *most terrifying trade association on earth* when it can thwart the will of Congress.

Additionally, you have learned of the new emerging research studies that have determined back surgeries are mostly unnecessary and ineffective. The editors of ^The^BACK*LETTER* told us, "The world of spinal medicine, unfortunately, is producing patients with failed back surgery syndrome at an alarming rate." This is quite an admission from prestigious medical editors from the Georgetown University Medical Center who speak the truth about the epidemic of unnecessary back surgeries.

The proof is positive and research studies cannot be clearer that chiropractic stands at the top of spinal treatments as Anthony Rosner, PhD, testified before The Institute of Medicine: "Today, we can argue that chiropractic care, at least for back pain, appears to have vaulted from last to first place as a treatment option."[746]

You have also learned from Scott Haldeman and John Mennell how chiropractic care may help visceral problems via the spinovisceral reflex phenomenon. Joseph Janse and Virgil Strang mentioned that spinal subluxations may impair the homeostasis of the body, and Heidi Haavik-Taylor and Bernadette Murphy showed us that a chiropractic adjustment is equivalent to rebooting the brain's circuitry. Most interesting, we learned that back pain may cause the brain to degenerate as A. Vania Apkarian's research team showed.

DD Palmer was correct when he said chiropractic was ahead of its time, and these modern researchers now substantiate his early beliefs in new ways by using high-tech electronic scanners and imaging devices. From bones to brains, scientists are finding new discoveries about chiropractic spinal care that were unknown to this early visionary. Fortunately, Palmer and his band of chiropractors survived the medical war to keep this ancient healing art alive today.

Certainly the AMA's evil schemes stemmed from the devious mindset of men filled with hate, greed, and bigotry. Their painful remarks are on the record. The more the AMA executives spoke, the more their testimonies appeared eerily reminiscent of the German Nazis. The similarity is shocking—the Jews were vilified by the Nazis and chiropractors were demonized by the AMA—with the same intention to contain and eliminate them both.

Let me be clear: the actions of the AMA's Committee on Quackery—the political dirty tricks and public slander against chiropractors—are not comparable to the Nazi atrocities during the Holocaust against the Jews and other minorities, and it is not my intent to even remotely attempt to equate them.

However, the *propaganda methods* used by the AMA against chiropractors were remarkably similar to what the Nazis employed. As if the AMA had taken a page from the Nazi's "Final Solution to the Jewish Question," the AMA's attorney Robert

---

746 Testimony before The Institute of Medicine: Committee on Use of CAM by the American Public on Feb. 27, 2003.

Throckmorton clearly spelled out his equivalence to the Final Solution in his article, "What Medicine Should Do about the Chiropractic Menace," labeling chiropractic an *"unscientific cult"* that deserved to be "eliminated."[747]

Quoting from their own words, let me reiterate their frightening plan. In 1962, the AMA Committee on Quackery issued a call to arms–its Iowa Plan–to demand the entire medical community "undertake a positive program of containment." As the AMA's Committee on Quackery executives testified, their goal was to watch chiropractors "wither on the vine" hoping the "chiropractic menace will die a natural but somewhat undramatic death."[748]

Let us pause to reflect upon this Iowa Plan strategy: I thought doctors were supposed to eliminate disease and suffering. I never imagined they were mostly concerned about the elimination of other healthcare providers. Tell me: does this sound like scientific men seeking the truth about health care in a scholarly debate or with scientific research?

Of course not; it speaks of medical bigots who wanted to eliminate a competitor at all costs by any means.

In spite of this horrendous language, Youngerman would still have you believe in the Good Samaritan image of MDs when he said: "The public does and should look to the medical profession for unbiased and authoritative information on this subject."

Indeed, has anything he said seem "unbiased" to you? His intention was for every honest American to embrace his evil mindset—the hatred, bigotry, and the lies. Sadly, too many did, just as many good Germans embraced the Nazi hatred after repeatedly hearing the same Big Lie—"Jews are bad, Jews are bad...kill the Jews," and six million European Jews were killed in death camps.

Likewise, too many MDs chanted the medical Big Lie—"chiropractors are quacks, chiropractors are dangerous, chiropractors are rabid dogs and killers," and thousands of chiropractors were arrested and imprisoned. The medical Nazis had no proof, and even after the *Wilk* trial where their lack of evidence was made public, that still has not stop them from provoking fear and skepticism in the public with their lies and hate propaganda.

These masters of deception had even deceived themselves. We heard H. Doyl Taylor admit, "I didn't know a chiropractor from an antelope." But when his superiors told him chiropractic was a menace, he reconsidered his ignorance and immediately recognized chiropractic as the "greatest hazard to the public health...I opposed whatever the Committee instructed me to oppose."[749] Like a good Storm Trooper, he blindly carried out his duty without question.

---

747 Ibid. PX-172 November 11, 1962.

748 G McAndrews, "Plaintiffs' Summary of Proofs as an Aid to the Court," Civil Action No. 76 C 3777, *Wilk*, (June 25, 1987):17.

749 Material relating to H. Doyl Taylor is based on a deposition in the case of *Wilk et al.* v. AMA et al., on 28 April 1987, in Phoenix, 15.

It became clear that many of the AMA's policies toward chiropractors paralleled those of the Nazi's. For example, it was well known the Nazis did not want any "race defilement" by the Jews with Aryans. Clearly the AMA played its own "race" card against chiropractors with Principle 3 of the Medical Ethics that declared it was unethical for any MD to associate with chiropractors. Likewise, its Principle 4 even demanded that AMA members spy on each other, just as Hitler had spies among the German people. [750]

With Principles 3 and 4, the AMA threatened their own members with professional "sterilization" if caught joined with chiropractors for the betterment of patients. It was professional death and financial ruin for MDs not to abide by both Principle 3 and 4 from 1963 until 1980. Regrettably, this fear of retribution lingers on among many MDs who remain afraid to refer patients to chiropractors for fear of professional disapproval.

Think of this possibility: if Fishbein and his ilk had lived in Germany at that time, there is no doubt that chiropractors would have found themselves in the same death camps with the Jews. Ironically, since Morris Fishbein was a Jew himself, he most likely would have been a victim of the same hatred he held toward chiropractors.

This Cold War continues today. Do not think this war to have chiropractic *wither on the vine* has ended just because of a favorable federal court decision or the passage of state scope laws to protect chiropractors. Medical tyranny continues to this day when chiropractors are omitted from hospitals, limited by health insurance, ignored by the media, or slandered whenever anyone says, "I don't believe in chiropractors."

During the *Wilk* trial, you heard the testimonies of honest MDs who knew that chiropractic helped patients and told the court these truths. You heard the judge remark how these medical-defendants' witnesses were actually testifying in behalf of the chiropractic-plaintiffs—the "admissions against interest." Just as not all Germans were Nazis, not all MDs toed the line of the evil men within the AMA. They were the "flowers in the desert" of medical depravity.

It may be difficult for some of you to think of your friendly neighborhood medical doctor as one who would harbor such awful sentiments. Here is one easy test to determine if your MD is a medical Nazi or a flower: simply ask him what he thinks of chiropractors. If he spews the medical propaganda, run from his office as fast as you can. If he responds positively, then you have found a flower in the desert—someone you can trust.

The Iowa Plan, in effect, acted as an herbicide for the medical mob that killed many of these flowers. This extermination plan resulted in a "lengthy, systematic, successful, and unlawful boycott"[751] described by the judge to eliminate the profession of chiropractic that has never been properly acknowledged.

---

750 PX-56, 156A

751 *Chester A. Wilk, James W. Bryden, Patricia A. Arthur, Michael D. Pedigo v. American Medical Association, Joint Commission on Accreditation of Hospitals, American College of Physicians, American Academy of Orthopaedic Surgeons,* United States District Court Northern District of Illinois, No. 76C3777, Susan Getzendanner, Judge, Judgment dated August 27, 1987.

Judge Getzendanner admitted in her Opinion that "The AMA has never made any attempt to publicly repair the damage the boycott did to chiropractors' reputations."[752] Restitution was never paid to the chiropractors who were unfairly imprisoned in the first half of the twentieth century. This atrocity included thousands of chiropractors who surrendered in the medical war, those who were spiritually broken, physically beaten, financially ruined, and those who finally decided to quit the fight. The fear of imprisonment was not that long ago considering the last chiropractor went to jail in 1975 for practicing chiropractic in Shreveport, Louisiana.

Sadly, we can still see evidence of medical bigotry. Just as the Nazis burned books, we saw the same academic tyranny as recently as 2005 at Florida State University when Raymond Bellamy and his medical mob sabotaged the will of the Florida state legislature that had voted 151-1 to implement a chiropractic program. Apparently the propaganda power of this medical mob superseded the will of the people and the state government in Florida.

Certainly, this medical tyranny at FSU was a travesty of academic freedom. We heard Bellamy call chiropractic "'pseudoscience" and "gobbledygook...not one shred of science," yet he failed to provide one shred of evidence to prove his accusations. Clearly these are not statements from a rational, scientific, or academic mind, but the ranting of a medical bigot hell-bent on spewing old propaganda from yesteryear. Once again, we heard Morris Fishbein speaking from the grave.

The fact remains this medical war has not ended and you could be its next victim. For example, if you or a member of your family is injured in a car accident and taken to a public hospital, your favorite chiropractor is still barred from entering that hospital to help you. Although he or she is licensed by the state government and you are in a public hospital paid by our public taxes, the medical staff holds the key to the door. This was the point of the *Wilk* trial, but for all intent and purposes, the doors to American hospitals remain locked to chiropractors.

Few people realize that only the local medical society holds the key to your hospital door, and most keep out all competition to maintain their stronghold on the medical Bastille. In spite of the *Wilk* trial ruling, this boycott is virtually still in effect since very few hospitals allow chiropractors on staff. The judge's ruling only stated a chiropractor could not be excluded because he is a chiropractor, but the court did not say any hospital was required to have a chiropractor on staff.

When only six percent of chiropractors have hospital privileges, it is obvious the medical society has no intention to integrate. If our public schools and universities only had six percent black students, the government would send in the federal troops to force integration. But, when public hospitals do the same, there is just too much prejudice, too much power, and too much money at stake to desegregate hospitals and to give patients a freedom of choice in their own healthcare matters. The medical industrial complex would not tolerate chiropractic competition.

---

752 S Getzendanner, US District Judge, *Permanent Injunction Order Against the AMA* (Sept. 25, 1987), published in JAMA, 259/1 (January 1, 1988):10

You heard the same frustration from Dr. Richard Deyo, a renowned spine researcher, when he said: "People say, 'I'm not going to put up with it,' and we in the medical profession have turned to ever more aggressive medication, narcotic medication, and more invasive surgery."[753] This is quite an admission from a spine researcher who found America does five times more back surgery per capita than Great Britain. [754]

What can be said of spine surgeons who know the research cannot support the vast quantities of spine fusions done today? Experts tell say that the disc theory is dead, but unethical surgeons still use disc abnormalities seen on an MRI image as selling points to scare unsuspecting patients. Surgical experimentation still exists, just as we once saw in the death camps with Drs. Josef Mengele and Eduard Wirths who practiced at Auschwitz.

Ultimately someone needs to ask: Where does the responsibility for these failures rest? Of course, it rests with not only the AMA leadership, but starts with the primary care providers who send patients to surgeons without using chiropractors first as the guidelines recommend. It also rests with spine surgeons, MRI owners, the hospitals, the surgical device manufacturers, and even the insurance companies who profit by these expensive surgeries by charging higher premiums to cover these huge costs.

This is a $100 billion industry that the medical industrial complex has no wish to lose to chiropractors who could help patients get well cheaply without drugs, shots, or surgery. This has been a failure of ethics as well as a failure of the lack of free enterprise in healthcare today when chiropractors are purposely excluded from the hospital marketplace to offer a cheaper and more effective treatment to patients who are denied the freedom of choice about their treatment options.

The evidence has shown that Fishbein's strategy did work to make his AMA incredibly powerful and wealthy, subsidized by dirty money initially from the tobacco industry and now from the drug companies. The AMA, Inc. marginalized competitors, influenced politicians, bribed the media, and taught the public to use only allopathic treatments, which has now led to a public addicted to tobacco, drugs, and surgery. And we wonder why Americans are so unhealthy today with medical leadership like this?

This is the real medical monopoly we have in America today, not the dramatic movies about medical heroism or the comedic medical shows you watch on television. Indeed, the current demise of the American healthcare delivery system is not a result of bad luck or unforeseen circumstances, but it is the result of the war by the medical industrial complex hell-bent to destroy competition and free enterprise.

Dr. Benjamin Rush, a Founding Father, warned about over two hundred years ago of the medical monarchy we have in America today. Just as post-war Germany was left in ruins by political demagogues, the American healthcare system today is in dire straits caused by this medical monarchy.

---

753 G Kolata, "With Costs Rising, Treating Back Pain Often Seems Futile," *NY Times* (February 9, 2004)

754 DC Cherkin, RA Deyo, *et al.* "An International Comparison Of Back Surgery Rates," *Spine*, 19/11 (June 2004):1201-1206.

A lot of evidence has been presented and reviewed. Now I ask the jury in the court of public opinion to be fair-minded in your appraisal of chiropractic. I simply want you to think about the evidence and the damage done by the medical monarchy to innocent chiropractors and patients:

- Think of the thousands of chiropractors over the past one hundred years who were constantly harassed and belittled because they helped sick people get well without drugs or surgery.
- Think of the thousands who were sent to prison for the crime of helping patients with the ageless art of spinal manipulation.
- Think of the broken hearts these chiropractic warriors endured in this medical war that they fought literally with only their hands. Like the Russian and Polish peasants who fought the Nazis soldiers with only their pitch forks, the medical war against chiropractors has been another lopsided battle.
- Think of the poor chiropractors who did not have the war chest funded by the tobacco and drug companies to defend itself from the medical propaganda. Chiropractors' only means of influence were satisfied patients telling their friends of their good results.

Now I ask you now to think of the damage done to innocent patients:

- Think carefully of the millions of people, perhaps yourself or family member, who have needlessly suffered from back pain, the most disabling condition in America today, when simple chiropractic care could have helped them.
- Think of the millions of Americans who suffered with unnecessary and ineffective spine surgeries as you heard the experts tell us.
- Think of the millions who are now addicted to strong medications for their chronic back pain from failed back surgeries.
- Think of the millions disabled from ever working again because they were misdiagnosed with a disc problem, mistreated by spine surgery, and misinformed that chiropractic care could help them.
- These people are also victims of this war who were never given a second opinion from a chiropractor—that freedom of choice in healthcare our Founding Father Benjamin Rush sought to guarantee in the Constitution.

Upon leaving today, I ask you to vote with your feet when you encounter medical bigotry. Walk out of the MD's office if he will not refer you to a chiropractor. Walk out of the hospital that only offers you drugs, shots, and surgery. Walk away from the medical bigot who demeans your local chiropractor.

There is more you can do by demanding your legal right to have chiropractic care. Just as Rosa Parks demanded her right not to sit in the back of the bus, you also should demand that a chiropractor be at your bedside when you want treatment. Brick by brick, we can kick down the medical Bastille.

- Demand that every local hospital employs chiropractors to help patients. As long as the medical society is in charge of the hospital, few chiropractors will be allowed on staff to help you. Plus, hospitals make much more money with spine surgeries, so they have no incentive to use the cheaper chiropractic treatment.

- Demand your insurance coverage gives chiropractors the same coverage they give MDs and physical therapists. You learned how the AMA sabotaged the initial Medicare legislation. Many Blue Cross/Blue Shield programs and Medicare coverage still limit only 12 visits a year to chiropractors, but give 60 or more for physical therapists. And there seems to be no limits for back surgery despite the loud calls for restraint. This inequality must end so you can have the best of both worlds and lower healthcare costs.

- Demand that all workers' compensation programs fully utilize chiropractic care for work-related injuries. Low back pain is the number one work-related injury, but patients are routinely denied access to chiropractors. Chiropractic care is legally included, but claims adjusters often refuse to authorize it because of the perverse motivation of these for-profit insurance companies that make more money by using more expensive treatments.

- Demand all public universities have a chiropractic curriculum to insure academic freedom. It is unconscionable that the third-largest physician level profession has been excluded from the curricula of major public universities. As we learned at FSU, political medicine will fight hard to keep chiropractic withering on the vine and to deny academic freedom to students.

- Demand an increase in research funding to chiropractic colleges to conduct extensive research to learn how chiropractic care might help people with Type O and Type B disorders as the researchers have recently discovered. These initial studies have shown that DD Palmer was a man ahead of his time, and now is the time for chiropractic experts to have an equitable part of the billions in research money hoarded by the medical profession.

In other words, everyone should demand that doctors of chiropractic are entitled to the same rights as medical doctors. That's fair enough, isn't it? That's the American way!

Let me add one more important point for you to consider on a personal level.

While you cannot change the morality of a medical bigot with a blackened heart toward chiropractors, what does this mean in terms of your own personal morality? I assume not everyone on this jury believes in chiropractic care; if this group is like those polled, there is a good chance some of you are skeptical. Indeed, if the information you've learned during this trial has not changed your mind, what will?

Just as the German population after the war had to accept the Nazi dogma against the Jewish people was perverted, and just as Southerners in America had to learn after the Civil War that racism was unacceptable, now every American who has been tainted by the medical propaganda needs to learn their blanket skepticism of chiropractors is unjustified, too.

When you hear a distasteful racist joke or hear a sexist comment about a woman, it is morally-incorrect to encourage such bigotry. The same can be said about derogatory comments by medical chauvinists. If you hear an MD call a chiropractor a quack, just recall that is the Medical Mussolini speaking from the grave.

If you hear someone say chiropractic is ineffective, recall the trial evidence and testimonies from medical experts that support chiropractic care. Recall the comparative studies and international guidelines that say spinal manipulation is preferable to drugs, shots, and back surgeries for most cases.

The next time you meet a chiropractor, rather than letting the suspicious slander enter your mind to prejudge him, instead I suggest you ask him or her about themselves, what it is like living under medical suppression, what it is like being a chiropractor in the medical war and, most of all, what he can do to help you feel better. It may be the most interesting conversation you've ever had.

Perhaps now you can understand that America cannot fulfill its American Dream until every chiropractor can work unfettered to help the millions of people who suffer daily. Now you can understand that all chiropractors want is the same civil rights, basic liberties, and professional respect they are due in a free society. They ask for no privileges as the medical brethren have. Chiropractors do not want to stand along them on the medical pedestal; all they ask for is a fair chance on a level playing field to help patients get well.

Finally, let me leave you with an uplifting comment by a former leader of the chiropractic profession. Despite the strafe from the on-going medical war, there were chiropractors who stood tall above the fray because they knew there was a bigger battle at hand. In 1993, Dr. Kerwin Winkler, chairman of the American Chiropractic Association's Board of Governors, spoke of the plight of chiropractic:

> It is time to tear down the walls of isolation, bridge the moats of prejudice, and work as a separate and distinct brigade of the same army. The enemy is not medicine; the enemy is disease."[755]

Dr. Winkler's comment is the most intelligent statement I've heard throughout this entire trial. I hope you take his wish to heart to bring an end to this senseless war. As he said, "It is time to tear down the walls of isolation..." It's time for every American to help tear down the walls of the medical Bastille for a healthier America.

Ladies and gentlemen of the jury, I ask that you find the medical profession guilty of war crimes against both chiropractors and unsuspecting patients. It is time to end the propaganda and it is past time to end the medical war against chiropractors. It is time to restore sanity in healthcare.

---

755 K Winkler, *Outlook* (Aug. 1993)

Index

8984563R0

Made in the USA
Charleston, SC
31 July 2011